PRESCRIPTIVE PLAY THERAPY

Also Available

Contemporary Play Therapy:
Theory, Research, and Practice
*Edited by Charles E. Schaefer
and Heidi Gerard Kaduson*

Essential Play Therapy Techniques:
Time-Tested Approaches
*Charles E. Schaefer
and Donna Cangelosi*

Play-Based Interventions
for Childhood Anxieties, Fears, and Phobias
*Edited by Athena A. Drewes
and Charles E. Schaefer*

Short-Term Play Therapy for Children,
Third Edition
*Edited by Heidi Gerard Kaduson
and Charles E. Schaefer*

Prescriptive Play Therapy

Tailoring Interventions for Specific Childhood Problems

edited by

Heidi Gerard Kaduson
Donna Cangelosi
Charles E. Schaefer

THE GUILFORD PRESS
New York   London

Printed in the United States of America

This book is printed on acid-free paper.

Last digit is print number: 9   8   7   6   5   4   3   2   1

The authors have checked with sources believed to be reliable in their efforts to
provide information that is complete and generally in accord with the standards
of practice that are accepted at the time of publication. However, in view of the
possibility of human error or changes in behavioral, mental health, or medical
sciences, neither the authors, nor the editors and publisher, nor any other party
who has been involved in the preparation or publication of this work warrants
that the information contained herein is in every respect accurate or complete,
and they are not responsible for any errors or omissions or the results obtained
from the use of such information. Readers are encouraged to confirm the
information contained in this book with other sources.

Library of Congress Cataloging-in-Publication Data is available
from the publisher.

ISBN 978-1-4625-4167-6 (paperback)
ISBN 978-1-4625-4168-3 (hardcover)

About the Editors

Heidi Gerard Kaduson, PhD, RPT-S, specializes in evaluation and intervention services for children with a variety of behavioral, emotional, and learning problems. She is past president of the Association for Play Therapy and Director of The Play Therapy Training Institute in Monroe Township, New Jersey. She has lectured internationally on play therapy, attention-deficit/hyperactivity disorder, and learning disabilities. Dr. Kaduson's coedited books include *Contemporary Play Therapy* and *Short-Term Play Therapy for Children, Third Edition*. She maintains a private practice in child psychotherapy in Monroe Township.

Donna Cangelosi, PsyD, RPT-S, maintains a private practice with children, adolescents, and adults in Wayne, New Jersey, where she provides psychotherapy, clinical supervision, and parent education. Dr. Cangelosi is coauthor of *Essential Play Therapy Techniques* and has published several chapters and professional articles on the theory and application of psychodynamic play therapy. She has lectured throughout the country on topics related to play therapy and loss issues in children.

Charles E. Schaefer, PhD, RPT-S, is Professor Emeritus of Clinical Psychology at Fairleigh Dickinson University. He is Cofounder and Director Emeritus of the Association for Play Therapy, which recognized him with its Lifetime Achievement Award. Dr. Schaefer is the author or coauthor of more than 100 research articles and author or editor of over 70 professional books, including *Play-Based Interventions for Childhood Anxieties, Fears, and Phobias* and *Essential Play Therapy Techniques*.

Contributors

Sue Ammen, PhD, Professor Emeritus, California School of Professional Psychology, Alliant International University, Fresno, California

Donna Cangelosi, PsyD, private practice, Wayne, New Jersey

Susan M. Carter, PhD, RPT-S, Registered Play Therapist, Center for Change and Growth PLC, Kalamazoo, Michigan

David A. Crenshaw, PhD, ABPP, Clinical Director, Children's Home of Poughkeepsie, Poughkeepsie, New York

Athena A. Drewes, PsyD, RPT-S, Child Psychologist, Parapsychologist, and Consultant, Rhine Research Center, Durham, North Carolina

Eliana Gil, PhD, Founder and Senior Clinical Consultant, Gil Institute for Trauma Recovery and Education, Fairfax, Virginia

Paris Goodyear-Brown, MSSW, LCSW, Founder and Clinical Director, Nurture House, Franklin, Tennessee

Robert Jason Grant, EdD, AutPlay Therapy Clinic, Springfield, Missouri

Heidi Gerard Kaduson, PhD, Director, The Play Therapy Training Institute, and private practice, Monroe Township, New Jersey

Erik Newman, PhD, Foothills Integrative Psychological Services, Lone Tree, Colorado

Charles E. Schaefer, PhD, Cofounder and Director Emeritus, Association for Play Therapy, Clovis, California; Department of Psychology (Emeritus), Fairleigh Dickinson University, Teaneck, New Jersey

Janine Shelby, PhD, Associate Clinical Professor, Department of Psychiatry and Biobehavioral Sciences, David Geffen School of Medicine, University of California, Los Angeles, Los Angeles, California

Quinn Koelfgen Smelser, LPC, NCC, therapist, Gil Institute for Trauma Recovery and Education, Fairfax, Virginia

Audrey D. Smith, undergraduate student, Department of Sociology, Samford University, Birmingham, Alabama

Alyssa Swan, PhD, Associate Clinical Director, Children's Home of Poughkeepsie, Poughkeepsie, New York

Lynn Louise Wonders, MA, Wonders Counseling Services, Marietta, Georgia

Laurie Zelinger, PhD, ABPP, RPT-S, private practice, Cedarhurst, New York

Preface

It is well known through empirical studies that a single play therapy theory has not proven equally effective with all the different psychological disorders of youth. Thus, prescriptive play therapists select from both directive and nondirective play therapy theories an intervention that has strong empirical support for the client's specific presenting problem. Therapists then modify it as needed for each client, based on his or her strengths, limitations, developmental status, and preferences. Such tailoring to address personal characteristics is necessary due to the amount of heterogeneity and variability that exists among individuals within the same diagnostic groups (Barlow, 1981; Rappaport, 1991). Metaphorically speaking, prescriptive play therapists believe that "one size does not fit all" and that "if the only tool you have is a hammer, you are likely to see every problem as a nail." Thus, a cardinal principle of this approach is that the more tools clinicians have in their therapeutic box, the more effectively they can prescribe a particular treatment that best meets the client's needs.

Although prescriptive psychotherapy is not new (Dimond, Havens, & Jones, 1978; Goldstein & Stein, 1976), the popularity of this approach has greatly expanded over the past 30 years, and it has evolved into a leading form of play therapy. The prescriptive play therapy model was first introduced to play therapists in the book *The Playing Cure: Individualized Play Therapy for Specific Childhood Disorders* (Kaduson, Cangelosi, & Schaefer, 1997). In order for prescriptive play therapy to continue to grow, there is a pressing need for a current, state-of-the-art book on this approach.

Part I of this book presents the rationale and practices underlying the prescriptive play therapy approach. In Parts II through V, prominent play therapists describe the application of their particular, tailor-made treatment for specific childhood disorders. Thus, each chapter offers a unique view of how prescriptive play therapy is practiced today. Specific assessment and therapy practices accompany illustrative case material in the chapters. Grounded in cutting-edge research, these clinical chapters provide a roadmap for selecting and individualizing play interventions for youth.

REFERENCES

Barlow, D. (1981). Editorial. *Journal of Applied Behavior Analysis, 14*(1), 1–20.

Dimond, R., Havens, R., & Jones, A. (1978). A conceptual framework for the practice of prescriptive eclecticism in psychotherapy. *American Psychologist, 33,* 239–248.

Goldstein, A. P., & Stein, N. (1976). *Prescriptive psychotherapies.* New York: Pergamon Press.

Kaduson, H. G., Cangelosi, D., & Schaefer, C. (Eds.). (1997). *The playing cure: Individualized play therapy for specific childhood disorders.* Northvale, NJ: Jason Aronson.

Rappaport, S. R. (1991). Diagnostic–prescriptive teaming: The road less traveled. *Journal of Reading, Writing, and Learning Disabilities International, 7*(3), 183–199.

Contents

PART I

Description of and Rationale for Prescriptive Play Therapy

CHAPTER 1

Basic Principles and Core Practices of Prescriptive Play Therapy

Heidi Gerard Kaduson
Charles E. Schaefer
Donna Cangelosi

History

Prescriptive psychotherapy is not new, and in recent years it has evolved into a leading form of psychotherapy (Goldstein & Stein, 1976; Dimond, Havens, & Jones, 1978). The fundamental goal of prescriptive psychotherapy is to tailor the intervention to the presenting problem and personal preferences/characteristics of the client. In formulating a treatment plan, prescriptive psychotherapists seek to answer Gordon Paul's (1967) important question: "*What* treatment, by *whom*, is most effective for *this* individual, with *that* specific problem, with *which* set of circumstances, and *how* does it come about?" Thus, the goal is for the treatment plan to be truly *client-centered* rather than focused on the personal preferences of the therapist.

The *prescriptive play therapy* model was first described by Heidi Gerard Kaduson, Donna Cangelosi, and Charles E. Schaefer (1997) in their book *The Playing Cure: Individualized Play Therapy for Specific Childhood Disorders*. They detailed the application of the therapeutic powers of play (Schaefer, 1993) to the common psychological disorders of youth. The popularity of prescriptive play therapy has mushroomed over the past two decades and is likely to continue to expand in the years ahead. The goal of the present, state-of-the-art volume is to describe the numerous advances in the theory, research, and clinical practice of prescriptive play therapy as it is applied to the broad spectrum of childhood disorders. The chapters are written by prominent play therapists with broad experience in the field of play therapy.

Conceptual Foundation

Basic Principles

Prescriptive play therapy is founded on a set of basic principles that serve as fundamental cornerstones of the approach and guide its practice. The five foundational principles of prescriptive play therapy follow.

Principle 1. Differential Therapeutics

Play therapy has been evolving over most of its 100-year history based on the "one true light" assumption. This is basically a nonprescriptive position which holds, in the absence of supportive evidence, that one's preferred treatment approach is equally and widely applicable to most or all types of client problems. Based on this belief, treatment is conducted essentially independent of diagnostic information. The difficulty with this "one-size-fits-all" assumption is that no one theoretical school (e.g., Rogerian, Adlerian, Jungian) has proven strong enough to produce optimal change across the many different and complex psychological disorders that have been identified (Smith, Glass, & Miller, 1980).

The prescriptive approach to play therapy (Kaduson et al., 1997) is based on the core premise of *differential therapeutics* (Frances, Clarkin, & Perry, 1984), which holds that some interventions are more effective than others for certain disorders and that a client who does poorly with one type of play therapy may do well with another (Beutler, 1979; Beutler & Clarkin, 1990). It rejects the Dodo bird verdict that all major forms of psychotherapy are equally effective for specific disorders (Beutler, 1991; Luborsky, Singer, & Luborsky, 1975; Norcross, 1995). Rather than forcing clients to adapt to one therapeutic approach (in a procrustean manner), prescriptive therapists adapt their remedies to meet the different treatment needs of individual clients.

Notwithstanding the "common" or "nonspecific" elements that characterize effective therapies of all types, increasing evidence has shown that specific interventions work better for specific disorders and problems (Chambless & Ollendick, 2001). Support for the efficacy of *disorder-specific treatment* is seen in the findings of meta-analytic outcome meta-studies, which indicate that the mean effect sizes of specific factors consistently surpass those of common factors (Lambert & Bergin, 1994; Stevens, Hyman, & Allen, 2000).

Principle 2. Eclecticism

Instead of strictly adhering to one particular school of thought, eclectic psychotherapists employ elements from a range of theories and/or techniques, with the aim of establishing an intervention tailored to a particular client's characteristics and situation. Prescriptive, eclectic therapy is a flexible and multifaceted approach that allows the therapist to select the method that has proven most effective in resolving a client's problems. A single theory does not prepare therapists to treat the ever-expanding range and complexity of psychological problems that clients present with today.

Prescriptive, eclectic therapists believe that the more remedies you have in your repertoire, coupled with the knowledge about how to apply them differentially, the more effective you'll be in meeting a particular client's needs (Goldstein & Stein, 1976). Using more than one change agent in therapy helps clinicians avoid the trap that Abraham Maslow has described: "If the only tool you have is a hammer, every problem starts to look like a nail."

According to Norcross (1987), "synthetic eclecticism" involves combining various theories into one coordinated treatment intervention. This differs from "kitchen-sink eclecticism," in which practitioners apply techniques from various schools of thought in a manner that ignores the theory that underlies them. Norcross warns that this atheoretical approach is haphazard and ineffective at best, and may, in fact, be harmful to some clients.

Surveys of clinicians have indicated that most clinicians identify themselves as eclectic, making the eclectic, "meta-theory" approach the modal theoretical orientation across disciplines (Norcross, 2005; Prochaska & Norcross, 1983). Similarly, a poll of play therapists (Phillips & Landreth, 1995) found that an eclectic, multitheoretical orientation was, by far, the most common approach reported by the respondents. Although eclectic psychotherapy is still not widely taught in graduate schools, it is likely to remain the treatment of choice by most practitioners in this country (Norcross, 2005).

As Goldfried (2001, p. 229) observed, "Most of us as therapists eventually learn that we cannot function effectively without moving outside of the theoretical model [to] which we had originally been trained, recognizing that the strength of another orientation may at times synergistically complement the limitations of our own approach."

The widespread eclectic movement (Kazdin, Siegel, & Bass, 1990) reflects a decisive departure from the aforementioned "purist," one-size-fits-all orthodoxy, together with a much greater openness by psychotherapists to adapt to differing contexts of the client's life, and thus tailor their strategies to the circumstances and needs of individual clients.

Principle 3. Integrative Psychotherapy

Since prescriptive play therapists are not confined by single-school theories, they often combine different theories and/or techniques to strengthen and/or broaden the scope of their intervention. Integrative play psychotherapy refers to the blending together of healing elements from different schools of play therapy into one combined approach in the treatment of a client. Thus, individual, group and family play strategies may be integrated to treat a particular case or psychodynamic and humanistic play theories. An integrated, multicomponent intervention reflects the fact that most psychological disorders are complex and multidimensional, caused by an interaction of biological, psychological, and social factors. Because most disorders are multidetermined, an integrated, multifaceted course of treatment is needed. The fact that there is high comorbidity among many psychological disorders, such as conduct disorder and attention-deficit/hyperactivity disorder, also points to the need for an integrative treatment approach.

Although prescriptive therapists seek to be both integrative and eclectic, many prefer to call themselves integrative rather than eclectic (Norcross & Prochaska, 1988). The type of integrative psychotherapy practiced by most prescriptive play therapists is termed *assimilative–integrative*. This means that therapists begin their training with a firm grounding in one primary orientation, typically child-centered, and then, over the course of their career, gradually incorporate or assimilate a number of practices from other schools (Messer, 1992).

Although prescriptive play therapists are often integrative, they are not always so. At times, the implementation of a single theory (e.g., child-centered play therapy) will be found to be the most effective prescription for a child's particular disorder.

Principle 4. Prescriptive Matching

Since the rate of improvement varies among different treatment procedures, prescriptive play therapists seek to match the most effective play intervention to each specific disorder or presenting problem (Norcross, 1991). It makes intuitive sense that treatment should be tailored to the needs of each individual child. However, prescriptive matching at the optimum level goes beyond this simple acknowledgment. It differs from the typical basis in the following way.

The typical basis of matching is a theory of psychotherapy rather than a direct matching of a specific change agent to the particular cause of the disorder. Optimally, in formulating a treatment plan, the clinician selects a therapeutic change agent that is designed to reduce or eliminate the cause of the problem. Thus, by treating not only the symptoms but also the underlying cause, the problem will be less likely to reoccur in the future. For example, an attachment-oriented play intervention such as Theraplay (Munns, 1992) would be a logical match for a child exhibiting disruptive behaviors where the underlying cause of the problem is the child's lack of a secure attachment. In a similar vein, abreactive/reenactment play therapy—a trauma-focused intervention—would be indicated for a fearful child whose symptoms are the result of an unresolved trauma experience.

One goal of a comprehensive assessment prior to treatment selection is to pinpoint the underlying cause of the disorder so that the therapist can then select a change agent (a therapeutic power of play) that is most likely to remedy this causal factor.

The 20 therapeutic powers of play identified by Charles Schaefer and his colleagues (Schaefer, 1993; Schaefer & Drewes, 2013) are listed in Table 1.1. The heart and soul of play therapy is contained in these therapeutic powers of play. They are the specific, essential ingredients in play that produce therapeutic change. Thus, prescriptive matching for a play therapist focuses on selecting the specific change agent(s) in play that will best resolve the client's presenting problem. For example, the "directing teaching" power of play would be indicated for a child who has difficulty making friends because of his or her lack of social skills or anger control skills. The "stress inoculation" power of play would be a good match for

TABLE 1.1. Therapeutic Powers of Play

Facilitates communication	Increases personal strengths
• Self-expression	• Creative problem solving
• Access to the unconscious	• Resiliency
• Direct teaching	• Moral development
• Indirect teaching	• Accelerated psychological development
	• Self-regulation
Fosters emotional wellness	• Self-esteem
• Catharsis	
• Abreaction	Enhances social relationships
• Positive emotions	• Therapeutic relationship
• Counterconditioning fears	• Attachment
• Stress inoculation	• Social competence
• Stress management	• Empathy

a child with medical related-fears or anxieties. Likewise, the "moral development" power of play would be a logical match for a child with conduct disorder. Prescriptive play therapists continually strive to acquire a deeper understanding of the multiple therapeutic powers of play and the disorders for which each of the change agents is most effective.

Principle 5. Individualized Treatment

The overarching aim of prescriptive play therapy is to tailor the intervention to meet the needs of a specific client. The goal is not just to treat the presenting problem but the person who is suffering from it.

The main idea behind individualized therapy is that each client is unique, and what works for many with the same disorder may not work for this particular individual. Research has found that therapy is more effective when it is adapted to the client's personal characteristics, in particular, culture, resistance, preferences, spirituality, therapy expectations, attachment style, environmental circumstances, and motivation to change (Norcross & Wampold, 2011). An important goal of the initial assessment is not only to determine a diagnosis, but also to highlight such important personal variables. It is important to remember that we are treating a *person* with a disorder, not just a disorder.

Core Practices

Principle 1. Comprehensive Assessment

The prescriptive approach to treatment planning begins with a comprehensive assessment of the symptoms and determinants (internal and external) of a client's problem. The assessment typically involves (1) multiple informants (i.e., parents, child, teachers) and (2) multiple methods (i.e., clinical interview or standardized instruments, such as behavior checklists) (Achenbach & Edelbrock, 1983), rating scales (Conners, Sitarenios, Parker, & Epistein, 1998), and projective techniques. In addition, direct observations of the child as well as parent–child interactions (Schaefer, 2014) are often used to gather data. Based on this information, an individualized case formulation is conducted before initiation of therapy. The case formulation is a descriptive and explanatory summary of the client's most important issues/problems (as well as strengths), and of the probable causal or contributory factors. A case formulation also includes the treatment goals and strategies, possible obstacles, and a means for evaluating progress.

The object of this assessment and case formulation is an individualized intervention tailored to the specific presenting problem and unique characteristics of the client. Chapter 2 of this book contains detailed guidelines about conducting a comprehensive initial assessment of the child.

As the treatment proceeds, additional assessment data and insights will be collected about the client and utilized to enhance the intervention.

Principle 2. Monitoring of Progress

The ongoing monitoring of change in a client's presenting problem(s) enables play therapists to determine if the client's symptoms are getting better, the same, or worse. This feedback is crucial in deciding whether to maintain or adjust the prescribed treatment plan so as to prevent premature termination and enhance the likelihood of success. Studies have shown that the monitoring of symptom change is most effective when it is done on a *weekly* basis throughout all phases of treatment (Schaefer & Gilbert, 2015).

This routine of monitoring symptoms ensures that the tailoring of treatment will be a continuous process. This allows for midcourse corrections and successful outcomes in treatments that had been producing negligible or negative results (Lambert et al., 2003; Harkin Webb, & Chang, 2016).

Principle 3. Empirically Supported Treatments

In the past, the field of psychotherapy relied too heavily on practices that had little supporting evidence or, at worst, had shown poor outcomes. Therapeutic interventions have been provided based on a belief in tradition (i.e., "that's what we've always done") rather than evidence-based information regarding what truly works. Research reviews reporting the empirical base for effective practice of play therapy are now available to assist therapists in expanding evidence-informed interventions (e.g., Baggerly, Ray, & Bratton, 2010; Reddy, Files-Hall, & Schaefer, 2005, 2016). In summary, prescriptive play therapists are committed to applying interventions that have been scientifically proved to be most effective in alleviating psychological pain in children.

Principle 4. Treatment Selection

The treatment selection procedure most compatible with prescriptive play therapy is the evidence-based practice model developed by the Presidential Task Force of the American Psychological Association (2006). According to this model, the therapist selects a treatment for a client by integrating three main sources of information: (1) empirically supported treatments for the disorder, (2) client needs and preferences, and (3) therapist variables, such as therapist expertise and clinical judgment. This model, which values *both* science and practice information, has become the dominant model across the field of psychotherapy. For the prescriptive play therapist, it provides the necessary flexibility to tailor the intervention to the specific disorder and unique preferences and situation of the client.

Principle 5. Role of the Therapist

Prescriptive play therapy requires the therapist to be competent in more than one theoretical orientation and technique of play therapy. At the minimum, he or she should develop skills in at least one directive and one non-directive form of play therapy because both will be needed to treat a wide variety of presenting problems and determinants. Moreover, since prescriptive play therapy is, at its core, a person-centered approach, the therapist must become knowledgeable of the personal, social, and cultural characteristics of the client that can boost or impede the efficacy of the treatment.

The role of the therapist in the prescriptive approach will vary depending on the specific play intervention selected for the client. For example, the therapist will be directive and structured when implementing a behavioral or Theraplay treatment plan but nondirective when adhering to a child-centered orientation. Often, the therapist trains a child's parents to be partners in treatment, while such parent involvement may be contraindicated in other cases. Thus, the prescriptive play therapy approach is best suited to therapists who are open, flexible, and pragmatic, as well as skillful in adapting a particular treatment protocol to their own personal style.

Summary and Conclusions

This chapter contains an overview of the basic premises and core practices of the prescriptive approach to play therapy. Prescriptive play therapists draw from a number of play therapy theories and techniques to select an intervention best suited to overcome the client's presenting problem. They then tailor this therapeutic intervention to the characteristics and preferences of the individual client to achieve a truly individualized approach.

The field of psychotherapy therapy today has evolved so that there are few, if any, "purists" who strictly and dogmatically adhere to a single theoretical orientation (Kazdin, Bass, Ayers, & Rogers, 1990). If the impressive growth and development that the field of play therapy experienced in the 20th century is to continue throughout the 21st century, it will likely be because the prescriptive (eclectic, integrative, evidence-informed) approach has become more fully and widely implemented by practitioners across the world.

REFERENCES

Achenbach, T., & Edelbrock, C. (1983). *Manual for the Child Behavior Checklist.* Burlington, VT: Queen City Publishing.

American Psychological Association. (2006). Evidence-based practice in psychology. *American Psychologist, 6*(4), 271–285.

Baggerly, J., Ray, D., & Bratton, S. (Eds.). (2010). *Child-centered play therapy research: The evidence for effective practice.* Hoboken, NJ: Wiley.

Beutler, L. E. (1979). Toward specific psychological therapies for specific conditions. *Journal of Consulting and Clinical Psychology, 47,* 882–897.

Beutler, L. E. (1991). Have we all won and must all have prizes? *Journal of Consulting and Clinical Psychology, 59,* 226–232.

Beutler, L. E., & Clarkin, J. (1990). *Systematic treatment selection: Toward targeted therapeutic intervention.* New York: Brunner/Mazel.

Chambless, D. L., & Ollendick, T. H. (2001). Empirically supported psychological intervention: Controversies and evidence. *Annual Review of Psychology, 52,* 685–716.

Conners, C., Sitarenios, G., Parker, J., & Epstein, J. (1998). Revision and restandardization of the Conners Teacher Rating Scale. *Journal of Abnormal Child Psychology, 26*(4), 279–291.

Dimond, R., Havens, R., & Jones, A. (1978). A conceptual framework for the practice of prescriptive eclecticism in psychotherapy. *American Psychologist, 33,* 239–248.

Frances, A., Clarkin, J., & Perry, S. (1984). *Differential therapeutics in psychiatry.* New York: Brunner/Mazel.

Goldfried, M. R. (2001). *How therapists change: Personal and professional reflections.* Washington, DC: American Psychological Association.

Goldstein, A. P., & Stein, N. (1976). *Prescriptive psychotherapies.* New York: Pergamon Press.

Harkin, B., Webb, T., & Chang, B. (2016). Does monitoring goal progress promote goal attainment?: A meta-analysis of the experimental evidence. *Psychological Bulletin, 142*(2), 198–229.

Kaduson, H. G., Cangelosi, D., & Schaefer, C. E. (Eds.). (1997). *The playing cure: Individualized play therapy for specific childhood problems.* Northvale, NJ: Jason Aronson.

Kazdin, A., Bass, D., Ayers, W., & Rogers, A. (1990). Empirical and clinical focus of child and adolescent psychotherapy research. *Journal of Consulting and Clinical Psychotherapy, 58,* 729–740.

Kazdin, A. A., Siegel, T. C., & Bass, D. (1990). Drawing on clinical practice to inform research on child and adolescent psychotherapy: Survey of practitioners. *Professional Psychology: Research and Practice, 21*(3), 189–198.

Lambert, M. J., & Bergin, A. (1994). The effectiveness of psychotherapy. In S. L. Garfield & A. E. Bergin (Eds.), *Handbook of psychotherapy and behavior change* (4th ed., pp. 143–189). New York: Wiley.

Lambert, M. J., Whipple, J., Hawkins, E., Vermeersch, D., Nielsen, S., & Smart, D. (2003). Is it time for clinicians to routinely track patient outcome?: A meta-analysis. *Clinical Psychology: Science and Practice, 10,* 288–301.

Luborsky, L., Singer, B., & Luborsky, E. (1975). Comparative studies of psychotherapies: Is it true that "everyone has won and all must have prizes"? *Archives of Abnormal Psychiatry, 32,* 995–1008.

Messer, S. B. (1992). A critical examination of belief structures in integrative and eclectic psychotherapy. In J. C. Norcross & M. R. Goldfried (Eds.), *Handbook of psychotherapy integration* (2nd ed., pp. 130–165). New York: Basic Books.

Munns, E. (1992). *Application of family and group theraplay.* Lanham, MD: Rowman & Littlefield.

Norcross, J. C. (1987). *Casebook of eclectic psychotherapy.* New York: Brunner/Mazel.

Norcross, J. C. (1991). Prescriptive matching in psychotherapy: An introduction. *Psychology, 28,* 439–443.

Norcross, J. C. (1995). Dispelling the Dodo bird verdict and the exclusivity myth in psychotherapy. *Psychotherapy, 32,* 500–504.

Norcross, J. C. (2005). A primer on psychotherapy integration. In J. C. Norcross & M. R. Goldfried (Eds.), *Handbook of psychotherapy integration* (2nd ed.). New York: Oxford University Press.

Norcross, J. C., & Prochaska, J. O. (1988). A study of eclectic (and integrative) views revisited. *Professional Psychology: Research and Practice, 19*(2), 170–174.

Norcross, J. C., & Wampold, B. E. (2011). What works for whom: Tailoring psychotherapy to the person. *Journal of Clinical Psychology in Session, 67*(2), 127–132.

Paul, G. (1967). Strategy of outcome research in psychotherapy. *Journal of Consulting and Psychology, 31,* 109–119.

Phillips, R. D., & Landreth, G. L. (1995). Play therapists on play therapy: A report of methods, demographics and professional practice issues. *International Journal of Play Therapy, 4,* 1–26.

Presidential Task Force of the American Psychological Association. (2006). Evidence-based practice in psychology. *American Psychologist, 6*(4), 271–285.

Prochaska, J. O., & Norcross, J. C. (1983). Contemporary psychotherapists: A national survey of characteristics, practices, orientations, and attitudes. *Psychotherapy: Theory, Research, and Practice, 20,* 161–173.

Reddy, L. A., Files-Hall, T. M., & Schaefer, C. E. (Eds.). (2005). *Empirically based play interventions for children.* Washington, DC: American Psychological Association.

Reddy, L. A., Files-Hall, T. M., & Schaefer, C. E. (Eds.). (2016). *Empirically based play interventions for children* (2nd ed.). Washington, DC: American Psychological Association.

Schaefer, C. E. (1993). *The therapeutic powers of play.* Northvale, NJ: Jason Aronson.

Schaefer, C. E. (2014). *Play observation of mother–child interaction style.* Unpublished manuscript.

Schaefer, C. E., & Drewes, A. A. (2013). *The therapeutic powers of play: 20 core agents of change* (2nd ed.). Hoboken, NJ: Wiley.

Schaefer, C., & Gilbert, J. (2015). How to assess a child's progress in play therapy. *Play Therapy, 12*(3), 16–19.

Smith, M. L., Glass, G. V., & Miller, T. I. (1980). *The benefits of psychotherapy.* Baltimore: Johns Hopkins University Press.

Stevens, S. E., Hyman, M. T., & Allen, M. (2000). A meta-analysis of common and specific treatment effects across the outcome domain of the phase model of psychotherapy. *Clinical Psychology: Science and Practice, 7,* 275–290.

CHAPTER 2

Comprehensive, Individualized Assessment for Prescriptive Play Therapy

Sue Ammen

Rationale

Prescriptive play therapy is a transtheoretical and therapeutically integrated approach (Schaefer & Drewes, 2016) where

> play therapists . . . choose which approach to use with a given client based on the client's unique presentation. The child's symptomatology, diagnosis, developmental needs, and natural leanings are matched with appropriate treatment goals and then matched to the most helpful interventions. The appropriate interventions, which may run the gambit from nondirective to directive, can then literally be prescribed at various phases of treatment, for various lengths of time, and in a flexible clinician informed order. (Goodyear-Brown, 2010, p. xiv)

The task of the prescriptive play therapist is to develop a coherent problem formulation that can be used to codevelop with the client and family a treatment plan with achievable goals tailored to the client's specific problems and situation (Schaefer & Drewes, 2016). In order to accomplish this task, the prescriptive play therapy must complete a comprehensive, individualized assessment. Schafer and Drewes describe a prescriptive play therapy assessment as providing in-depth understanding of the child, the family, and origins of the child's presenting problem. The assessment includes multiple informants, multiple methods, and ongoing assessments throughout treatment to measure progress. Through this process, the treatment is customized to the client's individual needs and problems. It is cost-effective because it focuses on the cause of the problem, not just the symptoms. The case formulation is a descriptive and explanatory summary that helps parents understand the origins of the child's presenting problems and leads to an individualized treatment plan—that is, a prescriptive plan that specifies treatment goals and strategies.

Prescriptive play therapy derives from prescriptive psychotherapy models with adults (Beutler, Consoli, & Lane, 2005) that describe treatment decision making as based on the conditions that tend to be present when therapeutic change occurs. This prescriptive matching process leads to a treatment plan by selecting therapeutic change agents that have the potential to address the underlying causes of the problem. Extrapolating to play therapy, the therapeutic powers of play (Drewes & Schaefer, 2016; Schaefer & Drewes, 2016) provide a frame for identifying therapeutic change mechanisms in prescriptive play therapy. These include (1) facilitates communication and teaching, (2) fosters emotional wellness, (3) enhances social relationships, and (4) increases personal strengths. (See Drewes & Shaefer, 2016, for an expanded description of these major categories and the specific therapeutic powers within each of them.)

Consistent with evidence-based practice recommendations (Spring, 2007), prescriptive play therapy treatment goals consider empirically supported treatments, client and family needs and preferences, and therapist clinical judgment and experience (Schaefer & Drewes, 2016). For example, Goodyear-Brown's (2010) prescriptive approach focuses on treating children with trauma, so she uses a flexibly sequenced course of play therapy treatment that is grounded in trauma-informed treatment goals. While these goals incorporate therapeutic powers of play (e.g., increase emotional literacy, assess and augment coping skills), they also integrate trauma treatment mechanisms (e.g., soothing the physiology, integrating linguistic with somatosensory content through creation of coherent trauma narrative). Play therapy interventions are customized to resolve the specific problems that brought the client to treatment within the context of the individualized needs of the child and family. A coherent problem formulation is based on a thorough assessment of why the presenting problem exists and what is contributing to it. The focus of this chapter is on the process of completing a comprehensive, individualized assessment to support prescriptive play therapy treatment planning.

A Comprehensive Individualized Assessment Approach for Use with Prescriptive Play Therapy

The following model of a comprehensive prescriptive play therapy assessment is adapted in large part from *Play Therapy Treatment Planning and Interventions: The Ecosystemic Model and Workbook* (EPT Workbook; O'Connor & Ammen, 2013). This book was written specifically for play therapists to facilitate their collection, organization, and understanding of case data, development of a comprehensive case conceptualization, and creation of a detailed, goal-oriented treatment plan.[1] While ecosystemic play therapy (EPT) is not specifically a prescriptive play therapy approach, the model has considerable overlap as an "integrative metatheory that allows play therapists to pull concepts and strategies from many other theories and to employ a wide variety of techniques, including empirically supported treatments (O'Connor, 2016, p. 223). Core components of EPT include being developmentally organized, relationship-focused, strengths-based, and grounded in an ecosystemic context of multiple interacting systems that change over time, including family systems, social systems, and metasystems such as cultural and sociopolitical contexts (Ammen & Limberg, 2005; Limberg & Ammen, 2008; O'Connor, 2016). These concepts are also compatible with prescriptive play therapy, which uses development and systems, as well as individual needs and preferences, in its conceptualization process (Gil & Shaw, 2009). At the same time, EPT is not a prescriptive play therapy model, as it emphasizes theoretical integration into a meta-theory. To understand the EPT model more fully, the reader is referred to the EPT Workbook or O'Connor (2016). For the purposes of this chapter, the focus is more generically on those aspects of the comprehensive assessment model that support the development of a prescriptive play therapy treatment plan. The key components of this prescriptive play therapy comprehensive assessment model are (1) intake and assessment data gathering; (2) case formulation; and (3) treatment planning. Rather than presenting a complete case vignette, brief case examples are used to illustrate aspects of the assessment model. For the purposes of this discussion, the term *caregiver(s)* is used to refer to a parent, foster parent, or other significant adult in a primary caregiving role with the child.

---

[1] The EPT Workbook (O'Connor & Ammen, 2013) contains detailed instructions and downloadable forms for completing all of the components of the intake, case formulation, and treatment plans.

Data Gathering: Intake and Assessment[2]

The data-gathering process often takes several sessions and typically includes an interview with the caregiving adults to gather a detailed history, a play interview with the child, a dyadic session(s) with the child and each caregiver, and/or family session with significant family members, and baseline assessments. It may include observations in other settings if relevant, such as school, review of records or consultation with other professionals, and more extensive play-based or standardized assessments. Child–Parent Psychotherapy (Lieberman, Ghosh Ippen, & Van Horn, 2015), a dyadic, empirically supported, play-based trauma treatment for young children, describes this as the *foundational phase* of treatment. In addition to gathering information, we are also initiating an important therapeutic process that includes engaging the family, instilling hope, and facilitating reflection on the issues that brought them to treatment. Hirshberg (1996) describes this as "history making, not history taking." When we invite parents to carefully tell the story of their child and family, we are helping them to hold their child in mind, and we are holding that family and child in our own mind. "When a child is held in mind, the child feels it, and knows it. There is a sense of safety, of containment, and, most important, existence in that other. . . . One of life's greatest privileges is just that—the experience of being held in someone's mind" (Pawl, 1995, p. 5).

Specific aspects of the intake and assessment process include:

1. Defining the presenting problem(s) from multiple perspectives, including the caregivers, the child, and other relevant systems.
2. Gathering a comprehensive developmental ecosystemic history from multiple informants and sources.
3. Observing the child in multiple contexts, including unstructured play, interactions with caregiver(s), family system(s), and other systems (e.g., school) when relevant.
4. Assessing the child's mental status.
5. Completing play-based developmental, relationship, and clinical assessments as relevant.
6. Gathering formal assessment data, including baseline documentation of symptoms and concerns.
7. Organizing information into a comprehensive intake report.

---

[2] See Chapter 3 in the EPT Workbook for the logistics of structuring the data-gathering process, including initial contact, interview with caregivers, interview with child, and interview with families. Examples of specific questions to gather the intake information and mental status are included in Chapter 4 of the EPT Workbook.

Defining the Presenting Problem

Effective treatment begins with the process of engaging the child and family as motivated participants, and one way to do this is to truly "see and hear" the problem from multiple perspectives. Parents and others may experience and understand the problem very differently from how it is experienced and understood by the child. Each participant's view of the problem is critical because each is making decisions and acting based on his or her own perception.

> Six-year-old Jose was being sent home from school due to aggressive behavior and refusal to do classwork. From his mother's perspective, the problem was that his behavior problems at school were interfering with her ability to work because she had to leave work to get him. The teacher saw him as oppositional and disruptive and affecting the learning of other children. Through the play interview, Jose shared that his father had been deported over the summer and he was terrified that his mother might also be deported while he was at school.

It is important to define the problem in terms of how it adversely impacts the child and/or others. These impacts can include causing distress to the child or others, interfering with relationships, limiting participation in developmentally expected activities, and/or limiting the family's participation in activities (Zero to Three, 2016). The task is to define the current problem(s) as specifically as possible, understand the historical origins of the problem, and identify each of the systems that is or was impacted by and continues to impact the problem. It is also helpful to explore what has been attempted both in the past and present to resolve the problem (response to interventions) and what it would look like if the problem (behavior, feelings, attitude) was better (solution-focused). This information not only helps define specific treatment goals, but is used to develop hypotheses about the etiology of the problem, factors maintaining the problem, and resources for resolving the problem.

Comprehensive Developmental Ecosystemic History and Observations[3]

The developmental ecosystemic history is organized around the child's and family's experience at different points in the child's development, and within the context of the relevant ecosystems surrounding the child and

---

[3] Refer to the EPT Workbook in Chapter 4 for a thorough discussion of the information that can be targeted relative to each of the systems.

family. The recommended structure is to have the caregivers reflect on each stage of their child's development, gathering current and historical information about each of the relevant systems as the opportunity presents itself. The developmental review starts by asking the caregivers to describe life in their family at each developmental stage, beginning with family life before conception of this child. At each stage it may be helpful to ask about their feelings about the child, difficulties, joys, worries, and any critical environmental events or traumas that occurred during that stage. Look for opportunities to understand the cultural context of the child and family, including cultural stressors, as well as resources and sources of resilience. The following is an outline of specific issues that may be addressed at each stage:

1. Prepregnancy (couple/marital history and other children).
2. Pregnancy (feelings, hopes, fears and images of baby during pregnancy, physical problems, depression/anxiety in either parent during and after pregnancy, alcohol, cigarette, or drug use, including marijuana and prescription drugs, stressors, and support system).
3. Birth (first memory of child, birth experience, support system, and any problems during delivery).
4. First year of life (primary caregivers, type of baby, caregiver experience of baby, parenting, and relationship, and any disruptions in caregiver–infant relationship).
5. Ages 1–3 years (type of toddler, developmental milestones—sitting, walking, talking, toilet training, developmental concerns, how caregiver(s) handled toilet training and limit-setting, and how child responded, attachment relationships with caregivers, day care and separations/reunions, relationship with siblings and extended family).
6. Ages 3–5 years (type of preschooler, preschool experiences, relationships with family members and with peers).
7. Ages 5–11 years (school history with emphasis on adjustment to kindergarten, first, third, and sixth grade—academic, behavioral, and social adjustment, close friends, self-esteem, gender role and identity, family relationships).
8. Adolescence (relationships with family, peers, authority figures, legal system if relevant, drug and alcohol use/abuse, beginning intimate relationships, future goals).
9. Adults in family (caregiver developmental levels and roles, coparenting system).

When the developmental interview is complete, follow up on any specific points or events relative to the specific ecosystems not covered in response to the open-ended developmental probes. Although the developmental history process generally covers the child's individual development and behavior, dyadic system with caregivers, family system, and school system, it is important to ask specifically about any risk behaviors (covered in the next section, "Mental Status Examination"), as well as any legal, medical, or mental health system involvement affecting the child, including direct and indirect impacts. For example, having asthma may mean taking a medication that affects the child's attention and behavior as well as ability to participate in physical activities (direct), which may affect the child's self-perception and the caregiver's perception of the child as less capable or more vulnerable (indirect). Finally, the degree to which the broader sociopolitical context affects the family should be explored, such as the impact of immigration stress or historical trauma and ongoing experiences of racism. Other potentially relevant diversity issues affected by the sociopolitical context include sexual orientation and gender identity, differently abled, and religious identity and affiliation.

The play interview with the child provides the opportunity to gather his or her perceptions of past and present events, as well as observe developmental functioning and mental status behavior. Observations of the child in the home or school setting may also be important, depending on the presenting problem concerns. The family interview provides the opportunity to observe the interactions between family members, particularly as they relate to the child client. In addition, the family interview allows the therapist to gather information about (1) different family members' individual perceptions of the problem; (2) strengths, supports, and sources of interference the family may provide to the treatment process; and (3) the ethnocultural beliefs and values of the family. A useful structure for completing a family interview (O'Connor & Ammen, 2013; Worden, 2003) includes (1) greeting and engaging, (2) defining the problem from each family member's perspective, (3) moving to an understanding of how the family functions as a system, (4) understanding the family culture, and (5) establishing goals and closure. Families can be described as being both a "represented family" within the minds of each participant and a "practicing family" as seen in how they interact with each other (Sameroff & Fiese, 2000). Using experiential activities with the family can help make the family aware of how they communicate and engage with each other. Useful activities include the collaborative drawing technique (Smith, 2000), family puppet technique (Ross, 2000), and family play genograms (Gil, McGoldrick, Gerson, & Petry, 2008). With younger children, families can be asked to play a game of Follow the Leader or build something together with a set of blocks. Asking each member to share something about the family that they value or want to keep provides cultural insight into the family members' beliefs, values, and understanding of their family.

Mental Status Examination

An important part of the intake is a play interview with the child to assess the child's mental status. The mental status exam (MSE) provides a structure for gathering very specific information that is helpful in understanding the child's individual cognitive and social emotional functioning. It is critical to consider the child's cognitive developmental level because it affects how the child organizes and processes information. We must consider both the child's actual developmental level and whether that developmental level is consistent with the child's age.

> For example, compare two 9-year-olds who demonstrate significant impairment in insight and judgment for their age. One is functioning at the Preoperational stage of development, and the other is functioning, as expected, at the Concrete Operations stage. In the first case, the child is not cognitively capable of age-appropriate insight and judgment. In the second case, the child is cognitively capable, but is experiencing interference from some other source. (O'Connor & Ammen, 2013, pp. 47–48)

The comprehensive MSE in the EPT Workbook[4] is designed to be used with children across the age span, including very young children (see Benham, 2000, for specific details about conducting an MSE with very young children). Because development significantly impacts how mental status abilities are assessed, many items, such as judgment or insight, are evaluated as being within or above or below normal limits relative to the child's normative age group. McConaughy (2005) and Greenspan and Greenspan (2003) provide helpful interview guidelines for evaluating developmentally typical differences in physical capacities, mood, relationships, affects, anxieties and fears, and organization of thinking. A comprehensive MSE should cover the following areas.

1. Behavioral observations (appearance, motor activity, speech, emotions, attitude, relatedness).
2. Cognitive development and functioning (level and functioning relative to chronological age).
3. Cognitive processes (orientation, memory, concentration, abstraction, intellect, judgment, insight, organization, self-regulation, and executive functioning).
4. Thought content (obsessions and compulsions, phobic thinking versus age-appropriate fears, somatic concerns, hallucinations, delusions).

---

[4]See Chapter 4 in the EPT Workbook for a detailed discussion of the MSE assessment process.

5. Trauma symptoms (reenactment behavior, nightmares, flashbacks, alexithymia, dissociative phenomena).
6. Subjective experience (self-concept, view of the world, three wishes, reality testing).

> Stefanni is a 10-year-old girl struggling with developmental delays and immature behavior. She describes herself as "stupid and ugly" and others/school as "wanting too much, it's too hard," and she wishes she could be Wonder Woman, who is strong and powerful. In other words, she experiences herself as not capable of dealing with the demands of her world—in particular, academic and social expectations. She experiences her self-image as "ugly" as she struggles with being overweight and her sense of disconnect from her body. Her wish to be Wonder Woman confirms her unmet needs to feel competent and in control. Her reality testing is immature and based in fantasy (adapted from O'Connor & Ammen, 2013, p. 54).

7. Dangerous behavior (accident proneness, self-injurious or suicidal behavior, aggressive or homicidal behavior, history of sexually inappropriate behavior, history of fire setting, family history of dangerous behavior).
8. Risk assessment and response plan (if positive response to any dangerous behaviors is exhibited or reported).

The MSE, when embedded in a more comprehensive intake evaluation, is one way of gathering information needed to make a traditional psychiatric diagnosis such as the DC: 0–5 diagnostic system for young children (Zero to Three, 2016) or the fifth edition of *Diagnostic and Statistical Manual of Mental Disorders* (DSM-5; American Psychiatric Association, 2013). The MSE data should be interpreted within a developmental framework, and areas of significant concern should be cross-validated with other sources of information.

Play-Based Assessments and Formal Assessment Data

Family Play History

Because cultural and family factors affect the content and form of the child's play (Westby, 2000), a play history is gathered from the family to get a sense of what types of play and toys the child prefers and how family members view play and play together. Helpful questions include "What kind of toys does your child most enjoy (e.g., puppets, dolls, animals, books, action figures, cars, blocks, etc.)?"; "In your home what kind of toys are allowed or not allowed, and what kind of play is encouraged or discouraged/not allowed?"; "Who does the child play with most often, and what does the child's play look like with caregiver(s), siblings, peers?"; "What is your family's attitude or understanding about the value of play?"

Representational Play Assessment

Play is critical as a medium for helping children to reflect on their experiences and communicate with others, making it important for the play therapist to know that the child is capable of using play symbolically. A significant developmental shift occurs between ages 3 and 3½ with the emergence of meta-linguistic thinking and the ability to recognize internal mental states in themselves and others. Concurrently they begin to project feelings and thoughts into the toy figures. While most children have well-developed representational play skills by age 5, many children in play therapy may have had experiences of trauma or neurodevelopmental problems that interfere with these skills. Children who haven't yet developed symbolic play skills (including developmentally typical very young children) will need direct modeling and structuring support from the play therapist. Children who have experienced trauma may engage in repetitive play sequences that do not reduce their anxiety, while others may avoid representational play (Drewes, 2001). In these cases, the focus needs to be on building a secure therapeutic relationship before working symbolically. Westby's (2000) assessment of representational play development is a valuable part of an initial intake when providing play therapy to younger children, children with neurodevelopmental concerns, or children with histories of trauma.

Parent–Child Relationship Assessment

Understanding the quality of the child's relationship with primary caregivers is often a core element in case conceptualization and treatment planning, either because the relationship needs to be a focus of treatment, or because it is a resource for the child that can facilitate treatment. The Marschak Interaction Method (MIM) (DiPasquale, 2000; Lindaman, Booth, & Chambers, 2000; *www.theraplay.org*) is a valuable and well-developed play-based assessment for capturing the interactive processes between a caregiver and a child. The interpretation of strengths as well as areas of concern lends itself well to treatment planning.

Developmental Screening

Assessment of the child's cognitive and social–emotional development is relevant for two reasons. First, it helps anchor the child's behaviors to actual development levels, especially if they are different from the child's chronological age. Delays in cognitive functioning affect the way the child understands and processes information. Social–emotional delays are not unusual in children with histories of trauma or neglect. Second, by recognizing where the child is actually functioning, treatment can be designed to address the child's needs and understanding at that level and to promote developmental growth, especially social–emotional functioning. The *Developmental Teaching Objectives Rating Form—Revised* (DTORF-R; Wood, 1992; Wood, Quirk, & Swindle, 2007; *www.dtorf.com*) is a developmental assessment completed through an interview with a caregiver or teacher that focuses on social–emotional functioning. Once the therapist becomes comfortable using the DTORF-R, it can be completed in 10–15 minutes. It is particularly useful for treatment planning because it provides specific developmental objectives within the behavior, communication, and socialization domains, based on what skills the child needs to master next. These objectives can then be translated to treatment goals. The DTORF-R can also be helpful in establishing the child's baseline functioning and monitoring treatment efficacy. (Refer to O'Connor, 2000, for a detailed description of the DTORF-R and its use in treatment planning.)

> Stefanni's DTORF-R results were as follows (i.e., tasks to be accomplished):
>
> - Behavior Goal: B12—Participates in individual movement activities with a group without loss of control (e.g., waits turn, does not intrude).
> - Communication Goal: C12—Can describe characteristics of self to others.
> - Socialization Goal: S17—Engages in interactive play with peers.

All of these goals are in the upper end of the Stage II goals, indicating that even though Stefanni is 10 years old chronologically, her social–emotional functioning is similar to that of a 4- to 6-year-old child (adapted from O'Connor & Ammen, 2013, p. 96).

Other Play-Based Assessments

The book *Play Diagnosis and Assessment* (Gitlin-Weiner, Sandgrund, & Schaefer, 2000) is an excellent resource for play-based assessments. Gil (2011) has developed an *extended play-based developmental assessment* to be used over several sessions. Lowenstein's (2008, 2010, 2011) three-volume *Assessment and Treatment Activities* provides a wide range of play-based assessments for children and families developed by experienced play therapists.

Baseline Clinical Screening

The American Psychological Association Task Force on Evidence-Based Practice in Psychology (EBPP) defines EBPP as "the integration of the best available research with clinical expertise in the context of patient characteristics, culture, and preferences" (2006, p. 273). The Task Force definition of *clinical expertise* also entails the monitoring of patient progress. "If progress is not proceeding adequately, the psychologist [or play therapist] alters or addresses problematic aspects of the treatment (e.g., problems in the therapeutic relationship or in the implementation of the goals of the treatment) as appropriate" (pp. 276–277). This is in full alignment with prescriptive play therapy (Gil & Shaw, 2009; Schaefer & Drewes, 2016).

> For example, the Trauma Symptom Checklist for Young Children (TSCYC) was used with a parent after his 3-year old child was in a car accident resulting in brief hospitalization. The TSCYC facilitated the caregiver's recognition of the impact of trauma symptoms on the child's behavior and provided a baseline for treatment. The TSCYC was completed again 2 months later, revealing improvement in several areas (sleeping better, not afraid of cars) and some remaining areas of concern (around dysregulated arousal). These concerns were then targeted in the treatment (adapted from O'Connor & Ammen, 2013, p. 103).

The codevelopment of goals and an explicit treatment contract with the child and the family provides a way to qualitatively track progress in treatment. The DTORF-R and MIM also can be used to monitor treatment efficiency through observation of changes in developmental goals or patterns of dyadic behavior. Clinical rating scales provide a quantitative way to measure target symptoms or concerns as a baseline measure and to monitor treatment outcomes. Many rating scales, however, require a level of training in measurement and the interpretation of tests. The following five assessments target specific issues that often are of concern in the initial assessment process. Many other assessment tools are available, depending on the clinical issues and focus of treatment.

The *Child Behavior Checklist* (CBCL) and *Teacher Report Form* (TRF) of the Achenbach System of Empirically Based Assessment (ASEBA; Achenbach, 2009; *www.aseba.org*) and the *Behavior Assessment System for Children* with both teacher and parent reports (BASC-3; Reynolds & Kamphaus, 2015; *www.pearsonclinical.com*) are comprehensive assessments of behavioral, emotional, and social problems. The *Trauma Symptom Checklist for Young Children* (TSCYC; Briere, 2001), is a caregiver-report rating scale for children ages 3–12. It includes posttraumatic stress intrusion, avoidance, and arousal scales, as well as anxiety, depression, anger/aggression, dissociation, and sexual concerns if relevant. The *Parenting Stress Index, Fourth Edition Short Form* (PSI-SF; Abidin, 2012), as reported by the child's caregiver, captures stress in the parenting role, the caregiver–child relationship, and as it relates to the child's emotional and behavioral difficulties. The *Adult–Adolescent Parenting Inventory–2* (AAPI-2; Bavolek & Keene, 2005); *www.assessingparenting.com*) assesses parenting and child-rearing attitudes and behaviors and provides an index of parenting risk in five specific domains: developmental expectations of children, parental empathy toward children's needs, use of corporal punishment, parent–child family roles, and parent's respect for children's power and independence.

Organizing Information into a Comprehensive Intake Report

In summary, the comprehensive intake assessment process involves multiple sources of information and multiple methods, including interviews, observations, play-based and clinical assessments, and review of records as relevant for the individual needs and concerns of the child client and family. The problem has been considered from many different perspectives, and information has been gathered about the child's current and past functioning in each of the relevant systems. The data-gathering process is nonlinear and complex. The information must then be organized into a traditional intake format, including identifying information, presenting problems, developmental, family, and other systems, mental status, assessment results including baseline data, and diagnostic formulation.

Diagnosis classifies clinical problems into well-defined, empirically supported categories and is often required for traditional mental health practice and third-party payers. It is also helpful in communicating with other professionals and may be useful in identifying evidence-informed treatments. At this time, DSM-5 (American Psychiatric Association, 2013) is the predominant system for psychiatric diagnosis. For children 5 and under, the DC: 0–5 diagnostic system for young children (Zero to Three, 2016) is recommended, particularly as more states are accepting it for payment purposes or cross-walking it to DSM-5. Interestingly, the DC: 0–5 system has retained its multiaxial system, which includes consideration of (1) physical health conditions/impacts, (2) psychosocial stressors and resources, (3) developmental competence across multiple dimensions, (4) relationship context, including parent–child relationship(s) and caregiving/coparenting environment, and (5) cultural considerations, including the importance of self-reflection on the part of the clinician to minimize bias by examining subjective responses to the child, family, and information gathered. Cultural considerations should be addressed throughout the assessment, diagnosis, and clinical formulation process.

Prescriptive Play Therapy Case Formulation

The prescriptive play therapy "case formulation is a theoretically grounded, descriptive, and explanatory summary of the client's most important issues/problems (as well as strengths) and of the probably causal and/or contributory factors" (Schaefer & Drewes, 2016, p. 231). The formulation helps the family and play therapist understand why the presenting problem exists (etiology) and the current contributions and context of the problem. These include the relative contributions of family relationships, psychosocial stressors, constitutional–maturational challenges in the child, and the cultural and socioeconomic ecology of the family.

The following structure provides one way to think about and integrate the intake and assessment data (adapted from O'Connor & Ammen, 2013). It is a basic framework only. In order to theoretically ground it, the play therapist needs to approach this conceptualization from the theoretical frames that are consistent with the prescriptive approaches identified as most appropriate for this individual client and family's needs.

1. Impact of the problems—on the child and on others in the child's ecosystem.
2. Comprehensive description of the child's (a) developmental functioning across several domains including cognitive, social, relational, emotional, language–communication, and sensory–motor, as well as representational play level if relevant; (b) pattern of strengths and difficulties; and (c) sense of overall adaptive capacity and resilience.
3. Etiological factors: How did the child come to be the child he or she is today? What factors contributed to the child's presenting problems and symptoms?
   a. Child factors: What role did factors inherent in the child (e.g., neurodevelopmental concerns, temperament, and cognitive strengths) play in the development of the current pattern of functioning and related problems?
   b. Ecosystemic factors: How have family, peers, and other systems contributed to difficulties as well as strengths in the child's current functioning? In particular, consider the nature of primary attachment relationships with caregivers, sibling and extended family relationships, and the coparenting context. Significant other system influences may include peers, school, medical experiences (of both self and others in the family), etc., as well as the sociopolitical system impacts (e.g., deportation of family member, parental job loss due to factory closing).
   c. Psychosocial stressors and trauma history: How have signifi-

cant stressful events in the child's life contributed to the child's present functioning? In particular, note that the child's developmental level when an event occurred will affect the ways in which they understand that event and themselves in relation to the event.

4. Maintaining factors: What factors are maintaining the present problems, and what factors/resources are available to help resolve the problem?

   a. Child factors: What role do factors inherent in the child continue to play in the current pattern of functioning and related problems?

   b. Ecosystemic factors: How do family, peers, and/or other systems maintain the problem or resist its resolution, or how are they a resource and support for change?

5. Cost/benefit ratio: What does the client gain or lose by functioning the way he or she is currently functioning, and to what degree is the child aware of both these gains and losses.

   Using the example mentioned earlier, 6-year-old Jose's disruptive school behavior interferes with his learning and causes his mother, teacher, and peers to be irritated with him. At the same time, his anxiety is lessened because he is able to be with his mother. Unless the intervention addresses his anxiety about losing his mother, as he did his father, his behavior is unlikely to change, as the risk of losing her is a much greater motivator than not having others irritated with him.

6. Family needs, culture, and preferences that might impact decisions about treatment.

After reflecting on the above framework, the play therapist should have a comprehensive understanding of the case. A brief case formulation can then be developed that includes an overall description of the child, a clear, operationally defined description of the presenting problem(s) and its impact on the child and others; as well as descriptions of the origin of the problem, factors currently maintaining the problem, and the roles of the different systems. Finally, the overall goal and expected outcomes for treatment are outlined, taking into account the family's needs, preferences, and expectations (O'Connor & Ammen, 2013).

Prescriptive Play Therapy Treatment Planning

During the assessment, the play therapist begins to develop a "shared view" of the family's story and the concerns that brought the child to treatment.

The clinical formulation guides the play therapist and family in developing an individualized plan for intervention. "The "right" approach is one that best fits the family and the therapist, addresses the concerns identified by both, and provides . . . an avenue through which the therapist can enter the clinical (family) system to effect change" (Ammen & Limberg, 2005, p. 225).

Before developing the plan with the family, the play therapist engages in prescriptive matching. This includes the following processes: (1) Identify therapeutic approaches that have empirical support for addressing the presenting problems and, if relevant, the underlying causes; (2) link these approaches to specific therapeutic change agents, such as the therapeutic powers of play; (3) reflect on one's own preferred practice modalities and experience; and (4) integrate the various theories underlying the interventions into a coordinated treatment plan. See Schaefer and Drewes (2016, p. 214) for a table of play therapy interventions with research support connected to specific disorders. The Evidence-Based Behavioral Practice Project, *www.EBBP.org,* has up-to-date resources that can help bridge the gap between behavioral health research and practice.

The play therapist then works with both the child client and his or her caregivers to codevelop individualized treatment goals that balance the needs of the client, family, and all relevant systems. Treatment contracts are created with both the child and with the caregivers that apply the goals of treatment to the needs identified by each party. The treatment goals and treatment contracts are organized into a realistic and sequential prescriptive play therapy treatment plan. The goals of treatment are regularly reviewed so that everyone remains fully aware of the purpose and direction of the treatment process.

Treatment progress is monitored through ongoing evaluation of baseline assessments. If treatment is not progressing, adjustments are made using the prescriptive matching process to consider other approaches and modalities. Treatment success can be determined by the degree to which the therapist, child, and family agree that the treatment goals have been achieved.

Conclusion

This chapter presents a comprehensive assessment model, adapted from the Ecosystemic Play Therapy Workbook (O'Connor & Ammen, 2013), that can support the development of a prescriptive play therapy treatment plan. It is developmentally organized, relationship focused, and grounded in the child's ecosystemic context, as well as the family's individual needs and preferences. The assessment model facilitates collection, organization, and understanding of case data, development of a comprehensive case conceptualization, and creation of a detailed, individualized, goal-oriented treatment plan.

REFERENCES

Abidin, R. R. (2012). *Parenting Stress Index, 4th edition Short Form.* Lutz, FL: Psychological Assessment Resources.

Achenbach, T. M. (2009). *The Achenbach System of Empirically Based Assessment (ASEBA): Development, findings, theory, and applications.* Burlington: University of Vermont Research Center for Children, Youth and Families.

American Psychiatric Assoication. (2013). *Diagnostic and statistical manual of mental disorders* (5th ed.). Arlington, VA: Author.

American Psychological Association. (2006). Evidence-based practice in psychology. *American Psychologist, 61,* 271–285.

Ammen, S., & Limberg, B. (2005). Play therapy with preschoolers using the ecosystemic model. In K. Finello (Ed.), *Handbook of training and practice in infant and preschool mental health* (pp. 207–232). San Francisco: Jossey Bass.

Bavolek, S. J., & Keene, R. G. (2005). *AAPI online development handbook: The Adult–Adolescent Parenting Inventory (AAPI-2): Assessing high-risk parenting attitudes and behaviors.* Asheville, NC: Family Development Resources.

Benham, A. L. (2000). The observation and assessment of young children. In C. H. Zeanah, Jr. (Ed.), *Handbook of infant mental health* (2nd ed., pp. 249–265). New York: Guilford Press.

Beutler, L. E., Consoli, A. J., & Lane, G. (2005). Systematic treatment selection and prescriptive psychotherapy: An integrative eclectic approach. In J. C. Norcross & M. R. Goldfried (Eds.), *Handbook of psychotherapy integration* (2nd ed., pp. 121–143). New York: Oxford University Press.

Briere, J. (2001). *The Trauma Symptom Checklist for Young Children (TSCYC).* Lutz, FL: Psychological Assessment Resources.

DiPasquale, L. (2000). The Marschak Interaction Method. In E. Munns (Ed.), *Theraplay: Innovations in attachment-enhancing play therapy* (pp. 27–51). Northvale, NJ: Jason Aronson.

Drewes, A. A. (2001). Developmental considerations in play and play therapy with traumatized children. In A. Drewes, L. Carey, & C. Schaefer (Eds.), *School-based play therapy* (pp. 297–314). New York: Wiley.

Drewes, A. A., & Schaefer, C. E. (2016). The therapeutic powers of play. In K. J. O'Connor, C. E. Schaefer, & L. D. Braverman (Eds.), *Handbook of play therapy* (2nd ed., pp. 35–60). New York: Wiley.

Gil, E. (2011). *The extended play-based developmental assessment.* Royal Oaks, MI: Self Esteem Shop.

Gil, E., McGoldrick, M., Gerson, R., & Petry, S. (2008). Family play genograms. In M. McGoldrick, R. Gerson, & S. Petry, *Genograms: Assessments and interventions* (3rd ed., pp. 257–274). New York: Norton.

Gil, E., & Shaw, J. A. (2009). Prescriptive play therapy. In K. J. O'Connor & L. D.

Braverman (Eds.), *Play therapy theory and practice: Comparing theories and techniques* (2nd ed., pp. 451–487). New York: Wiley.

Gitlin-Weiner, K., Sandgrund, A., & Schaefer, C. (Eds.). (2000). *Play diagnosis and assessment* (2nd ed.). New York: Wiley.

Goodyear-Brown, P. (2010). *Play therapy with traumatized children: A prescriptive approach.* New York: Wiley.

Greenspan, S. I., & Greenspan, N. T. (2003). *The clinical interview of the child* (3rd ed.). Arlington, VA: American Psychiatric Publishing.

Hirshberg, L. M. (1996). History-making, not history taking: Clinical interviews with infants and their families. In S. J. Meisels & E. Fenichel (Eds.), *New visions for the developmental assessment of infants and young children* (pp. 85–124). Washington, DC: ZERO TO THREE Press.

Lieberman, A. F., Ghosh Ippen, C., & Van Horn, P. (2015). *Don't hit my mommy!: A manual for child–parent psychotherapy with young children exposed to violence and other trauma* (2nd ed.). Washington, DC: ZERO TO THREE Press.

Limberg, B., & Ammen, S. (2008). Ecosystemic play therapy with infants and toddlers and their families. In C. Schaefer, P. Kelly-Zion, J. McCormick, & A. Ohnogi (Eds.), *Play therapy for very young children* (pp. 103–124). New York: Jason Aronson.

Lindaman, S. L., Booth, P. B., & Chambers, C. L. (2000). Assessing parent–child interactions with the Marschak Interaction Method (MIM). In K. Gitlin-Weiner, A. Sandgrund, & C. Schaefer (Eds.), *Play diagnosis and assessment* (2nd ed., pp. 371–400). New York: Wiley.

Lowenstein, L. (Ed.). (2008). *Assessment and treatment activities for children, adolescents, and families: Practitioners share their most effective techniques* (Vol. 1). Toronto, ON, Canada: Champion Press.

Lowenstein, L. (Ed.). (2010). *Assessment and treatment activities for children, adolescents, and families: Practitioners share their most effective techniques* (Vol. 2). Toronto, ON, Canada: Champion Press.

Lowenstein, L. (Ed.). (2011). *Assessment and treatment activities for children, adolescents, and families: Practitioners share their most effective techniques* (Vol. 3). Toronto, ON, Canada: Champion Press.

McConaughy, S. H. (2005). *Clinical interviews for children and adolescents: Assessment to intervention.* New York: Guilford Press.

O'Connor, K. J. (2000). *The play therapy primer* (2nd ed.). New York: Wiley.

O'Connor, K. J. (2016). Ecosystemic play therapy. In K. J. O'Connor, C. E. Schaefer, & L. D. Braverman (Eds.), *Handbook of play therapy* (2nd ed., pp. 195–225). New York: Wiley.

O'Connor, K. J., & Ammen, S. (2013). *Play therapy treatment planning and interventions: The ecosystemic model and workbook* (2nd ed.). Waltham, MA: Academic Press.

Pawl, J. H. (1995). The therapeutic relationship as human connectedness: Being held in another's mind. *ZERO TO THREE, 15*(4), 1–5.

Reynolds, C. R., & Kamphaus, R. W. (2015). *Behavior Assessment System for Children (BASC-3)* (3rd ed.). Bloomington, MN: Pearson Clinical.

Ross, P. (2000). The family puppet technique for assessing parent–child and family interaction patterns. In K. Gitlin-Weiner, A. Sandgrund, & C. Schaefer (Eds.), *Play diagnosis and assessment* (2nd ed., pp. 672–681). New York: Wiley.

Sameroff, A. J., & Fiese, B. H. (2000). Models of development and developmental risk. In C. H. Zeanah, Jr. (Ed.), *Handbook of infant mental health* (2nd ed., pp. 3–19). New York: Guilford Press.

Schaefer, C. E., & Drewes, A. A. (2016). Prescriptive play therapy. In K. J. O'Connor, C. E. Schaefer, & L. D. Braverman (Eds.), *Handbook of play therapy* (2nd ed., pp. 227–240). New York: Wiley.

Smith, G. (2000). Assessing family interaction by the Collaborative Drawing Technique. In K. Gitlin-Weiner, A. Sandgrund, & C. Schaefer (Eds.), *Play diagnosis and assessment* (2nd ed., pp. 446–456). New York: Wiley.

Spring, B. (2007). Evidence-based practice in clinical psychology: What it is, why it matters: what you need to know. *Journal of Clinical Psychology, 63*(7), 611–631.

Westby, C. (2000). A scale for assessing development of children's play. In K. Gitlin-Weiner, A. Sandgrund, & C. Schaefer (Eds.), *Play diagnosis and assessment* (2nd ed., pp. 15–57). New York: Wiley.

Wood, M. M. (1992). *Developmental Teaching Objectives Rating Form–Revised user's manual.* Athens, GA: Developmental Therapy Institute.

Wood, M. M., Quirk, C. A., & Swindle, F. L. (2007). *Teaching responsible behavior: Developmental therapy—Developmental teaching for troubled children and adolescents* (4th ed.). Austin, TX: PRO-ED.

Worden, M. (2003). *Family therapy basics* (3rd ed.). Pacific Grove, CA: Brooks/Cole–Thomson Learning.

ZERO TO THREE. (2016). *DC: 0–5 diagnostic classification of mental health and developmental disorders of infancy and early childhood.* Washington, DC: Author.

PART II

Clinical Applications of Prescriptive Play Therapy for Internalizing Disorders

CHAPTER 3

Play Therapy for Children with Depression

Erik Newman

Description of the Disorder

According to the fifth edition of the *Diagnostic and Statistical Manual of Mental Disorders* (DSM-5; American Psychiatric Association, 2013), depressive disorders are defined as those that are predominantly characterized by sad and/or irritable mood, as well as feelings of emptiness. The DSM-5 depressive disorders category contains three diagnoses that affect children and adolescents. Major depressive disorder (MDD) and persistent depressive disorder (PDD; also known as dysthymic disorder) are the two most well-known of these. However, the DSM-5 also introduced a new depressive disorder, disruptive mood dysregulation disorder (DMDD). The addition of DMDD reflects the fact that children with severe mood swings and temper outbursts, who were too frequently being diagnosed with pediatric bipolar disorder, much more frequently develop unipolar depression than bipolar disorder. Common types of depression, common comorbidities, and assessment of depression in children are discussed in this chapter.

Types of Depression

Major depressive disorder (MDD) is estimated to occur in approximately 7% of individuals (American Psychiatric Association, 2013). However, this rate is believed to be closer to 2–3% in children and adolescents (Polanczyk, Salum, Sugaya, Caye, & Rohde, 2015), with rates increasing dramatically with the onset of puberty. The disorder is two to three times more common in female than male adults, though it is believed that the prevalence is at least as high in boys as in girls during childhood. A diagnosis of MDD requires the presence of at least five of nine possible symptoms during the same 2-week period that cause clinically significant distress or impairment and are not attributable to the physiological effects of a substance or other medical condition. Symptoms include (1) sadness, emptiness, hopelessness; (2) diminished interest or pleasure in activities; (3) significant change in diet or weight; (4) insomnia or hypersomnia; (5) psychomotor agitation or retardation; (6) fatigue or loss of energy; (7) feelings of worthlessness or excessive/inappropriate guilt; (8) concentration difficulties or indecisiveness; and (9) recurrent thoughts of death or suicidal thoughts/plans. Most symptoms (except for weight change and suicidal ideation) must be present nearly every day.

The defining feature of PDD is the persistence of sadness and depressed mood most of the day, more days than not, over a much longer period of time. In adults, depressed mood must persist for at least 2 years. However, in children, this symptom can manifest as irritability and must be present for at least 1 year. In addition, two of the following six symptoms must be present: (1) poor appetite or overeating; (2) insomnia or hypersomnia; (3) low energy or fatigue; (4) low self-esteem; (5) poor concentration or difficulty making decisions; and (6) feelings of hopelessness. Overall, PDD is believed to have a lower prevalence rate than MDD, though because it is chronic and requires fewer symptoms, it is more commonly observed beginning in childhood.

DMDD is characterized by severe and recurrent temper outbursts that are developmentally inappropriate and grossly disproportionate to the situation. These outbursts occur at least three times per week on average. A defining feature of DMDD is that, in between outbursts, mood is consistently irritable or angry. This is in contrast to what used to be labeled "pediatric bipolar disorder," where mood was said to fluctuate rapidly, but no guidelines were given as to the mood between outbursts. DMDD is not diagnosed before age 6 or after age 18, and retrospectively, symptoms must have been present before age 10. Symptoms also must have been present for at least one year. The prevalence of DMDD is estimated to range from 2 to 5%, and it is more common in males and school-age children than in females and adolescents.

Common Comorbidities

Depressive disorders commonly co-occur with other psychiatric diagnoses. In fact, all other psychiatric disorders increase the risk for depression.

One of the most common comorbidities for depression is anxiety, with estimates ranging from 21 to 91% (Cassano, Rossi, & Pini, 2003). Generalized anxiety disorder, panic disorder, separation anxiety disorder, social anxiety disorder, and obsessive–compulsive disorder have all been identified as commonly comorbid with depression. In addition, children with adjustment disorders, attachment disorders, and trauma-related disorders all commonly experience symptoms of both depression and anxiety. Furthermore, as depressed children emerge into adolescence and adulthood, concern increases for comorbid substance use disorders, disruptive behavior disorders, eating disorders, and personality disorders.

Children with neurodevelopmental disorders also frequently present with symptoms of depression. Children with autism spectrum disorder, attention-deficit/hyperactivity disorder, and specific learning disorders often become anxious about functioning with their disabilities, and the longer they go without appropriate services for their disabilities, the more helpless and depressed they feel.

Assessment of Depression

Depression should be assessed through clinical interview with parents, clinical interview and observation of the child, and behavior rating scales. The clinical interview with the parents allows the clinician to assess the presence, frequency, intensity, and duration of DSM-5 symptoms. In contrast, behavior rating scales allow the clinician to determine how deviant the child's symptoms are from most asymptomatic children. Rating scales also provide quantitative data that can be captured multiple times over the course of treatment to objectively assess treatment progress. Broadband rating scales may be used to survey all symptom domains, though a more fine-grained assessment of depressive symptoms can be acquired through a narrow-band measure that examines affective, cognitive, physiological, and interpersonal symptoms of depression separately.

Direct clinical interview of the child can be helpful, though depending on the age of the child, he or she may not be able to verbalize concerns. In these cases, play-based assessment is likely to yield more useful information. However, behavioral observations are also critical to the assessment phase. For example, the clinician should note the child's weight, energy level, psychomotor rate, mood, and facial affect. In addition, cognitive and neuropsychological assessment data can provide useful information when available. For example, evidence of slow processing speed and concentration difficulties can add to the symptom presentation, particularly when previous assessment data is available to demonstrate a change in functioning over time.

Rationale for Cognitive-Behavioral Play Therapy

The play therapy approach illustrated in this chapter is predominantly modeled on cognitive-behavioral therapy (CBT), an approach that aims to alter mood by first altering behaviors and thought patterns. CBT is universally recognized as an evidence-based treatment for depression in individuals of all ages. However, CBT is very structured, and it is important to recognize that school-age children are often quite savvy and sensitive. Many children recognize when their therapist is too concerned with their own agenda to effectively respond to their concerns and needs. As such, it is necessary to find ways to genuinely join with children in their distress, their joy, and their curiosity to effectively lead them toward more optimal processing of their emotions. Internal family systems (IFS) is an approach that provides a nice framework for doing this. Relevant concepts from these CBT and IFS approaches are discussed below, followed by descriptions of the applications of these concepts within a play therapy framework.

Cognitive-Behavioral Therapy

CBT has its roots in the 1950s and 1960s (Meichenbaum, 2017), and provides a relatively structured approach to the treatment of many psychiatric disorders, including depression. There are many variants of CBT (Beck & Alford, 2009; Ellis, 1957), some of which place greater emphasis on the role of thoughts in psychopathology and others of which place greater emphasis on behavior. However, the core idea behind CBT is that thoughts, behaviors, and emotions are all related. We feel the way we do, and we often act the way we do, because of beliefs we hold about things that happen in our lives. It is difficult to simply decide to *feel* differently. However, we can alter how we *think* about ourselves, others, and the world by challenging or disputing our *beliefs*. Our new beliefs, in turn, result in new emotional and behavioral experiences. In addition, we can choose to change our behavior directly, which can also change how we feel. The implications of these ideas for depressed children are that, if we teach them skills that will help them effectively understand, think about, interpret, and respond to events in their world, they will escape the negative thought and behavior patterns that resulted in their depression. This objective is accomplished through focusing on many different goals and concepts that will be described below.

　　The first goal of this approach is to provide *psychoeducation* with both the parents and the child. It is important to identify the type of depression the child suffers from, as the symptom presentation is quite different for the various types. For example, a child with MDD or even PDD may primarily evidence sadness, hopelessness, low self-esteem, and lack of energy. These children may be quite aware that they are struggling emotionally, though they have little motivation to engage in treatment or in daily activities that could improve their mood. On the other hand, a child with DMDD will likely present as persistently irritable but may have limited awareness or vocabulary to communicate that awareness. This distinction is critical for parents to understand as they begin to wrap their heads around the specific challenges their children are facing. Most importantly, both the parents and the child should come away with the understanding that the child is not to blame for the disorder, that the symptoms are separate from who he or she is as a person, and that all stakeholders (e.g., child, parents, teachers, therapist) take some responsibility for addressing the current struggles.

The second goal of CBT for depression is to develop *emotion regulation* skills. This is a multistep process that begins with appropriately identifying emotions, advances to monitoring emotional experiences in a variety of situations, and culminates with accurately identifying triggers for emotional experiences.

The third goal of treatment is to develop and strengthen *coping skills*. This includes being able to identify the maladaptive skills currently being used, the consequences of those strategies, and more adaptive skills that can replace them. Effective development of coping skills involves identifying a variety of physical, creative, social, and solitary outlets that can be used appropriately depending on the situation.

A fourth goal of CBT is to develop more effective *problem-solving* skills. This involves evaluating the coping skills and possible solutions that are available in a given situation, weighing the pros and cons of each, and choosing the best one. It also involves evaluating the success or failure of the chosen solution to determine whether, and in what circumstances, it should or should not be used again in the future. A specific challenge for children who exhibit chronic or extreme irritability is that they are likely to struggle to make effective decisions, particularly when they are emotionally distressed, even if they have the tools available to them under less activating circumstances.

Behavioral activation is a critical concept in the behavioral treatment of depression. A key component of depression is the lack of desire and/or energy to participate in activities that are typically enjoyable for the child. Comorbid anxiety often strengthens avoidance of those activities. Behavioral activation focuses on identifying activities that are likely to improve mood and then lead to actual engagement in those activities. This process can be tricky, and it is often necessary to work through many factors that serve to maintain depression, anxiety, and avoidance. For children, this will typically involve parents (parent involvement will be discussed in greater detail below). However, play therapists have the perfect tools at their disposal to aid in this process. Simply by offering children options of fun activities and letting them guide their play, the therapist is creating an environment that is likely to improve mood. This improvement may be only temporary at first, but therapeutic change is a learning process. The more opportunities children are given to experience positive emotions, the more they learn that life can be enjoyable, and the more hopeful they become about the future.

Internal Family Systems

IFS is a framework that has been developed over the past 20–30 years by Richard Schwartz, a marriage and family therapist (see Schwartz & Sweezy, 2020). Schwartz brought his family systems perspective to the treatment of individuals by conceptualizing their challenges as the conflict between multiple "parts" or subpersonalities. IFS treats each part as a separate entity with valuable functions, voicing their own valid points of view and interacting with one another in an attempt, albeit not always successfully, to protect the client and allow him or her to function.

The goal of IFS is to achieve *self-leadership*. The *self* is defined as the core and innate presence within each of us that promotes healthy functioning. When individuals are self-led, they exhibit many transformative qualities, which are referred to as the "eight C's": curiosity, confidence, creativity, courage, calmness, connectedness, clarity, and compassion. In addition, the self allows people to be present in the moment, adopt an appropriate perspective, accept that which cannot be changed, and be playful. However, we each have additional parts that blend with the self and sometimes overwhelm its capacity to function adequately. These parts fall into three categories. The first category is referred to as *exiles*. Exiles are parts that have been hurt in some way (e.g., abused, neglected, shamed, humiliated, scared), and they carry the intense emotions that go along with those experiences and memories. In order to allow the individual to function without being overwhelmed by the emotional pain of these experiences, exiles are banished by the two other parts, which are referred to as *protectors*. There are proactive protectors called *managers* and reactive protectors called *firefighters*. Managers focus on being vigilant and prepared. They take action to prevent exiles from being triggered, and they often cause us to act in rigid and avoidant ways, including avoiding connections with others and avoiding prioritizing our own well-being. Despite the hard work of the managers, exiles sometimes become triggered nonetheless by unpredictable environmental factors. This is when the firefighters go to work. They use extreme measures to once again banish the exiles. In adults, this often takes the form of substance abuse, binge eating, or self-harm. In children, it is often reflected in aggression, meltdowns, and complete shutdowns. Therapeutic change occurs by acknowledging, validating, and honoring these parts, and by unburdening them and inviting them to take on new qualities.

For those not familiar with IFS, this concept may still sound familiar because similar ideas were popularized in the Disney Pixar film *Inside Out*. This film features subpersonalities living inside the head of a young girl, each representing the emotions she is capable of experiencing (joy, sadness, fear, anger, disgust), reacting accordingly to situations the young girl is experiencing, and guiding her behavior. Fortunately, the popularity of this movie gives children a concrete framework within which to understand otherwise complex ideas. The concepts of self, exiles, managers, and firefighters are a bit advanced for many children. However, subpersonalities that encompass specific emotions are more developmentally appropriate.

At first glance, it may seem that the principles of IFS are in some ways antithetical to the principles of CBT. After all, CBT aims to challenge perspectives, while IFS seeks to validate them. However, by the very nature of depression, many depressed children come to therapy defended and with no motivation to participate. IFS validates these emotional experiences and invites clients to participate when they are ready. This approach serves to soften their protectors and allow more of their self to lead their interactions, thereby making them more curious and playful. This in turn increases not only their willingness to engage in therapeutic play, but also their ability to enjoy it more fully and make use of it.

Application of Evidence-Based Principles to Play Therapy Interventions

Psychoeducation

The principles described above allow for many opportunities to utilize the therapeutic powers of play to maximize the benefits for children. In the initial phase of therapy, it is often helpful to engage in psychoeducation and to set expectations for what play sessions will look like. The *teaching* powers of play are used consistently throughout this intervention, and they can be used from the very beginning in an effort to set the right tone and engage children in the process.

With regard to psychoeducation, it is important for both the child and the parents to understand the relationship between the child and his or her symptoms. One way of doing this is to draw two separate figures on a white board or a sheet of poster paper. One figure represents the child, while the other represents depression. Once these figures are drawn, the therapist enlists the child and parents in generating positive qualities of the child that are written inside the "child" figure and symptoms associated with the depression that are written inside the "depression" figure. This helps to illustrate the fact that the child has many positive qualities and that he or she is not defined by the depressive symptoms.

With regard to setting therapeutic expectations, the child should be told that the initial phase of therapy will be focused on getting to know one another. In the service of building rapport, the therapist should allow the child to explore the playroom and identify fun activities. This puts less pressure on the child to conform to the therapist's agenda in the beginning, and it utilizes the principle of behavioral activation to allow for positive emotions to develop in relation to the therapeutic process. However, the therapist should also prepare the child for the fact that, after a few sessions, the therapist will begin to invite the child to participate in fun activities and games of the therapist's choosing in order to achieve the necessary therapeutic goals. If necessary, the therapist can make a deal with the child in which the child gets to choose an activity after participating in the therapist's activity.

Emotion Regulation

Once sufficient rapport is established to engage in a variety of playful activities of the therapist's choosing, the *emotion regulation* powers of play can be used to develop a variety of emotional competencies. The first of these competencies is emotion identification. Depending on the child's age and the presence or absence of other comorbid conditions, this skill may already be developed. However, it is important to be sure, as it is difficult to process emotions in a more complex way and effectively cope with them if the child does not have those basic building blocks. Simple techniques can be used to confirm that these skills exist and to develop them if they do not. The child should be asked to list several emotions and playfully make faces for those emotions. The child can also be asked to identify the emotions of faces in drawings or pictures and to draw his or her own pictures of faces with a variety of emotions.

Once the child has demonstrated the ability to accurately identify emotions, concepts from the IFS model can be used to promote *self-expression* and *self-actualization,* two other therapeutic powers of play. In general, the IFS model promotes these powers through an emphasis on allowing the parts to communicate their concerns and allowing the self to take a larger role in guiding the child's behavior and perspective. The self is then able to lead the healing process. However, the IFS model also allows for tools that can be used throughout treatment to achieve many of the CBT goals described earlier. This begins with creating the child's parts. He or she should be asked to create puppets that represent a variety of emotions.

These puppets can be made in many different and creative ways. As suggested in the Puppet Characters with Feeling Names technique (Fall, 2001), sock puppets can be made with different-colored yarn, buttons, beads, and markers. Alternatively, they can be made with brown or white paper bags. The child should be encouraged to personalize them so that they are meaningful representations of those parts or emotions. Giving each puppet a name, personality, background, and specific concerns can help the child feel more connected to the process. These puppets can then be used throughout the therapeutic process to check in with each part about what they are experiencing in the moment in relation to current activities and the memories they elicit. This may seem foreign to the child at first, and it may be necessary for the therapist to model use of the puppets in this way.

Other play techniques can also be used to monitor the child's emotional experiences and to help the child connect these emotions to the contexts in which they occur. For example, the Color-Your-Life technique (O'Connor, 1983) involves asking the child to color in a circle that is drawn on a sheet of paper. The child is asked to identify different emotions, assign a color to each emotion, and color different amounts of each emotion to reflect his or her feelings. This can be done for the child's general mood or for feelings associated with specific contexts (e.g., different times of day, school vs. home). The child can then be taught to further differentiate emotions related to contexts through techniques such as the Feeling Word Game (Kaduson, 1997). In this technique, the child is asked to identify feeling words that the therapist writes down on separate sheets of paper. Poker chips, pennies, beads, or other objects are placed in a jar and used to represent emotions. The therapist then tells a personal story and asks the child to place different amounts of chips on each feeling word for how he or she would feel during that scenario. This helps children to develop an understanding of what kinds of situations trigger different emotions, as well as an understanding that people can have different amounts of different emotions all at the same time. The therapist and child should take turns with different scenarios so that the therapist can model the process for the child. When children are depressed, they tend to focus only on negative emotions, so it may be helpful for the therapist to highlight the positive emotions that can be experienced even during sad and challenging scenarios. Throughout each of these techniques and scenarios, the child should be asked to check in with the various puppets (i.e., internal parts) about their perspectives.

Coping Skills

Another set of therapeutic powers of play that are utilized in this model are the *ego-boosting* powers. Because depression is often associated with low self-esteem and self-efficacy, it is important to ensure that the depressed child develops skills that increase confidence, competence, and empowerment. This can be accomplished by focusing on developing coping skills and problem-solving skills. Coping skills are the variety of tools that children use to manage their emotions and deal with their problems. As a general organizing theme, it may be useful to adopt a concrete representation of a toolbox to sort their different types of coping skills. For example, Goldberg-Arnold and Fristad (2003) suggest using a drawing of a toolbox with four different compartments for physical outlets, social outlets, creative outlets, and relaxation skills. Each time the child practices a new skill, it can be added to the toolbox as a concrete way of tracking what skills are available to him or her.

Before introducing and practicing new coping skills, the child should be asked to generate (with the therapist's help as necessary) a list of skills he or she is already using. This can increase a sense of confidence by allowing children to feel they are already bringing certain skills to the table. It may also serve to highlight the fact that they currently have very few options. The therapist can then initiate a discussion about how each of the child's puppets makes use of those few strategies and what else might be helpful to them. Then the therapist can invite them to use other tools as well through a variety of playful demonstrations. For example, deep breathing can be illustrated through the use of the relaxation training technique, Bubble Breaths (Cabe, 2001). In this technique, the therapist illustrates that blowing a big bubble requires a deep breath in and a slow breath out (as opposed to shallow and fast breaths). The therapist then challenges the child to see who can blow the biggest bubble. Through this process, the child learns not only to take deep breaths, but also to associate deep breathing with the cue, "bubble breaths," which makes it easier to remember to use it when cued in the future.

Depressed children often have low self-esteem and self-efficacy. They receive messages from peers, teachers, and even parents that they are worthless, that they can't do anything right, and that things will never get better. Eventually, they internalize those messages. An important skill for children to have is the ability to turn off those messages and choose to take in other messages instead. One way to do this is to allow their puppets and other toys to be characters in TV shows about them that air on different channels. The therapist can either use a large black picture frame or just cut a black border out of a large piece of poster board and create a flat-screen TV frame. The therapist and the child create stories that send various types of messages, both pessimistic and hopeful ones, and the child can practice fully listening to their messages and then asking their permission to turn down their volume or temporarily change the channel.

Some depressed children, for example, those with DMDD, struggle to control their frustration and display tantrums, meltdowns, and even aggressive behavior. These children will benefit from techniques aimed at processing and coping with anger. The Anger Wall technique (Sribney, 2003) uses Post-it notes on the wall to distinguish anger triggers that result in levels of anger ranging from "frustrated" to "mad" to "steaming." Once the child is effectively able to process his or her anger, effective coping can be illustrated with balloons. In the Balloons of Anger technique (Horn, 1997), the therapist discusses many frustrating events and blows into a balloon each time an event is discussed. The therapist explains that, if air is only blown into the balloon without air being let out, eventually it explodes. Using a second balloon, the therapist discusses the same events, but also illustrates the use of various coping skills, letting air out of the balloon each time a coping skill is used. In this way, the anger never reaches the threshold for explosion.

Problem-Solving Skills

Problem solving is a complex process requiring evaluation of the factors that contribute to problems as well as decision making about adopting the appropriate course of action to address the problem or the factors that caused the problem. Straightforward techniques can be used to illustrate the problem-solving process, including a technique called Hand-ling the Decision-Making Process (Bertoia, 2003), in which a hand is traced on a sheet of paper, a problem is written in the middle of the hand, and possible solutions are written on each finger. Pros and cons are then written in the spaces between the fingers. Having the puppets engage in the process is a useful way of honoring the concerns of each of the child's parts. In addition, techniques such as Broadcast News (Kaduson, 2001) can be used to frame "ask-the-expert" news segments where children get to guide listeners navigating problems they are familiar with.

A nice tool that can be used to assist more complex social problem solving is the Closeness Circle. This technique was devised as a way of assessing and mapping relationships in the interpersonal psychotherapy for depressed adolescents (IPT-A; Mufson, Dorta, Moreau, & Weissman, 2011) model, another evidence-based treatment for depression. The Closeness Circle involves using concentric circles drawn on a sheet of paper, writing the client's name in the innermost circle, and then writing the names of family members and friends in the outer circles depending on how close they are to the client emotionally. However, with preadolescent children, it is often helpful to make this concept even more concrete. One way of doing this is to create an oversized Closeness Circle. Instead of drawing concentric circles on a piece of paper, it can be helpful to use duct tape to tape several pieces of poster paper together, large enough to cover the entire floor, and then draw the innermost circle in the center, large enough for the child to stand inside it. The outer circles can be drawn feet apart (as space provides), creating plenty of space for each circle. The names of various people within the child's support circle can be written on individual sheets of regular paper and placed in their appropriate places within the concentric circles, based on how close the child is to each person emotionally. The therapist can then role-play interactions with those people, demonstrating how challenging it can be to effectively communicate with those farther away. In addition, when a social problem or conflict involves a parent or other family member who is able to participate in the therapeutic process, this can be used as a concrete way of relating to that parent. The pros and cons of the current dynamic can be processed, and negotiations can take place about social roles. The child and therapist can also choose fun activities for the child and parent to engage in together in an attempt to bring them closer emotionally, which would in turn bring the parent into a closer concentric circle.

Parent Involvement

Parent involvement is a critical component of successful child therapy. This starts at the very beginning of the therapeutic process with psychoeducation and setting expectations for therapy. It is essential that parents of depressed children understand the factors that contribute to the child's symptoms, environmental cues and events that trigger mood changes, and behavior management strategies that improve self-esteem rather than shaming the child. For example, parents need to understand that depression results in low motivation to participate in activities and that lack of participation in activities worsens depression because it decreases opportunities for new learning. Parents should engage their depressed child in warm and supportive ways that send the message that they understand that the symptoms are not the child's fault, while at the same time providing a variety of fun, creative, social, and relaxing activities for their child. In a supportive tone, they should maintain firm expectations that the child participate in these activities.

One trap that often occurs in these situations is that depressed children refuse to participate in activities. Parents often misinterpret the function of this behavior and assume the children are doing so to be defiant. It is essential that they understand that this behavior is part of the child's depressive symptoms and that punishing it is likely to further shame the child for his or her symptoms. Parents should set the child up for success by beginning with very few demands, catching the child meeting those demands, and using positive reinforcement strategies to increase the likelihood of that behavior occurring again in the future. In the beginning, this may take the form of a token economy or other extrinsic reward system wherein the child earns points that can be traded for various items on a reward menu. Over time, it is hoped that expectations can be increased and that consistent extrinsic rewards can be faded out as the benefits of participation become more intrinsically rewarding.

Parents should also be taught how to model emotion regulation, coping, and problem-solving skills at home. They should be encouraged to label their own emotions, and to notice and comment on when the child is expressing emotions. They should comment on the reason for the emotion, as well as options for dealing with those feelings. They can also set up regular times for family members to play together using activities of the child's choosing.

For children with DMDD or explosive/aggressive tendencies, parents should be taught the principles of the collaborative problem-solving approach (Greene, 2014), an evidence-based approach to parenting "explosive" children. This approach allows both parent and child to express their wishes and needs, and models a problem-solving method that respects both points of view in reaching a solution. Using skills such as empathy, defining the problem, and inviting the child to participate, parents act as a "surrogate frontal lobe" in modeling how to effectively think through the pros and cons of possible solutions. This approach also emphasizes the importance of proactive problem solving as opposed to reactive problem solving. Parents should not try to reason with children during a tantrum or meltdown, as the logical brain is flooded by the emotional brain. Parents should instead wait until a time when the child is calm, address what occurred previously, and discuss the application of that lesson in future instances.

Finally, parents need to be aware of additional types of interventions that should be considered when the child's symptoms are not sufficiently improving through therapy alone. They need to understand the importance of consulting with a psychiatrist to determine whether medication might be helpful. They also need to understand the role that school can play in both maintaining the child's depression and potentially alleviating it. Some children, especially those with severe mood symptoms or comorbid neurodevelopmental disorders, may need an individualized education program to ensure adherence to therapeutic goals across settings. Others may simply need minor modifications of classroom structure or homework expectations in order to ensure that challenges in school do not continue to affect their self-esteem.

Case Vignette: Johnny

Johnny is a 10-year-old Caucasian male who was brought to play therapy by his mother due to significant changes in his mood and behavior following his parents' divorce when he was 9. Johnny and his brother, who is 3 years younger, witnessed frequent conflict between their parents in the year leading up to the divorce, and Johnny became tense and seemed to worry a lot. He still enjoyed spending time with both parents, but he was reportedly cautious about his own behavior for fear of upsetting them and stressing them out even more. However, once his parents separated and his father moved out of the house, Johnny's mood declined rapidly. At first, he cried a lot and seemed sad most of the time. He stopped responding to his parents' attempts to engage him in activities they used to enjoy together (e.g., going out for ice cream, riding bikes together). He seemed to blame himself for not doing enough to bring joy to his parents, and he began to doubt his self-worth all around. The crying lessened after a few months, but he became increasingly angry and irritable. He started eating more and sleeping less. Johnny clearly met the criteria for MDD. His frustration tolerance was diminished, and although he did not meet the criteria for DMDD, he began displaying periodic explosive outbursts.

When Johnny arrived for his first session, he was quite resistant to therapy. He did not want to speak to the therapist, and he sat in a corner while his mother spoke with the therapist. As the therapist explained the core symptoms of depression to his mother, it was not clear if Johnny was listening. However, as the therapist began describing depression as something separate from who Johnny was as a person and as something that was not his fault, it became clear that Johnny was listening because he began periodically looking at the therapist in response to specific statements. Mom and the therapist agreed to offer Johnny a special dinner at his favorite restaurant after the session for participating in the remainder of the discussion. As a result, Johnny began reluctantly interacting. He was asked to think of things to draw on poster paper to represent him and his symptoms. He chose to draw a dog to represent him and a big, angry wolf to represent his symptoms. With the help of his mother, he wrote words such as "smart," "kind," and "generous" inside the dog, and he listed many of the symptoms described previously, such as worrying, feeling sad, crying frequently, feeling angry, and having tantrums inside the wolf. As the therapist began to describe everyone's responsibility for calming the wolf, he began to smile and nod at his mother as if to say, "See, you're responsible for helping me too." He begrudgingly agreed to come back again to meet with the therapist alone, and said goodbye.

Over the course of the next three sessions, the therapist let Johnny explore the playroom and identify games and toys that he found interesting, with the understanding that after a few meetings in which they would get to know each other, they would slowly transition to other kinds of activities. Johnny gravitated toward superhero characters and games. He also wanted to show the therapist his drawings of some of his favorite superheroes. Throughout these sessions, Johnny and the therapist chatted about his life, about his relationship with his brother, and briefly about how he missed his father. He began to evidence subtle smiles on occasion, and by the third session Johnny was no longer resistant to participating, but his affect remained fairly restricted.

By the end of the third session, the therapist began making silly and playful emotion faces with Johnny and asking him to make faces as well. It was clear that Johnny had an adequate emotional vocabulary and understanding of a variety of emotional experiences. The therapist concluded the third session by introducing the idea of the puppets to represent his emotional responses. At first, Johnny seemed hesitant about the idea, but he agreed to make the puppets because he enjoyed creative arts projects and it seemed that it would at least be fun to make the puppets. During the fourth session, he used small white paper bags to create the puppets, drawing their faces and coloring in their clothes with markers, and then gluing yarn to the heads for hair. His happy puppet had rosy cheeks, bright green clothes, and yellow hair, and he named him Chip. His sad puppet had brown hair and wore all blue, and his name was Mopey. His angry puppet had red hair and red clothes, and his name was Torchy. His scared puppet had green hair and wore purple clothes, and his name was Mouse. The therapist also made his own puppets along with Johnny so that they could communicate with one another through the puppets.

After making the puppets, the therapist also introduced the Color-Your-Life technique. The therapist modeled the technique by coloring mostly yellow in the circle for happy, with a little area of red for mad. The therapist modeled discussion of the colors using the puppets, with his happy puppet saying, "Yay, I get to hang out and play with Johnny for a while. This is great! I just want to sing and play all day long!" Then he modeled the angry puppet saying, "Yeah, but my team lost the baseball game this afternoon. I just want to scream!" Johnny laughed at the therapist's demonstration. The therapist then asked Johnny to color in the circle with different colors for different emotions based on how he was feeling in that moment. He colored mostly yellow for happy, with a small section of blue for sad. After a prompt from the therapist, he picked up Chip and said, "Making puppets is much better than doing homework." Next he put Mopey on his hand, but he struggled to figure out what to say. With coaching from the therapist on expressing sadness and the reasons he felt that way, he was able to say, "I'm sad because I want to see my dad." The therapist then picked up his own sad puppet and said to Chip, "Yeah, it sounds like you're having fun making dolls instead of doing homework," and then turned to Mopey and said, "But you kinda want to see your dad. It can feel really strange to feel both good and bad at the same time." The therapist then had Johnny make Color-Your-Life drawings for that morning, the night before, the last time he spent time with his mom, and the last time he spent time with his dad.

The Color-Your-Life technique and puppet play became a regular part of therapy, occurring at the beginning of each session. In addition, the Feeling Word Game was used several times, with both the therapist and Johnny sharing stories that evoked various emotions. Over the next few sessions, Johnny became more familiar with the routine and learned to express his emotions through the puppets. More importantly, through developing the puppets' personalities and using them to engage in other tasks, he learned to identify the triggers that activated those personalities as well as the "go-to" behaviors that those personalities preferred. For example, one of his nighttime drawings had a lot of sadness and anger expressed in it, and he identified that he was not able to speak to his father on the phone that night. Torchy wanted to scream at his mom, while Mopey just wanted to go to his room, not talk to anyone, and sleep forever. After receiving consistent therapist validation of those different parts, Johnny was even able to express anger through Torchy at both of his parents for "ruining his life" because they couldn't get along with each other. The therapist then asked Johnny if it would be alright to invite Chip into the conversation to see if he had anything to add, and Johnny responded with, "Well, Chip doesn't like it either, but he's happy that at least mom and dad are still nice to me even if they're not always nice to each other."

The therapist introduced the topic of coping skills using the toolbox in about the seventh session, while still consistently using the puppets to process emotions. Various ideas for coping strategies were introduced, but Johnny did not engage enthusiastically at first. He acted as though the ideas were dumb, and he expressed resentment at the notion that he should be the one to change his behavior, especially after developing the ability to voice anger toward his parents. However, as the therapist continued to invite the perspectives of each puppet and validate them in turn, he began to soften. He was able to hear that perhaps Mopey shut everything down because that was his go-to response, but that maybe it was okay for him try out other responses as well. He began to engage in the Bubble Breaths technique, and he enjoyed challenging the therapist to see who could blow the biggest bubble. He also created TV shows with Chip and Mopey on different channels, and he practiced changing the channel to his puppets' different messages. At the therapist's suggestion, he let Torchy express anger at his parents and Mopey express sadness about the former life he was grieving when he had both of his parents together. He gave those puppets permission to speak, but he also asked them if it would be okay if he switched over to the "Chip channel" for a while. He then voiced interesting new experiences that he never had before, such as meeting other kids his age in two separate neighborhoods and getting to go out for dinner more often. His affect was noticeably improved during those discussions.

Around the 10th session, the therapist introduced more complex problem-solving ideas. By then, Johnny's protectors had softened significantly, and he was willing to engage in any activity suggested by the therapist. The therapist discussed the steps to problem solving and used the Closeness Circle to illustrate the nature of the problems he was facing. Six sheets of poster paper taped together with duct tape were used to create one large "canvas" for the circle. He was placed in the middle circle, and three outer circles were drawn. He wrote "MOM," "DAD," and "BRO" on three separate sheets of paper. He was first asked to place those sheets in the appropriate circle to show how close he used to feel to them before his parents separated. He placed all three family members in the closest concentric circle to him. Then he was asked to place them in the appropriate circles based on how close they were now. He moved his mother and brother to the middle circle and his father to the outer circle. A brief discussion took place with the puppets to validate how awful that felt, and then he was asked to place the papers in the appropriate circles for where he would like them to be. He moved his brother back to the innermost circle, left his mother in the middle circle, and moved his father into the middle circle. After processing that change with the puppets, he was able express that he wanted to be close with all of them, but that he was also still resentful of his parents and lacked trust that they would not hurt him again.

The Broadcast News technique was then used to put Johnny in the expert role of figuring out how to feel close to his family without getting hurt. During this news segment, he allowed the therapist to use his puppets to call in and ask questions of the expert. The puppets all asked questions to address their concerns, and Johnny generated relevant responses. For example, Mouse expressed worry that Johnny's parents would upset him and asked how he could make sure that wouldn't happen, and Johnny said he could either stay away from them altogether or tune them out (a "manager" response). Mopey asked what would happen if he did get really upset, and he said he could lock himself in his room away from everyone else (a "firefighter" response). Chip asked if he would ever be able to be happy and achieve his goal of bringing his family closer toward his inner circle if he was always tuning others out and locking himself away, and he said he could also talk to them about how he was feeling (a "self-led" response).

The therapist worked with Johnny's mother to ensure that she was aware of the kind of progress he was making and the openness he was showing. The therapist also wanted to encourage her to be patient and look for opportunities to validate Johnny's emotional experiences. His mother also relayed this information to his father and reported that he was quite receptive to those suggestions. Within about 6 months, Johnny's mood was markedly improved. He still had moments of feeling sad and angry, but he also had many more moments of joy with both parents. The therapist ended treatment by helping Johnny to identify more individuals he could add to his Closeness Circle that he could use for support when he needed it.

The therapist also reminded Johnny that Chip, Mopey, Torchy, and Mouse were all inside the innermost circle with him, and that he should respect all of their wishes and look to them for help as well whenever he was feeling distressed, overwhelmed, or out of control.

Conclusion

Depression is a relatively common disorder in children, particularly when the new diagnosis of DMDD is taken into consideration. Depression in children can take the form of sadness, low self-esteem, hopelessness, and lack of motivation, but it can also manifest as significant irritability and aggression. The treatment for depression with the most empirical support in children is CBT. However, aspects of IFS and other evidence-based treatments such as IPT-A can also be helpful. This chapter describes an approach to play therapy that utilizes the therapeutic powers of play to achieve CBT-derived therapeutic goals, including psychoeducation, emotion regulation, coping skills, and problem-solving skills. It also incorporates principles from IFS that can be useful in treating children with depression, as well as suggestions for how to implement those principles in a play-based format. This includes the use of puppets to represent various "parts" within the child that need to have their voices heard and validated before they are willing to work toward change. By using these puppets consistently throughout the therapeutic process, the child develops a relationship with, and an acceptance of, each of these parts, and learns how to meet their needs in a way that promotes healthier functioning.

REFERENCES

American Psychiatric Association. (2013). *Diagnostic and statistical manual of mental disorders* (5th ed.). Arlington, VA: Author.

Beck, A. T., & Alford, B. A. (2009). *Depression.* Philadelphia: University of Pennsylvania Press.

Bertoia, J. D. (2003). Hand-ling the decision-making process. In H. G. Kaduson & C. E. Schaefer (Eds.), *101 favorite play therapy techniques* (Vol. 3, pp. 14–18). Northvale, NJ: Jason Aronson.

Cabe, N. (2001). Relaxation training: Bubble Breaths. In H. G. Kaduson & C. E. Schaefer (Eds.), *101 more favorite play therapy techniques* (pp. 346–349). Northvale, NJ: Jason Aronson.

Cassano, G. B., Rossi, N. B., & Pini, S. (2003). Comorbidity of depression and anxiety. In S. Kasper, J. A. den Boer, & J. M. Ad Sitsen (Eds.), *Handbook of depression and anxiety* (2nd ed., pp. 69–90). New York: CRC Press.

Ellis, A. (1957). Rational psychotherapy and individual psychology. *Journal of Individual Psychology, 13,* 38–44.

Fall, M. (2001). Puppet characters with feeling names. In H. G. Kaduson & C. E. Schaefer (Eds.), *101 more favorite play therapy techniques* (pp. 248–251). Northvale, NJ: Jason Aronson.

Goldberg-Arnold, J. S., & Fristad, M. A. (2003). Psychotherapy for children with bipolar disorder. In B. Geller & M. P. DelBello (Eds.), *Bipolar in childhood and early adolescence* (pp. 272–294). New York: Guilford Press.

Greene, R. W. (2014). *The explosive child.* New York: HarperCollins.

Horn, T. (1997). Balloons of anger. In H. G. Kaduson & C. E. Schaefer (Eds.), *101 favorite play therapy techniques* (pp. 250–253). Northvale, NJ: Jason Aronson.

Kaduson, H. G. (1997). The feeling word game. In H. G. Kaduson & C. E. Schaefer (Eds.), *101 favorite play therapy techniques* (pp. 19–21). Northvale, NJ: Jason Aronson.

Kaduson, H. G. (2001). Broadcast News. In H. G. Kaduson & C. E. Schaefer (Eds.), *101 more favorite play therapy techniques* (pp. 397–400). Northvale, NJ: Jason Aronson.

Meichenbaum, D. (2017). *The evolution of cognitive behavior therapy.* New York: Routledge.

Mufson, L., Dorta, K. P., Moreau, D., & Weissman, M. M. (2011). *Interpersonal psychotherapy for depressed adolescents* (2nd ed.). New York: Guilford Press.

O'Connor, K. J. (1983). The Color-Your-Life technique. In C. E. Schaefer & K. J. O'Connor (Eds.), *Handbook of play therapy* (pp. 251–258). New York: Wiley.

Polanczyk, G. V., Salum, G. A., Sugaya, L. S., Caye, A., & Rohde, L. A. (2015). Annual Research Review: A meta-analysis of the worldwide prevalence of mental disorders in children and adolescents. *Journal of Child Psychology and Psychiatry, 56*(3), 345–365.

Schwartz, R. C., & Sweezy, M. (2020). *Internal family systems therapy* (2nd ed.). New York: Guilford Press.

Sribney, K. M. (2003). Anger Wall. In H. G. Kaduson & C. E. Schaefer (Eds.), *101 favorite play therapy techniques* (Vol. 3, pp. 118–121). Northvale, NJ: Jason Aronson.

CHAPTER 4

Play Therapy for Children with Fears and Phobias

Laurie Zelinger

Description of the Disorder

Fears

A feature distinguishing between fear and anxiety is related to the timing of the impending threat and its physiological response within the body. Fear is the emotional response to a real or perceived *imminent* threat and is associated with surges of increased autonomic arousal, whereas anxiety is anticipation of *future* threat and is more often linked to muscle tension and vigilance (fifth edition of the *Diagnostic and Statistical Manual of Mental Disorders* [DSM-5]: American Psychiatric Association, 2013). Rachman (1976) indicates that fear can energize behavior and is a "decisive causal factor in avoidance behavior."

Childhood fears are a given. A literature review by Augustyn and Hermann (2017) reports that "children between ages two and six years were found to have approximately four fears, whereas children between ages 6 and 12 years had an average of seven." A large-scale study of nearly 8,000 children ages 5–16 in Great Britain conducted by Meltzer et al. (2008) revealed that nearly one-third of children in that national sample (32.1%) were assessed by their parents as having one of the 12 fears commonly seen in children including animals (11.6%), blood/injection and injury (10.8%), medical or dental procedures, the dark (6.3%), dentists/doctors, the natural environment, vomiting/choking diseases, loud noises, imagined or supernatural beings, small enclosed spaces, and specific types of people and specific phobias (see Figure 4.1).

- Animals
- Loud noises (e.g., sirens, machines, thunder)
- The dark or being left alone
- Medical or dental procedures
- Blood/infection/injury
- Weather events
- Vomiting/choking/acquiring diseases
- Supernatural beings (e.g., ghosts and monsters)
- Stangers
- Particular types of people in unfamiliar clothing or uniform
- Small, enclosed spaces
- Using toilets away from home
- Certain types of transportation, bridges, or tunnels

FIGURE 4.1. Common childhood fears. Data from Schaefer and Drewes (2016) and Schowalter (1994).

Lewis, Amatya, Coffman, and Ollendick (2015) estimate that 20% of children have severe nighttime fears and sleep problems. They note that 58.8% of children between ages 4 and 6 and 84.7% of children between 7 and 9 years of age report at least mild nighttime fears. Several studies report that girls tend to experience more fears and with greater intensity than boys do, and that they are more comfortable expressing their fears (Bauer, 1976; Kendler et al., 2008; Meltzer et al., 2009; Muris, Ollendick, Roelofs, & Austin, 2014; Schowalter, 1994).

Fear has a function related to survival. Evolutionarily speaking, animals and humans most attuned to threats in their environment used their increased vigilance to activate coping mechanisms for survival. Thus, there was greater probability that those "survival genes" would be passed down to future generations to boost their endurance. While some of those fears are no longer needed or relevant and may even be a nuisance in our modern everyday existence, they nevertheless remain coded in our genes, a gift from our ancestors. Some of these fears appear to be inborn, such as the common fear of snakes and rats, and lay dormant until triggered. "Prepotent fears refer to those which are inborn but not necessarily present at birth. They include separation anxiety, aversion to the unfamiliar, discomfort with abruptly changing stimuli and wariness of strangers" (Evans, Gray, & Leckman, 1999). Yet other fears are attributed to one's direct or indirect experience with a frightening situation.

Certain fears occur with regularity among the human species at specific stages in the developmental process. The "ontogenetic parade" (Augustyn & Hermann, 2017) posits that normal childhood fears develop and resolve in a predictable pattern throughout childhood. For example, infants are often swaddled to counteract an inherent fear of loss of support, while children

6 months to 3 years of age are often afraid of strangers, loud noises (e.g., vacuum cleaners, flushing toilets, machines, thunder, and sirens), sudden movement, looming objects, and separation from caretakers (Schaefer & DiGeronimo, 2000). Toddlers may be afraid of people who do not resemble others within their regular sphere of experience, such as people in uniforms or costumes, or storied figures such as ghosts and monsters. Particular animals may also engender fear if the child perceives they represent danger.

Fears change with the maturity of a child's cognitive structures and the ability to differentiate reality from fantasy. Children in the 3- to 5-year-old range experience fears related to things they can see and hear such as unfamiliar noises, animals, masks, and the dark, as well as those that can be imagined. They are now entering an expanding world of possible robbers, bad guys, kidnappers, and monsters that are most surely lurking under the bed or in the closet.

Once children reach ages 6–11, they may still maintain some of their previous fears and are likely to encounter additional new ones. Common fears include snakes (even when there is no likelihood of seeing one), spiders, vomiting, and major weather events, while their growing awareness of the world may now give rise to fears of scary television shows, movies, or the news. Children at this age may be afraid to be left alone, worry about death, and have increased concerns about injections and medical issues. As part of a healthy growth process, this age marks a time where greater importance gets assigned to peer affiliation and acceptance. Any anticipated fear of failure, rejection, or ridicule by friends or teachers may become so intense as to override their confidence and cause anguish.

Fears typically come and go throughout the developmental process of childhood and can usually be managed with little more than attentive parenting, safe and uneventful contact with the feared stimulus, and reassurance. However, about 10% of fears do not resolve and instead develop into greater issues of significant proportion (Muris et al., 2014). When there has been an excessive and persistent fear of an object, situation, or experience that is not normally considered dangerous, which has lasted for at least 6 months and causes extreme distress in the individual, that person is considered to have a phobia. The longer a phobia persists, the harder it is to eradicate. Phobias are an extreme form of anxiety that produce feelings of terror and dread that activate the fight-or-flight response and do not respond to logic or reassurance. They tend to affect females more than males at a rate of 2:1.

Phobias

DSM-5 (American Psychiatric Association, 2013) includes fears and phobias within its classification of anxiety disorders and identifies three types of phobias: *agoraphobia, social anxiety disorder* (also known as *social phobia*), and *specific phobia*.

Agoraphobia is a marked fear or anxiety about two or more of the following situations: using public transportation, being in either enclosed places or open spaces, standing in line or in a crowd, and being outside of the home alone.

Social anxiety disorder (formerly called *social phobia*) is a marked fear about one or more social situations in which the individual is exposed to possible scrutiny by others (American Psychiatric Association, 2013). Common social interactions such as having a conversation, eating, being observed, using a public restroom, or performing in front of others are mere examples of the countless activities that might raise one's anxiety, promulgated by the fear that the person will be negatively evaluated, humiliated, or rejected. Prevalence rates for childhood social anxiety disorder range from 3 to 6.8% in pediatric primary care samples, from 0.5 to 9.0% in community samples, and from 29 to 40% in clinical samples, and this disorder has a high comorbidity rate with other psychiatric disorders (Hitchcock, Chavira, & Stein, 2010). Selective mutism, an anxiety disorder in which one is unable to speak in certain social settings despite having full expressive verbal language in more familiar, comfortable surroundings, has a comorbidity rate with social anxiety disorder of 70–95%.

Specific phobia (or *simple phobia*) is the catchall category for any phobias other than agoraphobia and social phobia, and covers five areas: *animal* (e.g., spiders, insects, dogs); *natural environment* (e.g. heights, storms, water); *blood–injection–injury* (e.g., needles, invasive medical procedures); *situational* (e.g., airplanes, elevators, bridges, enclosed places); and *other* (e.g., situations leading to vomiting, loud sounds, or costumed characters).

Symptoms of Fears and Phobias

There is agreement that symptoms of fear fall within three domains: physiological, cognitive, and behavioral, with variability in expression across cultures and ethnic groups.

Physiological

Physiological responses are usually tied to autonomic arousal and may include increased heart rate, trembling, sweating, shortness of breath, a feeling of choking, chest pain or discomfort, muscle tension, upset stomach/nausea/abdominal problems, a feeling of dizziness or fainting, numbness, chills or hot flashes, and a flushed appearance (Children's Hospital of Philadelphia, 2018; Hitchcock et al., 2010) Although rare in children under age 5 but more common in teens ages 14–18, some people faint at the sight of blood, needles, injury, or medical procedures. This condition, known as vasovagal syndrome or vasovagal syncope, is the result of an overreaction of the autonomic nervous system arising from a sudden increase in heart rate and blood pressure, followed by a slowing of the heart, a drop in blood pressure, and reduction in blood flow to the brain (Orenius, Säilä, Mikola, & Ristolainen, 2018). This is important information for the treating clinician, as some relaxation exercises would be contraindicated for use with this population.

Cognitive and Behavioral

A person in the throes of a panic or anxiety attack is often preoccupied with thoughts of possible contact or demise from the feared situation. Heightened anticipatory anxiety is fueled by a fear of losing control, going crazy, or dying and is accompanied by dread or terror. Internal scenarios swarm with "what–if" possibilities, all confirming that an encounter will be beyond tolerable. If left to run rampant, these thoughts become all-consuming and can lead to a panic attack, described as a sudden surge of intense fear that reaches a peak within minutes. Children usually make valiant attempts to structure their lives in order to avert any possible link to the feared experience, or they may rigidly adhere to behaviors they believe will stave off the threat. Evans et al. found that "some normative ritualistic behavior[s] that appear during middle childhood are probably carried out with the child's belief that he or she is averting some awful disaster or is warding off imaginary terrors" and is tied to the magical thinking of the preoperational period, where action and thought are relatively undifferentiated. While compulsive-like rituals and behaviors give the child a sense of control, they unwittingly strengthen avoidance patterns. More and more time and attention are required to maintain the rituals, creating a focus of avoidance that actually disrupts the process of extinction and serves to empower the ritual, whereby the fear is never faced. When a child is powerless to fend off the objectionable crisis, however, and the situation must be endured, children will often ask their parents to check that the feared situation is absent. Infinite numbers of caretakers have served the role of bodyguard, inspector, taste tester, and monster chaser as their child's fears change through the developmental process.

Genetics

While some fears are correlated with one's prior experience or exposure to a frightening situation, other fears are considered to be genetically linked and passed down through the generations. Over thousands of years, animals and humans who were most adept at using survival skills were those who managed to thwart constant threat and produce offspring with the genetic endowment better equipped to survive.

Certain fears appear to be inborn and remain dormant until triggered.

> It is argued that a heritable predisposition to needle phobia may have its roots in evolution, given that humans who avoided stab wounds and other incidences of pierced flesh would have a greater chance of survival. . . . a heritable predisposition to abruptly increase vagal tone and collapse flaccidly rather than freeze or attempt to flee or fight in response to an approaching sharp object or the sight of blood may have evolved as an alternative survival reaction. . . . Approximately 80% of adults with a needle phobia reported that a first-degree relative exhibits the same fear (Orenius et al., 2018)

Rachman (1977) indicated a high incidence of shared fears among children in the same family, with correlations ranging between .65 and .74, as well as a correlation of .67 between the number of fears exhibited by children and their mothers.

While genetics may account for the inheritance of characteristics, Kendler et al. (2008) posited a "developmentally dynamic" hypothesis which suggests that genetic effects on fear susceptibility may vary over a lifetime. In their longitudinal twin study assessing fear of animals, situations, and blood/injury in children as they developed from 8 to 20 years of age, it was found that "fear mechanisms can be altered by hormonal changes occurring during puberty" and that "it cannot therefore be assumed that genes that influence a trait during one age period will be entirely the same as those that impact the same trait in a later developmental phase" (p. 428).

Temperament

Temperament appears to play a role in the emergence and maintenance of specific phobias. It has been hypothesized that shy, inhibited children have a low threshold for arousal in the amygdala and hypothalamus pathways, especially for unfamiliar events, and that they react with sympathetic arousal noted as high heart rate and acceleration of heart rate under stressful conditions (Ollendick, Hagopian, & Huntinger, 1991). In the review of a longitudinal study by Bierderman and colleagues, Ollendick et al. report that "the rates of all anxiety disorders were higher in inhibited than uninhibited children" (i.e., generalized anxiety disorder, separation disorder, avoidant disorder and phobic disorders) (p. 103).

Causes

The etiology of phobia formation is not fully understood at this time. Schowalter, in his historical context of understanding phobias, states that in the early 1900s, the psychoanalytic interpretation underlying phobia development was based on intrapsychic conflict. Since then, other theories have dominated the research, with unanimous agreement that genetics is at least one factor, but perhaps not the only one, in the development of fears. A seminal piece by Rachman (1977) posits the concept of three pathways to fear—*conditioning, vicarious acquisition,* and *transmission of information*—with a tendency among individuals toward a specific avenue.

Direct behavioral conditioning refers to a child's personal experience with a frightening situation. In a conditioning model, any neutral stimulus that had impact on the child at the same time that a fear response was evoked would acquire the ability to trigger that fear in the future. For example, if a child were pushed into a swimming pool unexpectedly during a family barbeque, any neutral stimuli (e.g., the smell of frankfurters cooking or the sight of lounge chairs) might engender the same fears at a future time if they were present at the time of the original event. Fears that arise in an acute manner seem best explained by this conditioning theory. Although phobias can result from direct terrifying experiences, they can also be due to indirect contact; by observing others showing fear.

Vicarious learning occurs when a child observes, and is consequently influenced by, someone responding in pain or fear to a stimulus or situation. For example, when a child sees that a parent's behavior reflects a fear of dogs (i.e., trembling in its presence, avoidance), he may develop the same symptoms of fear that his parent has effectively modeled. Anxious parents tend to have difficulty exposing their children to the situations that cause them personal discomfort, and they often insulate them from the wider range of experience the world has to offer. When a child shows inherent traits of anxiety and parents model their own fearful reactions, it validates for the child that the situation must be dangerous and is to be avoided. The child's world becomes restricted, and he is then robbed of the opportunity to develop healthier response patterns. Conversely, positive modeling can "immunize" children against future vicarious fear learning (Askew, Reynolds, Fielding-Smith, & Field, 2016).

Information transmission is the third pathway in the tripartite model of fear acquisition and occurs constantly throughout a child's life via parent, teacher, peers, media, or others. Instruction reveals which situations are to be feared, which are not. These fears are typically mild rather than severe (Rachman, 1977).

Fears that arise suddenly may have their genesis during "critical moments" when one's psychological state is most vulnerable. Predisposing factors include emotional upset, physical illness, and associated feelings of weakness, nausea, or dizziness. "The diathesis-stress model asserts that if the combination of the predisposition and the stress exceeds a threshold, the person will develop a disorder" (Augustyn & Hermann, 2017).

Incidence

Askew, Reynolds, Fielding-Smith, and Field (2016) found that anxiety disorders are the most common psychological disorder in the United States, with a prevalence rate of over 25%. Generalized anxiety disorder, separation anxiety, and specific phobia are nearly always the most commonly diagnosed anxiety disorders, occurring in 5% of community samples of children and 15% of outpatient clinic-referred samples (Ollendick, King, & Muris, 2002). According to Lewis, Amatya, Coffman, and Ollendick (2015), 15% of referrals for the treatment of childhood phobias are related to the dark, and Orenius et al. (2018) report that within the general population, needle phobia can be diagnosed in 19% of children ages 4–6 years and in 11% of children ages 10–11 years. Data from the National Comorbidity Survey conducted by the National Institute of Mental Health (2017) estimated that 19.3% of adolescents had specific phobia, with higher rates recorded among females (22.1%) than males (16.7%).

Rationale for Prescriptive Play Therapy Intervention

Children love to play. When interventions for anxiety and fear incorporate play as the vehicle for service delivery, children become engaged. In a review of the literature, Augustyn and Hermann (2017) state that "fears can often be managed through reassurance, education, experience and/or exploration through play (e.g., games involving monsters, scary animals or ghosts)" (p. 7). The goal of play therapy with fearful children is to help them manage their fears and return to a state of emotional, behavioral, cognitive, and physical well-being. When enjoying the therapeutic powers of play, children are able to access opportunities for communication, self-expression, emotional regulation, a sense of control, and a sense of well-being, leading to positive change. The prescriptive play therapist must draw upon her knowledge and experience and consider the individual characteristics of the child in order to determine which empirically based treatment strategy or combination of approaches would best fit the youngster and the presenting problem (Schaefer & Drewes, 2016). The use of standardized assessments should also be considered as part of a treatment plan, as they can be pivotal in making a differential diagnosis that would dictate best practice, as well provide measurements of the effect of an intervention when used in a pre- and posttreatment design.

Step-by-Step Details of the Intervention

Because fear is the motivating behavior underlying avoidance, all of the empirically based strategies for fears and phobias are designed to foster safe contact with the feared stimulus. According to Lewis, Amatya, Coffman, and Ollendick (2015), cognitive-behavioral therapy (CBT), systematic desensitization, graduated *in vivo* exposure, cognitive restructuring, reinforced practice, and participant modeling are empirically based methods of choice in treating anxiety disorders. As such, the integrative approach used with a child named Olivia (see the case vignette below) incorporated these techniques in order to address her fear of insects.

The first step in the process of reducing a fear of insects with Olivia required that a hierarchy of fear be created with her input, ranging from hearing the word *bug,* ranked as a "1," to getting stung by a bee, which earned a ranking of "10." Next, relaxation and mindfulness exercises were taught in order to provide a competing cognitive, behavioral, and physiological response that would interfere with the fear response. When Olivia's high biological activity levels were unresponsive to relaxation efforts, child-centered play activities were activated instead as a competing emotion, bringing comfort and relief, an alternative to relaxation.

The next step in the therapy process introduced graduated fear situations, which were done through play. Plastic facsimiles of bees, wasps, dragonflies, spiders, grasshoppers, beetles, and flies were selected for exposure purposes and placed around the playroom. Additionally, this psychologist has a homemade collection of dead bugs she found locally which were stored in clear plastic jars with magnifying covers, as well as a professionally prepared selection of exotic insects in clear cubes. An interactive educational game, Interactive Amazing Bugs, by Scientific Toys Limited, provided psychoeducation, and toy microphones were used to amplify the therapist's verbal praise and examples of positive statements that Olivia could rehearse. The goal of each session was to raise Olivia's anxiety levels at the same time that she was engaged in juxtaposing relaxation activities, whereby the fear reaction would become diluted and then extinguished.

Parent Involvement

Parents and caregivers are among the first to witness a child's fears, and their response may lay the groundwork for how a fear is managed. When a parent responds to the child's woes with compassion and offers to face the fear together, the child will trust that something can be tried to help him or her feel better. It is common, however, for parents to believe they are protecting their child when they offer comfort from distress and escape from things that scare them. While these parental acts of love bring immediate solace to the child, they do not have lasting effects. A child who is not helped to face a phobia will be plagued by it.

Parent education may be needed to help them understand that some fears and phobias appear to have a genetic basis, while others may arise directly from a child's terrifying experience, or even vicariously from watching others respond with fear in specific situations. It is also helpful to know that there is a high concordance of fears within families. Armed with this knowledge, parents should do their best to provide experiences for their children that would immunize against establishing the same fears they experience. This would involve observing other people who are not afraid as they interact with the situations that might be repelling and anxiety-producing for the parent. Parents would need to learn how to reinforce a child's effort to tackle his or her fears and recognize how misguided efforts to shield or comfort the child may interfere with extinction. Parents must also understand that the goal of any plan is to eliminate avoidance of the feared object and that any progress the child makes toward the feared situation should be reinforced. For parents to be active agents in the process, it is advised that they show understanding of the child's experience, even when those reactions may appear foreign to them.

Olivia's parents were instructed to be patient, to ask what she imagined would happen if she saw a bee, and to dispel the misconceptions she described. Interactive discussion, books, and videos were recommended to provide accurate information and challenge the schema maintaining Olivia's distorted understanding. Her parents were advised to take outdoor excursions and to play in their backyard so that Olivia would be forced to contend with nature, and were also told to praise her for taking steps in the right direction. They were asked to randomly play "Freeze!" both in and out of the house, helping Olivia learn to remain still when she unexpectedly encountered a flying insect. They were also urged to help Olivia do her "therapy homework" whenever it was assigned.

Case Vignette: Olivia

Nine-year-old Olivia is the oldest of four children in an intact family, where both parents work and child care is often provided by babysitters. Developmental milestones were acquired within typical time frames, and Olivia began a toddler program at age 2½ where she adjusted well but began to display focusing issues. Distractibility continued to be brought to the parents' attention, as were anxiety and concerns regarding a lack of awareness of her surroundings.

At age 5, Olivia was diagnosed with attention-deficit/hyperactivity disorder (ADHD), and at age 6 she was evaluated by her school district and classified as a "student with Other Health Impairment." An individualized educational program was developed which included resource room, counseling, and occupational therapy. An independent neuropsychological evaluation performed at age 8 revealed average to superior scores on both intelligence and achievement tests. Behavior surveys, however, illuminated many areas of difficulty. Clinically significant levels of maladjustment were confirmed on Olivia's self-report and parent and teacher versions of the third edition of the Behavior Assessment System for Children. Rankings in the Behavioral Symptoms Index depicted extremely serious concern, as did scores in the following areas: somatization, internalizing problems, atypicality, withdrawal, and anxiety. While teachers and parents endorsed significant rankings in the realm of hyperactivity, Olivia did not recognize those behaviors in herself. The neuropsychological report confirmed the diagnosis of ADHD (combined presentation) as well as generalized anxiety disorder. She was given medication for ADHD, which was administered only on school days.

At age 9, Olivia was frequently complaining of headaches and stomachaches and was becoming school avoidant. She began showing increased reluctance to leave the house and was developing an intense fear of bugs. Long sleeves were worn on a daily basis, she refused to play outside or go to the park, and any obligatory or unavoidable time outdoors was spent scanning the skies for flying insects and inspecting the sidewalks for their shadows. Her fear of bugs was on high alert during the warmer months, as insect life was just awakening from a cold dormant winter when she could forget her fears. Schowalter (1994) reports that the easier it is to avoid the feared stimulus and the less disruptive to the child's life, the less likely she will be to tell others about it. Augustyn and Hermann (2017) and Hitchcock et al. (2010) indicate that overcautiousness, avoidance, freezing, irritability, angry outbursts, crying, clinginess, tantrums, and running away are among a child's common behavioral responses to the feared stimulus. The deciding moment for her parents to seek therapy came when she and her family were taking a walk and Olivia suddenly, and blindly, flew into the street to avoid a bee.

Session 1

Olivia's first session used child-centered play therapy to orient her to the therapist and the therapeutic process. She announced that she wanted to be a science teacher or an animal rescuer when she grows up, and although she likes animals, she is afraid of bees; adding that the warm weather is beginning to bring them out. High-activity levels resulted in an active, fast-paced exploration of the playroom and the handling and discarding of toys after a brief investigation. When the session ended, Olivia's parting comment was, "You understand me."

Session 2

The mother participated in the session with Olivia and helped identify her fears in order to create a hierarchy for use in treatment.

Session 3

Whenever Olivia arrived at this psychologist's office for a play therapy session, she would frantically run from her car to the office with arms waving so as to keep possible winged creatures at bay. Once inside, she would inspect the waiting room for pesky insects. Olivia declared that she was "petrified of bugs, spiders, and flying bees." Discussion provided a form of imaginal exposure where she was encouraged to give details of her harrowing insect experiences. She asked this therapist to google which colors bees are most attracted to, so that she could avoid wearing clothing with those colors.

Session 4

Playful exposure utilized a systematic desensitization trial and reinforced practice, where this psychologist introduced plastic spiders and bees that were kept at an 8-foot distance from the table where she was working. Olivia's engagement in an arts and crafts project she chose served as a pleasant incompatible response, allowing the bugs, which she described as "gross," to gain closer proximity (e.g., successive approximations) throughout the session. Before leaving, Olivia was able to hold the plastic bugs in her hands.

Session 5

In vivo exposure was attempted in an outdoor session where Olivia and this psychologist walked around the block holding the plastic bugs from the week prior. When a flying insect cast a shadow on the sidewalk, Olivia grabbed the therapist around the waist. In order for exposure to be successful, it was critical that Olivia experience the anxiety, rather than being shielded from it or allowed to escape. Therefore, it was decided that the outdoor session would continue for an additional 10 minutes before returning inside to the office. Although the therapeutic technique referred to as "flooding" would have required Olivia to remain fully immersed in the activated fear situation until the fear and physiological responses had faded, this psychologist used a modified approach and maintained the outdoor experience for only 10 minutes. Once in the playroom, Olivia agreed to let the psychologist take the plastic bugs from her and hide them in the sandtray. She was instructed to dig them up with her hands; a task she resisted only marginally.

Session 6

In vivo exposure was repeated again; this time Olivia and the therapist went to the garden to look for bugs. Olivia was often startled by the slightest movement of a leaf, clutching the therapist for relief. The therapist did not return the embrace, particularly because she did not want to provide escape from the anxiety Olivia was experiencing. While Olivia insisted on using an implement to dig up soil, she was challenged to use her hands. Upon return to the playroom, Olivia was shown two real, but dead, bugs that were among a collection this psychologist accrued exclusively for this purpose. Olivia was asked to look through the magnifying cover in order to inspect them at close range and to discuss what she noticed.

Session 7 (the Same Week)

Olivia was brought in for treatment a second time that week, as summer was near, more bugs were about, and she was going to be attending day camp. A return to the garden was on the agenda to implement *in vivo* exposure, reinforced practice, and systematic desensitization. Although Olivia used a trowel for digging, her hierarchy required that she do so without gloves. She trembled at the thought of handling weeds. Modeling and verbal instruction were provided by the therapist: "I don't like dirt or bugs or things that move in the ground but I can do this and I will be okay" (Ollendick, Hagopian, & Huntinger, 1991). Positive reinforcement was given for each effort Olivia made. Upon return to the playroom, her task was to search for the 26 plastic insects hidden in the sand. Once accomplished, Olivia was challenged to repeat the assignment, but this time blindfolded! She did. Several times during the trial she screamed as her fingers wandered beneath the sand. After all 26 insects had been found, Olivia coyly offered that her shrieks were "half real and half fake." She also said that she had been sleeping in her own bed the past three nights; something she had not done in over a year.

Session 8

Olivia asked to play the game "Operation." While her choice could have been a purely child-centered one, this psychologist elected to continue the prescriptive model of exposure and moving up the hierarchy, placed a real dead bug from the collection on the game board. The goal of the game is for the players to perform an "operation" by removing small plastic body parts from the "patient" without setting off the vibrating buzzer that signals the player is "out." The effect of a player getting "out" created such a loud buzz and palpable vibration that the bug actually rambled across the board as though imbued with life. Olivia laughed and cringed at the sight of the moving corpse.

Session 9

With camp starting the next day, psychoeducational input was added to the treatment plan. The game called *Interactive Amazing Bugs* was introduced. This game offers auditory information about different insects, and button selections provide specific facts depending on one's area of interest. The game was used to challenge Olivia's cognitive distortions about the amplified dangers and powers of bugs. She was given homework to watch YouTube videos of bugs.

Session 10

Olivia did not tackle the homework assignment from the previous week and was urged to try again. Camp had started over a week earlier, and she was spending her days indoors with administrative staff. One day, when all campers were required to go outside for a group photo, Olivia was in such a hurry to get it over with that she ran and tripped. Managing her scraped knees and rising despair, she carefully wedged herself in a line between two of the tallest campers, thereby guaranteeing that any determined bee would find them first and she would be spared their dreaded sting. Once the photo was taken, Olivia quickly returned to her niche indoors and moved her things to the camp nurse's office for the remainder of the day.

During the session, Olivia sheepishly recounted an incident that had occurred over the weekend when her family was taking a short trip in their van. Olivia was sitting in the back row with one sibling, and two were in the middle row in front of her when she suddenly discovered, what she was convinced was a wasp; trapped, flying, and seeking its escape. Olivia panicked and tried to open the car door as her father was driving at a high speed on the highway. In her attempt to kill the dreaded creature, she unbuckled her seatbelt and wildly began swatting the air, injuring a younger sibling in the process. The commotion forced her father to pull off the road, and as Olivia leapt out of the car, the moth (apparently "disguised" as a wasp) followed. Embarrassment and humiliation followed as well.

As Olivia recounted this story, she absentmindedly began hiding bugs in the sand for the therapist to discover, and when that activity was over, she asked to play the interactive bug game again. Proudly, she announced that she had been sleeping in her own bed every night; a bonus that was accomplished with her reduced fear and anxiety.

Session 11

Olivia said that the videos made her more frightened, and so she stopped watching. She also stated that, while at camp, a bee came near her on the jungle gym. She closed her eyes, clung to the bars, used self-talk, fought the urge to jump off, and waited until it flew away. Cognitive restructuring at work!

Session 12

Olivia reported that during the week, when a bug flew near her, she closed her eyes and it left. If she had been in a therapy session at that time, she would have been instructed to keep her eyes open in order to prevent escape from the anxiety.

Session 13

Olivia observed the psychologist handle the crispy dead bugs from her personal collection and hold them in the palm of her hand. Olivia petted the cicadas, water beetle, and the disconnected tail of a dragonfly before deciding to make slime for the remainder of the session.

Session 14

Olivia reported that she was taking part in all family activities, both indoors and out. She reached the eighth level on her hierarchy; staying outside and remaining still with eyes open, in the presence of any flying insects. Her ninth level was to have a bug land on her, an occasion that could not be orchestrated during a session, and her tenth level was most certainly not advised: to be stung by a bee. Therefore, Olivia, her parents, and this psychologist agreed that her steady rise up the fear ladder was successfully completed.

Session 15

By Session 15, Olivia reported that she was no longer afraid of bugs and was still sleeping in her bed every night. The end of the summer coincided with significant therapeutic progress in both her fears and sleep hygiene, and as such, therapy sessions moved from weekly to every third week. At this time, progress has been maintained for over a year, and monthly sessions are primarily check-in opportunities to assess ongoing friendship issues.

Empirical Support for the Intervention

Cognitive-Behavioral Therapy

Determining the most efficacious treatment to use with a specific client requires that the clinician be knowledgeable about many of the recognized empirical approaches and choose the prescriptive model that is the best match for that patient's characteristics and particular fear. The goal of prescriptive play therapy using CBT for fears and phobias is to coerce a fear response and to challenge catastrophic thoughts so that new information and perspectives can be acquired to reframe the emotional network, leading to the extinction of the anxiety response. Hitchcock et al. (2010, p. 7), in their literature review of empirically supported treatments, report that "cognitive behavior therapy is often an effective first line of treatment for social anxiety disorder with response rates as favorable as pharmacotherapy treatments."

Systematic Desensitization

The primary goal of systematic desensitization is to reduce anxiety so that avoidance behavior can be eliminated (Davis & Ollendick, 2005). Desensitization is accomplished using three steps: (1) teaching the child to relax his or her thoughts and body, (2) developing a hierarchy of feared objects or situations, with those at the bottom representing the least provocative and those at the top the most upsetting, and (3) providing a trial of exposure with avoidance response prevention where the child is instructed to engage in a relaxation exercise while the therapist gradually and systematically introduces the feared stimuli (either imaginal or *in vivo*). When relaxation is not feasible, other forms of engagement such as humor or play can elicit competing, pleasant responses that become a counterconditioning obstacle to the anxiety response. A review of outcome research indicates that between 68 and 83% of participants achieved benefit from exposure with response prevention and that the gains were maintained long term (Rowa, Antony, & Swinson, 2007). The therapist using relaxation must be cognizant, however, that relaxation may be contraindicated in cases of vasovagal response due to the risk of a decrease in heart rate and blood pressure. Instead, graded exposure that includes applied muscle tension would be a safe alternative (Orenius et al., 2018).

Reinforced Practice

Reinforced practice is considered a well-established treatment for phobia (Davis & Ollendick, 2005). Repeated, controlled, graduated practices allow one to approach the feared object at first from a distance and then from closer vantage points, while recognizing that no ill has come from it. While reinforced practice may successfully induce behavioral change, the physiological and cognitive symptoms of the fear response may remain unchanged.

Participant Modeling

Participant modeling is a vicarious learning experience aimed at changing the behavioral and cognitive component of a phobic response through observation of a model. It is described by Davis and Ollendick (2005, p. 150) as having "well-established empirical status." It subsumes that learning can occur vicariously as a patient watches a relaxed model interact with the feared object without any resulting negative outcome. The therapist instructs the child in how to copy those interactions both verbally and physically, with the eventual realization that an aversive outcome was not produced.

Immunization refers to positive modeling interactions with the feared stimulus which can immunize children against future vicarious fear learning. Askew et al. (2016, p. 288) observe that "fear reduction was greater when the fear reversal pathway matched the acquisition pathway." The best prognosis can be achieved when the pathway of selected treatment (i.e., verbal learning, observational learning) matches the fear learning pathway that initiated the fear response.

Conclusion

Fears and phobias are ubiquitous in children. Some are inborn and have been ascribed to genetics. They are the result of ancestral influences where skills once needed for survival were passed down through the generations. They unfold at different points in a child's development and give rise to fears that are characteristic of children at specific ages. Other fears develop through experience, either directly or indirectly. A child may personally endure a frightening situation, or may vicariously witness somebody in distress. Each of these scenarios has the ability to impact the child and generate fear. When there is an excessive and persistent fear that interferes with daily functioning and has lasted at least 6 months, the child may be among the 10% of cases where a fear evolves into a phobia. The earmark of a phobia is that the child, at all costs, tries to avoid the dreaded object or situation and is consumed with thoughts about its danger.

Empirically based treatments aim to reduce or eliminate the avoidance associated with those fears. They focus on physiological responses of fear as well as one's thoughts and behaviors. Several empirical methods are available to the clinician, with most relying on exposure, relaxation, therapist feedback, and cognitive restructuring. Although many of these strategies have a verbal component, the experienced play therapist will find ways to engage the phobic child with playful interactions, toys as facsimiles of the actual feared objects, and humor. The therapist will also be in a position to support the parent, ensuring that clinical treatment is aligned with home expectations. When a parent understands the rationale behind the chosen methods and her role in the process, she will recognize how to help her child take the necessary risks to extinguish the fear.

REFERENCES

American Psychiatric Association. (2013). *Diagnostic and statistical manual of mental disorders* (5th ed.). Arlington, VA: Author.

Askew, C., Reynolds, G., Fielding-Smith, S., & Field A. P. (2016). Inhibition of vicariously learned fear in children using positive modeling and prior exposure. *Journal of Abnormal Psychology, 125*(2), 275–291.

Augustyn, M., & Hermann, R. (2017). Overview of fears and phobias in children and adolescents. Retrieved October 14, 2018, from *www.uptodate.com/contents/overview-of-fears-and-phobias-in-children-and-adolescents*.

Bauer, D. H. (1976). An exploratory study of developmental changes in children's fears. *Journal of Child Psychology and Psychiatry, 17,* 69–74.

Children's Hospital of Philadelphia. (2018). Phobias in children and adolescents. Retrieved September 12, 2018 from *www.chop.edu/conditions-diseases/phobias-children-and-adolescents*.

Davis, T. E., & Ollendick, T. H. (2005). Empirically supported treatments for specific phobia in children: Do efficacious treatments address the components of a phobic response? *Clinical Psychology: Science and Practice, 12*(2), 144–160.

Evans, D. W., Gray F. L., & Leckman, J. F. (1999). The rituals, fears and phobias of young children: Insights from development, psychopathology and neurobiology. *Child Psychiatry and Human Development, 29*(4), 261–276.

Hitchcock, C. A., Chavira, D. A., & Stein, M. B. (2010). Recent findings in social phobia among children and adolescents. *Israel Journal of Psychiatry and Related Sciences, 46*(1), 34–44.

Kendler, K. S., Gardner, C. O., Annas, P., Neale, M. C., Eaves, L. J., & Lichtensen, P. (2008). A longitudinal twin study of fears from middle childhood to early adulthood: Evidence for a developmentally dynamic genome. *Archives of General Psychiatry, 65*(4), 421–429.

Lewis, K. M., Amatya, K., Coffman, M. F., & Ollendick, T. H. (2015). Treating nighttime fears in young children with bibliotherapy: Evaluating anxiety symptoms and monitoring behavior change. *Journal of Anxiety Disorders, 30*, 103–112.

Meltzer, H., Vostanis, P., Dogra, N., Doos, L., Ford, T., & Goodman, R. (2009). Children's specific fears. *Child: Care, Health and Development, 35*, 781–789.

Muris, P., Ollendick, T. H., Roelofs, J., & Austin, K. (2014). The short form of the Fear Survey Schedule for Children—revised (FSSC-R-SF): An efficient, reliable, and valid scale for measuring fear in children and adolescents. *Journal of Anxiety Disorders, 28*, 957–965.

National Institute of Mental Health. (2017). Specific phobia. Retrieved August 19, 2018, from *www.nimh.nih.gov*.

Ollendick, T. H., Hagopian, L. P., & Huntzinger, R. M. (1991). Cognitive-behavior therapy with nighttime fearful children. *Journal of Behavior Therapy and Experimental Psychiatry, 22*(2), 113–121.

Ollendick, T., King, N. J., & Muris, P. (2002). Fears and phobias in children: Phenomenology, epidemiology, and aetiology. *Child and Adolescent Mental Health, 7*(3), 98–106.

Orenius, T., Säilä, H., Mikola, K., & Ristolainen, L. (2018). Fear of injections and needle phobia among children and adolescents: An overview of psychological, behavioral, and contextual factors. Retrieved August 19, 2018, from *journals.sagepub.com/doi/pdf/10.1177/2377960818759442*.

Rachman, S. (1976). The passing of the two-stage theory of fear and avoidance: Fresh possibilities. *Behavior Research and Therapy, 14*, 125–131.

Rachman, S. (1977). The conditioning theory of fear-acquisition: A critical examination. *Behaviour Research and Therapy, 15*, 375–387.

Rowa, K., Antony, M., & Swinson, R. P. (2007). Exposure and response prevention. In M. M. Antony, C. Purdon, & L. J. Summerfeldt (Eds.), *Psychological treatment of obsessive–compulsive disorder: Fundamentals and beyond* (pp. 79–109). Washington, DC: American Psychological Association.

Schaefer, C. E., & DiGeronimo, T. F. (2000). *Ages and stages: A parent's guide to normal childhood development.* New York: Wiley.

Schaefer, C. E., & Drewes, A. A. (2016). Prescriptive play therapy. In K. J. O'Connor, C. E. Schaefer, & L. D. Braverman (Eds.), *Handbook of play therapy* (2nd ed., pp. 227–240). Hoboken, NJ: Wiley.

Schowalter, J. E. (1994). Fears and phobias. *Pediatrics in Review, 15*(10), 384–388.

CHAPTER 5

Play Therapy for Children with Obsessive–Compulsive Disorder

Susan M. Carter

Description of the Disorder

Obsessive–compulsive disorder (OCD) is a neurobiological disorder that impacts young children through adults; in the absence of treatment, it can be debilitating and chronic (Rosa-Alcazar et al., 2017). It is characterized by repetitive, intrusive thoughts of excessive worry that cause an anxious response, followed by a behavior engaged to give relief to those repetitive thoughts, a behavior the child feels compelled to engage in (American Psychiatric Association, 2013). Although OCD is a neurobiological disorder of the child, it is also a disorder of the family (March, 2007). The pattern can be the basis of formed rituals that interfere with a child's academic performance, their social and emotional development, play and sleep, family gatherings, and functional activities of daily living. For many children and their families, these symptoms eat up valuable family time and cause significant emotional distress for the child, their parents, and their siblings (March, 2007). It is a highly stressful and emotionally disruptive experience for everyone in the child's life—parents, siblings, extended family, and teachers and peers at school. Often the situation becomes worse when adults attempt to intervene to hurry or dissuade the ritual process. Children become emotionally dysregulated, and more time may be spent managing meltdowns than on the ritual itself. Thus, many parents become enablers, accommodating the process rather than constructively aiding their child (Lebowitz, 2013).

OCD, an anxiety disorder, has been found in children and adolescents with prevalence rates of 1–2% of the population (Rosa-Alcazar et al., 2017; Myrick & Green, 2012) and is compounded by genetic factors, environmental exposure, and the child's own temperament (Hill, Waite, & Creswell, 2016). Often children of anxious parents or grandparents also suffering from OCD will be more likely to have the disorder. A child who has experienced a difficult life event—trauma, grief and loss, or vicarious trauma experiencing anxiety-producing information from television or the Internet—can be at risk of developing OCD symptoms. Additionally, a child's own temperament, being highly cautious, can be a risk factor for OCD (Hill et al., 2016). This chapter presents DREAM AWAY, a flexible, manualized prescriptive play therapy approach to treating young children with OCD, utilizing cognitive-behavioral play therapy (CBPT), considered the best practice for OCD treatment.

The most widely researched psychological treatment for OCD in children is cognitive-behavioral therapy (CBT), which integrates cognitive therapy (CT) with exposure and response prevention (ERP) (Barton & Heyman, 2016; Farrell, Schlup, & Boschen, 2010; March & Mulle, 1994, 1995, 1998; Myrick & Green, 2012; Strimpfel, Neece, & Macfie, 2016). CT involves identifying the irrational thoughts and beliefs leading to emotions and behaviors (Knell, 1998); ERP refers to exposure the stimulus for those thoughts, imaginary or *in vivo,* while inhibiting the irrational behavioral response (March & Mulle, 1995). However, though there is significant research showing the effectiveness of CBT with ERP as a treatment for OCD, many children and adolescents do not respond (Lebowitz, 2013). As many as half of the clients continue to suffer from OCD symptoms after participating in therapy. CBT has as its basis the *verbal* processing of beliefs, thoughts, and behaviors. It emphasizes the impact of irrational or maladaptive beliefs on thoughts and feelings, and the meaning from these beliefs that one ascribes to life events, to be at the core of the therapy (March & Mulle, 1998). For CBT to be effective, clients must be able to distinguish between what is illogical thinking and what is rational thinking (Knell, 1998, 2009). Young children may not be developmentally capable of making this distinction or able to verbally communicate their inner thoughts and beliefs, contributing to the lack of response to CBT by so many children. Knell (1998, 2009) recommends adapting CBT for young children into play therapy. "Cognitive Behavioral Play Therapy . . . is based on the cognitive theory of emotional disorders and cognitive principles of therapy, and it adapts these in a developmentally appropriate way. It is sensitive to the developmental issues of children and emphasizes the empirical validation of the effectiveness of interventions" (Knell, 2009, p. 119).

In research for evidence-based treatments, a manual format may be developed with prescribed goals and techniques, specific to each session or phase of treatment, to be used to ensure uniformity across therapists and to minimize variability, thus improving the reliability of outcomes. Several manualized approaches using CBT have been developed, studied, and found to be valuable in the treatment of OCD in children and adolescents (Kendall & Hedtke, 2006a; March & Mulle, 1998). In clinical practice rather than in research studies, however, some variability or flexibility in the application of the process may be needed. March and Mulle (1998) identify the importance of modifying the manualized therapy to the therapist's personal style and to the developmental stage of the child to increase positive outcomes from the intervention. Strimpfel et al. (2016) stress the need to attend to the unique characteristics of each individual child client when engaging in CBT manualized treatment for OCD. All children have their own OCD symptom manifestations and symptom clusters that are as unique as all children are themselves. Strimpfel et al. emphasize that the use of manualized approaches has merit, but that flexibility in application is also warranted. Kendall, Gosch, Furr, and Sood (2008, p. 987) stress "flexibility with fidelity," utilizing clinical expertise and judgment to modify, expand, or otherwise enhance an evidence-based approach to improve the outcome for a specific client. Understanding the child and his or her interests and passions can enhance the outcome of the therapy while still following the prescribed steps of the treatment protocol.

Rationale for Prescriptive Play Therapy

Prescriptive play therapy (Schaefer & Drewes, 2016; Schaefer, 2011; Gil & Shaw, 2009) is an approach to play therapy that customizes a unique treatment from a variety of techniques and supporting theories to meet the child's individual needs. It is a problem-focused intervention, specifically designed to address *the issue* that brought the child or adolescent to therapy, rather than being more globally focused on improved development or adjustment. Schaefer and Drewes (2016) offer six core principles or tenets of prescriptive play therapy:

1. *Individualized treatment:* for both the disorder and the child.
2. *Differential therapeutics:* play therapy inclusive of diagnostics; maintaining the premise that some play therapy modalities are more effective for certain children and for certain disorders than others.
3. *Transtheoretical approach:* eclectic, pulling together three criteria to avoid random eclecticism: empirical evidence, clinical experience, and the desires of the client.

4. *Integrative psychotherapy:* combining two or more theories of psychotherapy into a unified, comprehensive intervention.
5. *Prescriptive matching:* finding the best therapeutic intervention to reduce or remove the cause of the presenting problem. It is the initial diagnostic assessment that is undertaken to identify, when possible, the specific cause of the difficulty in order to select an appropriate theoretical match.
6. *Comprehensive assessment:* to provide clear understanding of the client, his or her family, and the source of the problem to inform treatment and parents.

Prescriptive play therapy is an approach to treating OCD in children that can map to CBT approaches through play. The mechanisms and change agents of play are engaged in a CBT structure to bring about the anticipated change in the child.

In play therapy, we look to the therapeutic powers of play (Drewes & Schaefer, 2011; Schaefer & Drewes, 2013) to identify what elements to weave into the play to affect the desired results. The four specific therapeutic powers of play have multiple core elements of change (Schaefer & Drewes, 2015, pp. 232–233):

1. Facilitates communication
   a. Self-expression/self-understanding
   b. Conscious thoughts and feelings
   c. Access to the unconscious
   d. Direct teaching
   e. Indirect teaching
2. Fosters emotional wellness
   a. Counterconditioning of negative affect
   b. Abreaction
   c. Catharsis
   d. Positive emotions
   e. Stress inoculation
   f. Stress management
3. Enhances social relationships
   a. Therapeutic relationship
   b. Attachment
   c. Social competence
   d. Empathy
4. Increases personal strengths
   a. Creative problem solving
   b. Resiliency

c. Moral development
d. Accelerated psychological development
e. Self-regulation
f. Self-esteem

Prescriptive play therapy, a useful, pragmatic approach (Schaefer & Drewes, 2016), invokes the therapeutic powers of play, along with best-practice guidelines, for optimal treatment results for young children. Best practices as an overlay to the play therapy theory or technique employed by the prescriptive play therapist can "get the job done with an individual case in the most cost-effective manner" (p. 233). In this context, Schaefer and Drewes listed best-practice guidelines with evidence-based support for multiple disorders, to direct prescriptive play therapy practice. They identified CBT with ERP, utilizing the March and Mulle (1998) manualized approach, as the best-practice intervention for OCD.

DREAM AWAY OCD in Young Children

DREAM AWAY OCD is a process specifically combining play therapy theory with best practices for treatment of OCD. It allows prescriptive play therapists to present interventions in an accessible format, to create a treatment foundation, and to clearly communicate the experience of managing OCD for their client families. It enables therapists to organize treatment plans and to enhance the process of planning for the prescriptive play therapy for OCD.

DREAM AWAY is an acronym for the therapeutic activities that a child and their parents may engage in to manage OCD. It is prescriptive in that it calls upon the basic tenets of prescriptive play therapy to accomplish the goals of the client. We have identified a library of interventions that engage the therapeutic powers of play, categorized by their specific anxiety management technique, and we have organized them under the acronym DREAM.

D: Deep breaths—fun and silly diaphragmatic breathing activities.
R: Relaxation techniques—focus games, mindfulness activities, yoga poses, and guided imagery.
E: Exercise—cardio activities to affect regulation.
A: Alter your thoughts—playful activities to change negative, repetitive thinking.
M: Manage your body—improve the mind–body connection and body posture through games and playful activities.

AWAY is an acronym to help clients and their families remember the steps to exposure response prevention.

A: Approach it; don't avoid it! Contradict the usual avoidance or enabling tactics children and parents engage in to manage OCD.
W: No WAY! Confront irrational, demanding, compelling thoughts.
A: About face! Do something *other* than what OCD is telling you to do.
Y: Yippee! You did it! Celebrate and reward efforts.

DREAM AWAY is also a mnemonic for the child, providing a way to enhance memory in times of OCD episodes that flood the problem-solving process and make choices more difficult. Mnemonics are an educational tool for remembering lists of information such as states and capitals, for example. Employing that device to enhance coping during the stress of treating OCD allows parents a coaching tool, as well as a memory tool for the child.

Designed as a prescriptive play therapy intervention for the child with OCD, DREAM AWAY OCD is an advanced play therapy process. Although most play therapists identify themselves as "eclectic" (Schaefer & Drewes, 2009), training to be a thoroughly eclectic, prescriptive play therapist takes time and investment. A versatile, prescriptive play therapist, in reference to the basic tenets of prescriptive play therapy detailed above, is required to be versed in most play therapy theories and associated techniques, appropriate child development, abnormal psychology and psychopathology (potentially inclusive of psychological testing), and the developmental assessment of interpersonal relationships, attachment, and neurobiological disruptions. One must be trained in differential diagnosis—that is, what distinguishes one diagnosis or syndrome from another. For example, trauma reaction (posttraumatic stress disorder) in children may have symptoms similar to ADHD, learning disabilities, depression, anxiety, oppositional defiant disorder, dysregulated mood disruptive disorder, or OCD. Therefore, one needs to be invested in staying current in the psychological literature. Finally, a prescriptive play therapist must develop keen clinical observation skills to take what is presented by parents, teachers, and the child, woven together with the knowledge, information, and experience gained in practice, to arrive at the underlying cause of the symptoms, which is at the core of prescriptive play therapy (Schaefer & Drewes, 2016).

Parent Involvement

At the core of prescriptive play therapy practice and DREAM AWAY OCD is parental involvement throughout the treatment process. It begins with an assessment process that is extended, developmentally appropriate, culturally informed, and inclusive of family members (Gil, 2011). Taking time to complete an exhaustive assessment of the child and the child's family system, the prescriptive play therapist obtains the information appropriate to complete a unique, individualized diagnosis and treatment plan that purports to be shorter in duration and more cost-effective overall (Schaefer & Drewes, 2009; Gil, 2011).

DREAM AWAY incorporates an initial parent-only consultation, a family dyadic assessment, a play-based assessment, and treatment plan consultation into the overall process. The initial consultation allows the therapist to collect valuable information about family history, child history, the history of specific symptoms manifested by the child, and the way the family currently responds to the child's needs. In this consultation, one can understand the role that OCD plays in the family system and how that role is enabled by family members. The prescriptive play therapist explains the assessment process and treatment planning to the family and gives the rationale for the process to gain their support.

A family dyadic assessment—parent and child—following the recommended assessment process from *Theraplay* (Gitlin-Weiner, Sandgrund, & Schaefer, 2000; Munns, 2000), observes interpersonal relationships, attachment, OCD symptoms, and parental accommodation of OCD symptoms. These are identified through the Marschak interactive method (DiPasquale, 2000; Lindaman, Booth, & Chambers, 2000). The therapist observes family dyads with the child and parent(s) or larger groups, including siblings, completing individualized, playful tasks assigned by the therapist that provide diagnostic information on the cause of the child's disorder. Individualization of the tasks is drawn from the initial consultation with the parents and the experience and training of the clinician. Creating a video of the assessment for review, possible supervision, and ultimate sharing with the parents in the treatment planning session are useful additions.

Another phase of assessment entails nondirected play time for play-based observation. Through the play, the prescriptive play therapist seeks affirmation of an hypothesized diagnosis from previous assessment encounters and assesses the child's ability to engage in play (Stagnitti, 2013), the manifestation of OCD in play, and any comorbid symptomology that may exist. The nondirective assessment time also furthers rapport and solidifies the therapeutic alliance.

In DREAM AWAY OCD, the therapist develops an individualized treatment plan and shares it with the parents, enlisting their cooperation and participation as cotherapists. Parents are the key determinant in the outcome of therapy with young children (Nash & Schaefer, 2010). Enlisting them as cotherapists ensures continued investment in the therapeutic process, practice of interventions at home, and a speedier decline of OCD symptoms.

Unlike the manualized CBT approach, DREAM AWAY encourages an active cotherapist role for parents in the treatment of OCD. With younger clients, parents may be invited to participate actively in the playroom. With school-age children, parents may be included after playtime and briefed on progress in session and on their role for the week ahead. With regard to playtime, there is a parent orientation that includes specific training in playroom interaction, communication, and demeanor, borrowed from filial therapy (Guerney, 1964). Parents are also taught how to be active participants in the modeling of coping skills and anxiety management techniques (Knell, 2009), including emotional regulation: noting their own emotional state, verbalizing those feelings, and then actively modeling physical and emotional regulation (Dion, 2018).

Case Vignette: Jake and the Big Feelings

Jacob (Jake) was a 4-year-old male, member of a family of four with one younger brother. Jake was not new to therapy: he had received physical therapy at age 9 months to aid in learning to crawl; tubes in his ears at 20 months due to infections; speech therapy at 3 years of age (and continuing) for pronunciation and expressive language; and occupational therapy at 4 years of age for sensory processing disorder and fine motor skills. His family revealed a history of anxiety disorders from both extended families. Parent consultation indicated a growing pattern of obsessing about "being frightened, refusing to return to usually visited places—school, tumbling, shopping, or to visit family." He was crying more, having frequent, public emotional meltdowns, and experiencing shame over his behavior ("Don't tell Daddy I cried"). When parents probed Jake about what was upsetting him, he responded, "I can't say it!" After the initial parent consultation, family dyad sessions with mom and dad, and two play-based assessment sessions, OCD was diagnosed. The therapist developed a prescriptive play therapy treatment plan incorporating DREAM AWAY and reviewed it with the parents. The therapist held an orientation meeting with the parents, in which they learned filial therapy techniques and synergetic play therapy techniques about emotional regulation for participating in the playroom.

The first session introduced OCD and self-regulation to Jake through puppets. Jake chose the pig as the client, and the therapist chose the fox to be the doctor. Jake became dysregulated at the "sight" of the fox ("He looks too scary!") and began to inch away and tear up; the therapist asked Jack that if we put the fox away for today could another puppet be the doctor? Jake nodded, still dysregulated, hugging his puppet and his mother. The therapist modeled regulation (Dion, 2018) by verbalizing the feelings in the room: "I am feeling nervous about the fox puppet; I'm going to take a deep breath." The, taking deep breaths, rocking back and forth sitting on the floor, the therapist taught Jake how to regulate. Jake began to mirror the rocking gently, and when directed, he chose a boy puppet to be the doctor. The puppets told a story about OCD and how it made a pig feel. Jake joined in with excitement: "I feel that way too!" Because of this self-awareness, the play therapist proposed that Jake give OCD a pretend name (usually a second-session activity). His mother suggested "Meanie," and Jake decided on "Poopyhead," which produced a round of giggles. He drew a poop emoji on the art board and called it "Poopyhead." Poop emojis were added to the *Playbook* activity sheets and deposited stickers of the same for use on his behavior sheets.

The first sessions involved direct teaching of anxiety management and self-regulating techniques, along with gentle exposure for Jake to practice them. His parents alternated bringing him to his therapy sessions and were highly coordinated in their communication with each other and with the play therapist. They engaged diligently in rehearsing each new skill and keeping track of progress. In Session 2, Jake helped identify his OCD stimulus and created the hierarchy. He coined the term *big feelings* and spoke about when he felt them. Again, this surprised his parents, as he couldn't talk about what troubled him before. It appeared that in the playroom he felt safe and confident enough to tell what was giving him big feelings. He identified four things that he obsessed about: scary pictures; the dark; being away from Mom and Dad; and going to preschool. He colored fear thermometers (Kendall & Hedke, 2006b) with animals marking the level of fear: as big as a mouse, as big as a dog, or as big as an elephant. He identified fear of the dark as between a mouse and a dog; fear of going to preschool as a dog; fear of being away from Mom and Dad as a dog; and fear of scary pictures in books as bigger than an elephant. Because his parents had reported somatic symptoms accompanying OCD, I had the doctor puppet come and explain why some pigs get stomach aches when they have big feelings and why sometimes when they are thinking about something that gives them big feelings, their tummy starts to rumble, telling them that big feelings are coming—get ready! The doctor puppet introduced the D of DREAM AWAY—"deep breathing as a way of listening to one's tummy and taking charge of big feelings"—with Bubble Breaths (Goodyear-Brown, 2002), the Smell the Flowers technique (E. Moberg, personal communication, 2014), and Bunny Breaths (Gruber & Kalish, n.d.). Jake chose Bunny Breaths but changed them to "dog sniffs" instead. It became the metaphor for "sniffing out OCD." His father picked up a dog puppet: "Let's sniff out what's going on in that tummy . . . " and "Let's sniff around like [their dog] and see if we find out what all these big feelings are about." It made practicing easy and fun at home using the family dog to sniff out OCD, and Jake talked about "big feelings" without being prompted. His parents reported progress immediately. Jake was still emotionally dysregulated and reactive, but he could speak of the feelings.

The play therapist encouraged more practice with ERP and introduced more DREAM elements in the following four sessions: relaxation techniques, exercise, and activities geared at altering his thinking. He chose yoga poses to practice with his mother and reading the book *The Boy and the Bear* (a guided relaxation for children) as his relaxation practice. Jake and his mother read *The Boy and the Bear* in the playroom and began exposure to darkness by turning off the lights with only natural light from a window. Jake became anxious, and we practiced relaxation with a bear puppet. When he was ready, he lit candles and turned off the lights. Mom read the story, while Jake and the play therapist each chose a puppet to be the boy and the bear. When we finished, Jake asked his mom to read the story again and then asked if they could take the book home. The book became the practice activity for the week, along with a link to the story for Jake to listen to whenever he liked.

Next session, yoga poses were chosen from two sources: *Yoga Pretzels* (Gruber & Kalish, n.d.) and *The ABCs of Yoga for Kids* (Power, 2010), both of which were child-oriented decks of cards. Jake and his parent practiced three poses—tree, dancer, and mountain—and made a routine to music as part of the prescriptive intervention. The therapist asked Jake to decide what fear he wished to work with, and he chose darkness. He began breathing slowly, "This is how the bear breathes," he said. With direction from the therapist, he closed the blinds on the window and shared that made him have big feelings, "but I can handle it," he said. He decided how many candles to put out, and then he turned out the lights, just briefly. With the lights back on, Jake and the therapist did the yoga routine, took deep breaths, and then repeated turning the lights out. Running to turn on the lights, Jake shouted with surprise, "My big feelings are gone!" Parents reported that by following the yoga routine, practicing breathing, and listening to *The Boy and the Bear,* Jake approached bedtime more easily.

Identifying cardio exercises—the E in DREAM—was next accomplished. Jake received a bicycle for his fifth birthday, so he decided he would ride his bike in their neighborhood "fast–fast" and Mom and Dad would run beside him. Also included in his team were mini-trampoline jumping and dance party with Mom for rainy days.

Altering negative thoughts—the A in DREAM—is a more complex topic for young children who may not be developmentally able to identify what they are thinking. Once Jake became involved in treatment, this was less and less of a difficulty for him. Jake made good use of "Poopyhead," getting sharing what OCD was telling him. The play therapist implemented several techniques—Change the Channel (Goodyear-Brown, 2002), My

Personal Remote (Copeland, 2013), and Talk Back to Poopyhead (Huebner, 2007)—that Jake could use when he was flooded with negative self-talk. His parents were prompted to state, "I spy Poopyhead," or "Do you hear Poopyhead?" They reported that after such prompts Jake would get his personal remote, point it at his head, and say, "I don't have to listen to you, I'm changing the channel!"

At Jake's suggestion, exposure now focused on going to preschool. Using both the sandtray and miniatures, he created a school setting and his house. The prescriptive intervention taught "magic words"—positive affirmations—about school, such as "School is fun"; "I like to see my friends and teachers at school"; "I feel safe at school." The therapist had Jake's mom announce, "Time for school, let´s go." Jake would say his magic words, and they pretended drive to school in the sandtray. Jake took deep breaths, said his magic words, and role-played separation from Mom to stay at school; she left and came back for him. Jake and his mother repeated the intervention multiple times. Both parents reported that the next Sunday evening Jake announced he was having big feelings about school the next day. He stated that Poopyhead was upsetting his tummy and he was not going to let him do it. Jake went to his room, said his magic words, and listened to the bear story. His parents indicated that there was no abreaction and no school refusal on Monday.

Jake was ready for the final activities related to anxiety management, those for M—managing your body. Jake had many somatic complaints, mostly stomach aches, that would be excuses for avoidance. A pattern of sensory processing disorder (i.e., being sensory overstimulated and becoming emotionally dysregulated as a result) was emerging as one trigger for his obsessions. Thus, it was important to have coping strategies related to sensory and physical management on his DREAM team and to incorporate sensory stimulus into the exposure activities. Jake chose Superman as his "power pose" (Cuddy, 2012). Not only did this give Jake the experience of *being* Superman, but it also set up a confident posture and opened his airways for deep breathing. Jake chose exposure activities that included puppets, loud noises, and other "scary" sensory inputs which allowed him to create his power pose, complete with cape, and manage the anxiety. For home practice, his parents created their own power pose and modeled times to "act brave so you feel brave" and to talk about what being powerful felt like to them. They were asked to have Jake "be Superman" before they gave him anxiety-producing directions, like "time for bed" or "tomorrow we go to Grandma's house."

Now that Jake's DREAM team was in place, in session he made DREAM cards with the coping strategies he preferred before tackling the most anxiety-producing stimulus, "scary pictures." Jake identified each kind of scary picture and each location where he saw scary pictures. Each picture was represented by a hierarchy—big as a mouse, dog, or horse. Work in sessions proceeded, with ERP using the least fearful picture. Jake got ready by choosing his anxiety management strategy from his DREAM cards. He approached the fearful picture; said, NO WAY! and did an about face to manage the emotional response. Practice at home graduated from returning books to his shelf and having him manage his feelings, to opening the books to look at one picture, to gradually looking at the pictures and reading the books. Within one week, Jake was tolerating the books at home. We alleviated his anxiety about attending preschool story time by allowing him to gradually participate in story time from a distance, managing his reaction, and slowly joining the group as he felt ready.

We celebrated the end of treatment with an exchange of handmade gifts, blueberry cake, and his family. Jake made a "scary" picture and wrote, "Don't be afraid!" on the bottom of it. The play therapist made him a DREAM AWAY bracelet to remind him to take his team wherever he went. After termination, one review session was held with Jake's parents 3 months later. They reported that although Jake was not entirely free of OCD symptoms, they were relaxed and coping as a family. They felt competent and confident as parents. Jake was happier and also more confident. He announced his OCD in a loud voice and indicated what he was going to do to manage.

Empirical Support for the Intervention

DREAM AWAY integrates CBPT with nondirected play to form the basis of play interventions added to the manualized program, and it allows time for unstructured, nondirected play, often enhancing the child's investment in play therapy. CBPT was developed to address the developmental difficulties children have engaging in CT (Knell, 1998, 2009). While the CT treatment process is goal-oriented, time-limited, and structured, CBPT strives to maintain a balance between spontaneous play and the teaching of skills and coping consistent with CBT. According to Knell (2009), this spontaneous–structured play balance in CBPT is a delicate dance. Unstructured play gives a wealth of information that informs and enhances the treatment process, without which "the therapist would lose a rich source of clinical information" (p. 124). However, when the play therapy is entirely child-driven, the therapist may lose the ability to meet identified goals (March, 2007). Movement toward a therapist-prescribed goal is often contrary to the tenets of play therapy modalities such as client-centered play therapy (Knell, 2009). DREAM AWAY OCD gives the child an explanation of "Sometimes I choose what we play and sometimes you choose," and the child decides who is first.

Building on the CBPT premise that therapy must include active, promoted generalization of learned coping strategies (Knell, 2009), DREAM AWAY increases positive outcomes by incorporating a *Playbook* of practice activities and promoting engagement in ERP outside of therapy. Parents are provided a *Playbook* in which they are given instructions for play-based practice activities each week, along with a copy of the treatment plan and working therapeutic agenda. The *Playbook* also contains worksheets for tracking obsessive statements and compulsive behaviors, and tools for measuring the intensity of intrusive repetitive thoughts. The *Playbook* then becomes the family's transition object for using and reinforcing skills from therapy in the child's world.

The CBT manualized approach developed by March and Mulle (1998) is considered the best practice for treating OCD in children and adolescents (American Academy of Child and Adolescent Psychiatry, 2012; Schaefer & Drewes, 2016). March, however, was not a fan of play therapy. In his book for parents, *Talking Back to OCD* (March, 2007), he recommends that parents avoid play therapy. I believe that March was referring to a nondirective modality of play therapy where diagnostics, specific goals, structure, and cognitive-behavioral techniques are not necessarily employed. DREAM AWAY as a prescriptive play therapy intervention follows CBPT and the format of the evidence-based manualized approach with flexibility.

March and Mulle (1998) identified their approach, with exposure being the catalyst for improved coping with OCD. The therapy was manualized to assure compliance by children and to improve the systematic and consistent application of CBT by therapists in the treatment of OCD (March & Mulle, 1995). Many therapists in clinical practice, including play therapists, avoid using a manualized approach, even though such interventions are clearly delineated as best practices (Vande Voort, Suvecova, Grown Jacobsen, & Whiteside, 2010). They cite concerns regarding the length of manual-prescribed treatment and inflexibility in application. In addition, many play therapists balk at the prep time, effort, and required inventory of materials essential in the planning and execution of interventions in CBPT compared to other play therapy modalities. Utilizing an organized system of interventions and props, coupled with the flexible application of a manual's structure, DREAM AWAY addresses these difficulties and integrates play therapy and the CBT/ERP manualized approach.

In the March and Mulle (1998) manualized treatment, the protocol takes place over 16 weeks, in four steps. Each session provides for review of the previous week, restatement of goals, presentation of new information, selection of exposure "targets" and practice relapse prevention, and then definition of homework for the coming week. The treatment consists of the following (March & Mulle, 1995, p. 178):

- Week 1: Establish a neurobehavioral framework.
- Week 2: Make OCD the problem; introduce map metaphors.
- Week 3: Generate a stimulus hierarchy; identify and teach transition zone; anxiety management training.
- Weeks 4–15: Anxiety management training; ERP.
- Weeks 1, 6, 12: Parent–child sessions.
- Week 16: Graduation ceremony.
- Week 22: Booster session.

March and Mulle encourage assigning OCD a "nasty nickname" (1995, p. 178) in Week 2 to externalize the problem. The transition zone in Week 3 refers to the stimulus hierarchy elements where the child will exercise response prevention. The level of anxiety the child experiences is measured in subjective units of discomfort (SUDs) and projected onto a fear thermometer with a scale of 1–10. It is recommended that a SUD be obtained at each session for each exposure target as well as at home for each homework target.

DREAM AWAY utilizes the framework of the above manualized process, weaves CBPT techniques into the context of the structure, and then individualizes the play interventions for the child. In the first session, for example, a doctor puppet might explain to a "client" puppet (chosen by the child) what OCD is and why we are talking about it, encouraging the child to express through the puppet ways that OCD manifests in his or her life (beginning stimulus hierarchy, rapport, and trust building). The child and play therapist then change places, the child becoming the explaining doctor puppet and the play therapist the client puppet: the child rehearses what has been taught about OCD and play therapy; the play therapist models for the child listing symptoms and sources of OCD. Bibliotherapy might be used to explain the what and why of OCD, with the parent reading and the therapist and child acting out the story with puppets or action figures. A nickname for OCD is encouraged, and then drawings can be made of the character, which can be used as an icon or watermark on the child's practice assignments.

Anxiety management training is done in the form of playful techniques and follows the DREAM elements, creating a manual of interventions from which to choose: D—deep, diaphragmatic breathing as a first-line calming strategy for anxiety and self-regulation (Goodyear-Brown, 2002, 2010; Lowenstein, 2016; Shapiro & Sprague, 2009); R—relaxation of mind and body through play-based yoga, mindfulness, and guided meditation; E—cardio exercise play (running, jumping, dancing); A—alteration of negative thoughts with prop-based interventions (Goodyear-Brown, 2002); and M—management of your body and becoming a superhero against OCD (Cuddy, 2012).

Anxiety management training proceeds with ERP to targets lower on the SUDs scale until the child has selected and mastered coping strategies in each DREAM category. When the child has completed his or her DREAM world or DREAM team (i.e., has developed skill in each of the DREAM categories from which to choose an anxiety management or coping strategy), ERP intensifies with higher SUDs targets, as identified in the manualized approach. We refer to the child as the "boss of their world" or "the coach of their team," and as such, the child determines which skills to employ to manage his or her response to the target. Staying in the metaphor and transferring responsibility to the child, parents are encouraged to coach the child, "I see [OCD nickname], your team needs a coach (or your world needs a boss)."

The playroom is an excellent resource for the imaginary or role-played exposure identified in the manual. Pretend situations, stuffed and miniature toys, drawings, and puppets can be employed to imitate the stimulus object. Each exposure provides an opportunity for the child to experience his or her response and to identify how he or she will manage that physical or emotional response in the safety of the playroom. As with the manualized approach, when the stimulus hierarchy is exhausted and parents are reporting age-appropriate coping with obsessive thoughts, hard work is celebrated and treatment is terminated.

To assist parents and children in the work outside of sessions, DREAM AWAY enlists the behavioral therapy technique of behavioral charts (Skinner, 1938, 1951). Several playful ways to create behavioral charts that reward progress toward a goal are available online and in play therapy technique books (Goodyear-Brown, 2002; Lowenstein, 2016). Websites like Free Printable Behavioral Charts (*www.freeprintablebehaviorcharts.com*) offer a huge selection of charts—treasure maps, stairs, superheroes, or animal pictures that build up visible and tangible rewards toward a grand prize. DREAM AWAY OCD encourages the special privileges as nonmonetary, goal-achieving grand prizes. Smaller ones can be positive reinforcements for interim achievements, set by the parent and child.

The CBT manualized approach identifies a duration of treatment of 16 sessions after assessment and diagnosis but indicates that the number is dependent on the client's needs (March & Mulle, 1995). DREAM AWAY mirrors the latter and is dependent on the client's needs, with the duration of treatment dependent on the unique progress of the child. Utilizing techniques and training from synergetic play therapy, the therapist can quantify each session as to change and progress toward the goal, watching for the child's empowerment to manage his or her inner experience and measuring progress toward treatment completion (Dion, 2018).

At the end of the final phase of the CBT manualized approach, clients are prepared for termination and graduation. DREAM AWAY also prepares the child and the parent for discontinuing treatment by reinforcing exposure response prevention techniques, building confidence in the child that "You can do it!" and preparing parents to coach and support ongoing mastery over OCD. Exposure to uncomfortable situations and events, *in vivo* and in the play room, continues with the tasks being chosen by the child and the playful interventions being devised by the play therapist and child together. In this way, integration of directive and nondirective techniques becomes more fluid and interchangeable as the client progresses toward ending treatment.

The last session marks graduation from play therapy. It is a celebration of the child's DREAM AWAY OCD work; the child's struggle and success are honored with food, friends, family, and fun. Children are engaged in planning the celebration, choosing the food, inviting friends and family, and determining what will be the "fun." The play therapist is responsible for providing the food and the fun. The child is asked to make a farewell gift for the therapist. The therapist makes a gift for the child as well to exchange at the closing session, as a way of honoring their relationship.

Conclusion

DREAM AWAY OCD, a flexible manualized treatment program for OCD in young children, combines CBPT and an evidence-based manualized approach in prescriptive play therapy. The treatment worked well for Jake and his family. Combining CBPT with an evidence-based treatment, coupled with parent inclusion as cotherapists, this prescriptive play therapy approach enhances the ability of younger children to gain control and manage OCD by overcoming many of the developmental issues limiting their ability to benefit from cognitive therapy. Through the therapeutic powers of play, other modalities of play therapy are efficacious in helping to resolve many childhood difficulties. However, as demonstrated, DREAM AWAY OCD combines CBPT with playful approaches to ERP, mirroring a manualized treatment, in a prescriptive play therapy modality, thereby creating a treatment method of choice for OCD in young children.

REFERENCES

American Academy of Child and Adolescent Psychiatry. (2012). Practice parameters for the assessment and treatment of children and adolescents with obsessive–compulsive disorder. *Journal of the American Academy of Child and Adolescent Pschiatry, 51*(1), 98–113.
American Psychiatric Association. (2013). *Diagnostic and statistical manual of mental disorders* (5th ed.). Arlington, VA: Author.

Barton, R., & Heyman, I. (2016). Obsessive–compulsive disorder in children and adolescents. *Paediatrics and Child Health, 25*(12), 527–533.

Copeland, L. (2013). *Hunter and his amazing remote control*. Chapin, SC: Youthlight.

Cuddy, A. J. C. (2012). Your body language may shape who you are (TED Talk). Retrieved from *www.ted.com/talks/amy_cuddy_your_body_language_shapes_who_you_are? Language=en*.

Dion, L. (2018). *Aggression in play therapy*. New York: Norton.

Dipasquale, L. (2000). The Marschak interaction method. In E. Munns (Ed.), *Theraplay: Innovations in attachment-enhancing play therapy* (pp. 27–51). New Bergen, NJ: Bookmart Press.

Drewes, A. A., & Schaefer, C. E. (2016). The therapeutic powers of play. In K. O'Connor, C. E. Schaefer, & L. D. Braverman (Eds.), *Handbook of play therapy* (2nd ed., pp. 35–60). Hoboken, NJ: Wiley.

Farrell, L. J., Schlup, B., & Boschen, M. J. (2010). Cognitive-behavioral treatment of childhood obsessive–compulsive disorder in community-based clinical practice: Clinical significance and benchmarking against efficacy. *Behaviour Research and Therapy, 48*, 409–417.

Gil, E. (2011). *Extended play-based developmental assessment*. Royal Oak, MI: Self.

Gil, E., & Shaw, J. (2009). Prescriptive play therapy. In L. Braverman, L. Schaefer, & C. O'Connor (Eds.), *Play therapy theory and practice* (2nd ed., pp. 451–488). Hoboken, NJ: Wiley.

Gitlin-Weiner, K., Sandgrund, A., & Schaefer, C. (Eds.). (2000). *Play diagnosis and assessment* (2nd ed.). Hoboken, NJ: Wiley.

Goodyear-Brown, P. (2002). *Digging for buried treasure*. (Self-published).

Goodyear-Brown, P. (2010). *The worry wars: An anxiety workbook for kids and their helpful adults!* (Self-published.)

Gruber, T., & Kalish, L. (n.d.). *Yoga pretzels: 50 fun yoga activities for kids and grownups*. Cambridge, MA: Barefoot Books.

Guerney, B., Jr. (1964). Filial therapy: Description and rationale. *Journal of Consulting Psychology, 28*(10), 304–310.

Hill, C., Waite, P., & Creswell, C. (2016). Anxiety disorders in children and adolescents. *Paediatrics and Child Health, 25*(12), 548–553.

Huebner, D. (2007). *What to do when your brain gets stuck*. Washington, DC: Magination Press:

Kendall, P. C., Gosch, E., Furr, J. M., & Sood, E. (2008). Flexibility within fidelity. *Journal of the American Academy of Child and Adolescent Psychiatry, 47*(9), 987–993.

Kendall, P. C., & Hedtke, K. A. (2006a). *Coping Cat: Cognitive-behavioral therapy for anxious children—therapist manual* (3rd ed.). Ardmore, PA: Workbook.

Kendall, P. C., & Hedtke, K. A. (2006b). *The Coping Cat workbook*. Ardmore, PA: Workbook.

Knell, S. M. (1998). Cognitive-behavioral play therapy. *Journal of Clinical Child Psychology, 27*(1), 28–33.

Knell, S. M. (2009). Cognitive-behavioral play therapy: Theory and applications. In A. A. Drewes (Ed.), *Blending play therapy with cognitive behavior therapy: Evidence-based and other effective treatments and techniques* (pp. 117–131). Hoboken, NJ: Wiley.

Lebowitz, E. R. (2013). Parent-based treatment for childhood and adolescent OCD. *Journal of Obsessive–Compulsive and Related Disorders, 2,* 425–431.

Lindaman, S. L., Booth, P. B., & Chambers, C. L. (2000). Assessing parent–child interactions with the Marschak interaction method (MIM). In K. Gitlin-Weiner, A. Sandgrund, & C. Sanefer (Eds.), *Play therapy diagnosis and assessment* (2nd ed., pp. 371–400). New York: Wiley.

Lowenstein, L. (2016). *Creative CBT interventions for children with anxiety.* Toronto, ON, Canada: Champion Press.

March, J. S. (2007). *Talking back to OCD.* New York: Guilford Press.

March, J. S., & Mulle, K. (1995). Manualized cognitive-behavioral psychotherapy for obsessive–compulsive disorder in childhood: A preliminary single-case study. *Journal of Anxiety Disorders, 9*(2), 175–184.

March, J. S., & Mulle, K. (1998). *OCD in children and adolescents: A cognitive-behavioral treatment manual.* New York: Guilford Press.

March, J. S., Mulle, K., & Herbel, B. (1994). Behavioral psychotherapy for children and adolescents with obsessive–compulsive disorder: An open trial of a new protocol-driven treatment package. *Journal of the American Academy of Child and Adolescent Psychiatry, 33*(3), 333–341.

Munns, E. (Ed.). (2000). *Theraplay: Innovations in attachment-enhancing play therapy.* New Bergen, NJ: Book-mart Press.

Myrick, A. C., & Green, E. J. (2012). Incorporating play therapy into evidence-based treatment with children affected by obsessive–compulsive disorder. *International Journal of Play Therapy, 21*(2), 74–86.

Nash, J. B., & Schaefer, C. E. (2010). Clinical and developmental issues in psychotherapy with preschool children: Laying the groundwork for play therapy. In C. E. Schaefer (Ed.), *Play therapy for preschool children* (pp. 15–29). Washington, DC: American Psychological Association.

Power, T. A. (2010). *The ABCs of yoga for kids.* Pacific Palisades, CA: Stafford House.

Rosa-Alcazar, A. I., Inesta-Sepulveda, M., Storch, E. A., Rosa-Alcazar, A., Parada-Navas, J. L., & Olivares Rodriguez, J. (2017). A preliminary study of cognitive-behavioral family-based treatment versus parent training for young children with obsessive–compulsive disorder. *Journal of Affective Disorders, 208,* 265–271.

Schaefer, C. E. (Ed.). (2011). Prescriptive play therapy. In K. J. O'Connor, C. E. Schaefer, & L. D. Braverman (Eds.), *Foundations of play therapy* (2nd ed., pp. 365–378). Hoboken, NJ: Wiley.

Schaefer, C. E., & Drewes, A. A. (2011). The therapeutic powers of play and play therapy. In C. E. Schaefer (Ed.), *Foundations of play therapy* (2nd ed., pp. 15–25). Hoboken, NJ: Wiley.

Schaefer, C. E., & Drewes, A. A. (2013). *The therapeutic powers of play: 20 core agents of change.* Hoboken, NJ: Wiley.

Schaefer, C. E., & Drewes, A. A. (2016). Prescriptive play therapy. In C. Schaefer,

L. Braverman, & K. O'Connor (Eds.), *Handbook of play therapy* (2nd ed., pp. 227–240). Hoboken, NJ: Wiley.

Shapiro, L. E., & Sprague, R. K. (2009). *The relaxation and stress reduction workbook for kids: Help for children to cope with stress, anxiety, and transitions.* Oakland, CA: Instant Help Books.

Skinner, B. F. (1938). *The behavior of organisms: An experimental analysis.* New York: Appleton-Century.

Skinner, B. F. (1951). *How to teach animals.* San Francisco: Freeman.

Stagnitti, K. (2013). *Learn to play: A practical program to develop a child's imaginative play skills.* West Brunswick, Victoria, Australia: Co-ordinates Publishing.

Strimpfel, J. M., Neece, J. G., & Macfie, J. (2016). Flexible manualized treatment for pediatric obsessive–compulsive disorder: A case study. *Journal of Contemporary Psychotherapy, 46,* 97–105.

Vande Voort, J., Svvecova, J., Brown Jacobsen, A., & Whiteside, S. P. (2010). A retrospective examination of the similarity between clinical practice and manualized treatment for childhood anxiety disorders. *Cognitive and Behavioral Practice, 17,* 322–328.

CHAPTER 6

Play Therapy for Children with Selective Mutism

Lynn Louise Wonders

Description of the Disorder

Classified as an anxiety disorder, selective mutism (SM) is characterized by a child's inability to speak in particular social situations where there is an ability to speak in other scenarios (American Psychiatric Association, 2013). It is common for children with SM to be highly verbal with family at home and for those same children to be silent and incapable of communication when they go to school or in other social places or events. Studies that use physiological indicators to measure severity of anxiety have shown that children with SM have higher chronic levels of arousal than children with other anxiety disorders (Beidel & Alfano, 2011). Children with SM may not appear to be overtly anxious because of their silence, so it is often misunderstood. It is important to differentiate SM from trauma-related mutism. Children's sudden mutism in all situations, followed by a trauma-tizing event, does not meet the diagnostic criteria for SM (Shipon-Blum, 2015). SM is a mechanism through which children avoid the otherwise overwhelming levels of anxiety they feel in specified social settings (Young, Bunnell, & Beidel, 2012). It is often accompanied by a variety of comorbid anxiety diagnoses, most commonly associated with social anxiety disorder or social phobia (Kristensen, 2000). Symptoms of SM are typically detected before the age of 5, but the disruption of a child's normal functioning most often begins when the child first enters school (Muris & Olldendick, 2015).

Rationale for Prescriptive Play Therapy

The research suggests that cognitive-behavioral therapy (CBT) and behavioral based methods are effective for treating SM in children (Campasano, 2011), but there are not many randomized control studies available specific to SM (Oerbeck, Stein, Wentzel-Larsen, Langsrud, & Kristensen, 2014). Given a child's cognitive developmental stage and the lack of verbal communication, Stallard (2005) explains that the methods of employing a CBT or behavioral approach with children are typically modified to adapt to the child's developmental stage and needs. The literature suggests that the integration of play-based interventions with a cognitive-behavioral approach is effective (Bergman, Gonzalez, Piacentini, & Keller, 2013; Busse & Downey, 2011) and that when young children with social and academic difficulties participate in play therapy, there is a significant decrease in social difficulties (Su & Tsai, 2016; Lin & Bratton, 2015, Wilson & Ray, 2018).

A number of approaches have been proposed to conduct play therapy based on a wide variety of theoretical orientations. The three main categories for play therapy approaches are nondirective, directive, and prescriptive.

Cognitive-behavioral play therapy (CBPT) is a directive play therapy approach that adapts the long-established and effective theoretical orientation of CBT used widely to treat anxiety in adults. CBPT helps children affected by anxiety disorders by using play-based techniques and interventions that address adaptive changes to thoughts, beliefs, and behaviors (Knell, 1993). When children diagnosed with SM exhibit the most severe symptom level, however, it is beneficial to begin treatment with a nondirective, child-centered play therapy (CCPT) approach. CCPT has been shown to yield significantly improved treatment outcomes (Lin & Bratton, 2015). Finally, a prescriptive play therapy approach enables the clinician to assess the severity of symptoms in order to selectively choose which theoretical orientation and which interventions may be most appropriate in helping children with SM over the course of treatment. It also enables the clinician to utilize a combination of nondirective and directive approaches as appropriate for the individual child's presenting challenges and developmental needs.

Assessment and Treatment Planning

A thorough assessment is crucial to ensure that the plan for treatment is appropriately designed for the individual needs of children with SM (Perednik, 2016). At the intake phase of treatment, it is important to gather as much information as possible from the child's caregivers through behavioral rating scales and consultation. The Selective Mutism Questionnaire (SMQ; Shipon-Blum & Stein, 2008) is a 17-item parent questionnaire that is useful in determining the child's diagnosis of SM and the level of severity (Letamendi et al., 2008). It is also important to engage in an initial observational session with the child to determine the severity of symptoms. It is within the framework of the clinical inquiries of a thorough intake process that the therapist is able to prescriptively assess and address the needs of each individual child. The SM-Social Communication Comfort Scale (SM-SCCS; Shipon-Blum, 2012) can be utilized to identify the level at which a child is verbally communicating. The SM-SCCS delineates four degrees of communication behaviors. Those degrees of communication behavior can be best conceptualized as a continuum of symptom severity. At the most extreme level of severity are children who are completely noncommunicative and fail to respond and to initiate communication in any manner in particular social situations. The SM-SCCS provides a lens through which the clinician can assess the level of symptom severity at both the start of therapy and throughout the course of therapy so that the appropriate prescriptive approach and relative interventions can be selected. The data collected from the behavioral indicators in the intake process (and throughout therapy) are a valuable point from which to best discern how severely the child's life and functioning are impaired by SM. This enables the clinician to develop the treatment plan accordingly. The course of treatment for children suffering with SM is a challenging process requiring a complex, multilayered approach with many considerations (Oerbeck et al., 2014). While the anxiety that causes the behavioral symptoms must be addressed and relieved, the behavioral symptoms themselves over time can become learned behaviors requiring an additional layer of interventions beyond those used to address the underlying anxiety (Shipon-Blum, 2010).

Interventions

When a Child Is Noncommunicative in Session

The most severe presentation of symptoms is the highly avoidant behavior of the child who does not make eye contact and does not respond or initiate communication either verbally or nonverbally in specific social situations. The most appropriate intervention when the symptoms are this severe while in session with the therapist is for the clinician to begin therapy with a CCPT approach, providing unconditional acceptance while using tracking, reflecting, and returning responsibility, while the child is given the freedom to explore the play room and to choose how the toys and play materials will be used. In the presence of the empathic and accepting therapist, the child has the opportunity to develop trust and connection with the therapist as a vital foundation (Landreth, 1991). When CCPT has been used to treat young children with other forms of anxiety, the literature shows a significant decrease in worry and overall anxiety (Stulmaker & Ray, 2015).

Building a culture of trust and forging a therapeutic bond in the play room is most likely to occur when the therapist uses this pure CCPT approach with weekly or biweekly sessions (Landreth, 1991). The child experiences the time in the play room as a safe and eventually familiar place to explore, experience, and express through natural, child-directed play. When a child is not communicating with words or gestures, he or she will communicate through the language of play, which a trained play therapist can observe and understand (Landreth, 1991). This child-centered approach provides a window through which the therapist can view the child's inner world. CCPT gives voice even to the child who does not speak, giving the child an experience of being seen, heard, and accepted without condition (O'Connor, 2000). The emotional safety cultivated through CCPT is needed before behavioral changes can be sought with more directive play therapy interventions.

The CCPT approach is continued until the clinician can see that the child is at ease in the play room, that the rapport between therapist and client is well established, and that the child is beginning to engage in gesturing or other nonverbal forms of communicating with the therapist. These observations provide assurance that a firm foundation of trust and connection has been established, which is essential when treating SM at this level of severity.

When a Child Uses Nonverbal Communication in Session

When the child makes eye contact with the therapist and uses gestures or sounds to connect and communicate with the therapist, this is an opening to begin introducing directive play-based activities to encourage engagement and communication while continuing to practice the unconditional acceptance, witnessing, tracking, and reflecting of CCPT. Eventually during this phase of treatment, the child will typically begin to use whispering, sounds, or verbalization to communicate with the therapist as treatment progresses.

Inside the Talking-Bubble

This intervention has been effective for treating children with SM using the metaphor of a bubble.

1. In the talking-bubble intervention, the therapist introduces the concept of bubbles with a bottle of bubble-blowing liquid, inviting the child to join the therapist in blowing bubbles of all sizes.
2. After blowing bubbles together, the therapist reflects aloud on how some bubbles are small, others are big, sometimes they can grow bigger, and sometimes they can be popped. The therapist animates the concept of an invisible bubble that belongs to the child called a "talking-bubble" explaining that inside this bubble a child feels safe, comfortable, and at ease with talking to certain people who are included inside the talking-bubble. The therapist explains that there are other people who are not included in the child's talking-bubble, people to whom the child does not talk.
3. On a large piece of paper, a big circle is drawn with a title at the top designating the circle as the child's talking-bubble. The therapist explains that inside the talking-bubble are the people the child talks to and then invites the child to write the names or draw pictures of other people who are inside the child's talking-bubble.

This intervention allows the child to externalize the reality of the delineation of situations in which the child feels at ease to speak freely and others where the child is uneasy and remains silent. It empowers the child to eventually choose who will be included inside the talking-bubble. This intervention continues to be referenced in future sessions, reflecting on how the bubble size can grow as the child adds more people and one day may even pop when the child decides to talk freely in most social situations.

When a Child Makes Vocal Sounds or Whispers in Session

As soon as a child begins communicating with the therapist using sounds of any kind, the next step in treatment is to engage the child, using that momentum with the introduction of behavioral-based directive play therapy techniques to reinforce and enhance the quality of the communication.

The WhisperPhone® Duet

This acoustical voice-feedback device can be used as an intermediary when a child is first beginning to connect through verbal communication with the therapist in session, reinforcing the verbal communication connection. The device allows a child to whisper into one end and be heard easily on the therapist's end with a plastic flexible tube in between (*https://whisperphone.com*). The device works as follows.

1. The device is introduced to the child in such a way as to elicit curiosity.
2. The therapist invites the child to hold one end and listen while the therapist whispers a fun message into the other end while sitting back to back.
3. The therapist then wonders aloud if the child would like to whisper something to the therapist.
4. The clinician can tell the child that this device will be available in the play room whenever the child may want to speak to the therapist.

When a Child Speaks to the Therapist in Session

When the child is including the therapist in the talking-bubble and is communicating with the therapist verbally, the goal of treatment at this phase is to help the child generalize this ability to other situations and people. Having now well established trust and the bond of the therapeutic relationship, the clinician can now safely employ more directive behavioral and CBPT interventions.

Superhero Superpower Skills

Using a resource that provides six Superhero Power Cards (Mendoza, 2013), the therapist can introduce an empowering intervention that helps children learn and practice relaxation and self-regulation (deep breathing and mindfulness, ignoring others' provocative behavior), and increase their self-confidence.

1. The intervention is introduced by inviting the child to share what superheroes he or she most admires and to reflect on their superpowers.
2. The therapist introduces the Superhero Power Cards one at a time. Each card teaches a powerful behavioral skill—for example: Use your super breath like Superman to breathe in strength and blow away worries and afraid feelings; stand like a superhero in the "power pose" to find your bravery and confidence; and use your super senses to be super present here and now by naming three things you can see, three things you can touch, three things you can hear, and three things you can smell.
3. Reference the newly learned superhero power skills to help the child remember and access his or her superpowers to overcome fear and anxiety.

When Treatment Goals Are Reached

Once a child is successfully speaking in most all social situations and has demonstrated an ability to self-regulate when feelings of anxiety arise, the course of treatment is systematically brought to a close through an appropriate process of termination. This process must take into consideration the risk of relapse, the age of the child, and the importance of having healthy goodbyes with appropriate closure (Vladair, Feyijinmi, & Feindler, 2017). A celebration of achieving the goals of therapy and emphasizing the effort the child has put forth is a crucial component of the termination process.

Celebration Station

Once the child has shown significant and consistent progress, it is beneficial to provide positive reinforcement of the new adaptive behavioral patterns reflecting the achievement of the treatment goals.

1. The therapist and child together create a colorful chart on a poster board with the title "Celebration Station" and decorate the outer edges with images or symbols of happy, joyful celebration.
2. They create 10 horizontal lines across the board. Each week over the final 10 weeks of therapy together, an achievement related to the therapeutic process on the chart worthy of celebration is recorded. Included can be high-five hand claps, special stickers, and maybe some celebratory music with dancing. At the conclusion of the final session, the child will take the chart home to keep as a reminder of all that was accomplished and of what can be done to self-soothe or self-empower should regression occur.

Parent Involvement

When there is parent involvement in the course of treating children with social phobia, children show significant and lasting improvement (Spence, Donovan, & Brechman-Toussaint, 2000). Social phobia (SOP) and SM are related disorders, with social phobia being more common in adolescence and SM more common among younger children (Crosby Budinger, Drazdowski, & Ginsburg, 2013). Treatment using CBT, behavioral techniques, and social learning interventions have been shown to be effective in treating social phobia (Crosby Budinger et al., 2013). It stands to reason that if parent involvement supports significant improvement in children diagnosed with SOP, then younger children with SM who have developmentally typical strong attachment to primary caregivers will also benefit from having parents involved in the therapy. Parent involvement begins in the initial parent intake consultation session. In addition to using the parent intake consultation to gather history and behavioral indicators, it is also a vital opportunity to provide the parents with psychoeducation about SM, the structure of the treatment process, and the importance of parent involvement throughout the course of therapy to ensure that parents are invested in the therapeutic process (Nock, Kazdin, & Kazdin, 2001). It is most advantageous for the therapist to meet with parents for consultation sessions after every four play therapy sessions to review progress in session, in school, and at home.

Case Vignette: Sienna

Sienna was 4 years old when her parents brought her to therapy after noticing that she refused to talk to anyone other than her mother, father, sister, and one of her grandparents who lived with the nuclear family. Sienna was in preschool, and her teachers expressed concern during the parent–teacher conference about her readiness for kindergarten. When Sienna attended birthday parties, she was completely socially withdrawn and eventually began expressing to her parents that she didn't want to go to parties anymore. In school she did not speak or communicate with either the teachers or the students. During recess, she sat by herself coloring, ignoring her peers' invitations to join in the playtime. Sienna's parents reported that she was verbose and openly expressive without reservation with her family at home.

In Sienna's intake observation session, she avoided eye contact with the therapist, showed no affect, and did not respond to or initiate communication. She walked around the play room looking at the toys but did not interact with the therapist at all as the therapist used tracking and reflection. According to the SM–SCCS (Shipon-Blum, 2012), Sienna's stage of symptom severity, at Stage 0, was the most extreme. The therapist knew it would be very important to use a pure CCPT approach in the beginning of the therapy process; given Sienna's age and stage of development, parent consultation sessions were scheduled for every 4 weeks, with brief phone consultations every 2 weeks throughout the course of treatment. The therapist developed regular consultation schedules with Sienna's teachers so that the teachers, therapist, and parents were all operating from a common plan and framework in order to best support Sienna's progress along the way.

The therapist provided CCPT for Sienna for 13 weekly sessions in the office play room, two sessions on site at Sienna's preschool, and one home visit. The home and school visits occurred in the second month of treatment to best assess whether there would be any difference in how Sienna related to the therapist in those environments. After 13 weekly CCPT sessions,

Sienna began making eye contact with the therapist, smiling and nodding or shaking her head in response to the therapist's statements. At this point, the therapist introduced CBPT-based interventions, including the talking-bubble and facilitative, interactive activities such as board games, gross motor games, and puppet play to encourage the connection and rapport the therapist had established. Sienna smiled and nodded when introduced to the idea of the talking-bubble and she delighted in the bubble-blowing activity. The therapist and Sienna observed it as a ritual to blow bubbles at the beginning of every session for the rest of her time in treatment, which provided a connective theme. At Session 25, Sienna whispered nervously to the therapist, patting her arm as they entered the play room. She whispered, "I want to tell you something." The therapist pulled out the WhisperPhone Duet and introduced how it works. Sienna responded by taking the WhisperPhone and using it to whisper to the therapist, "I'm almost ready for you to be in my talking-bubble—but not yet!" The therapist responded with delight and celebration and assured her that the therapist would wait until she was ready. In the next two sessions, Sienna regressed and did not want to communicate or interact with the therapist at all, so the therapist reverted to a CCPT approach to give Sienna the space and time she needed to process. In the 28th session, Sienna ran into the play room and grabbed the WhisperPhone, motioning for the therapist to join her. Using the device, she told the therapist in a whisper that she was ready for the therapist to be included in her talking-bubble. Sienna began talking to the therapist interactively, still whispering but both initiating and responding. The therapist allowed a few more sessions to progress using CCPT so as not to push her too quickly, risking another regressive incident. By the time the therapist and Sienna reached the 31st session, Sienna was speaking to the therapist as comfortably as she did with her parents, sister, and grandmother. A deep trust had been forged, and the summer break from school had begun. In order to help her transition to kindergarten, the therapist decided it was time to introduce a more directive level of CBPT since she was now speaking with her comfortably and consistently.

Over the following 10 weeks of treatment, the therapist provided age-appropriate psychoeducation, puppet role play, and Superhero power skills to teach Sienna relaxation skills, recognizing and externalizing her scared feelings and strategic coping skills. The therapist began a graduated exposure intervention beginning with Sienna rehearsing the practice of speaking to people outside of her talking-bubble through use of the puppets, then in the mirror in session, and eventually recording her practicing on a video so that she could watch and listen to herself speaking to the imaginary outside person. After six sessions of this activity, the therapist and Sienna agreed on a goal for Sienna to say "Hello" to at least one person outside of her talking-bubble each week.

By the time kindergarten started, Sienna appeared to feel equipped and ready with only minor signs of anxiety. The therapist met with her new teacher to bring her onto our team and prepare her with some suggestions for how to help Sienna feel at ease. The therapist continued to see Sienna on a weekly basis. Reports from teachers and parents indicated that Sienna was managing her anxiety well. They reported that she was at times very quiet but managed to speak to ask questions and respond when needed.

In October, the therapist began a 10-session termination process, building Sienna's Celebration Station each week to provide positive reinforcement of her achievements. Together the therapist and Sienna created a plan in the event of regression or relapse. Sienna graduated from therapy 2 weeks before the Christmas holidays. At a check-in consultation with her parents 3 months after termination, the parents reported that Sienna was doing very well with no relapses and appeared to be a happy, well-adjusted child with friends, parties, and positive reports from school.

Empirical Support for the Interventions

SM is considered a difficult disorder to treat in therapy. The most recent literature addressing the treatment of SM in children is relatively limited, with very few randomized control-led studies specific to SM, with those studies having very small sample sizes (Oerbeck et al., 2014). The literature prior to 2006 supports the use of behavioral and cognitive-behavioral interventions, with multimodal therapeutic interventions also showing promise. (Cohan, Chavira, & Stein, 2006). The little research that has been done specific to SM suggests that CBT and behavioral-based methods are effective in helping children suffering with SM (Campasano, 2011). Given the levels of severity of symptoms in children who are diagnosed with SM (Klein, Armstrong, Skira, & Gordin, 2017) and the literature showing that young children with anxiety benefit from CCPT (Stulmaker & Ray, 2015), it stands to reason that a substantial case can be made for the use of CCPT when the symptom severity is most extreme in young children. CCPT has been shown to yield significantly improved treatment outcomes (Lin et al., 2015) and specifically has been shown to be effective in helping preschool-age children with somatization (Schottelkorb, Swan, Jahn, Haas, & Hacker, 2015) which often occurs with underlying anxiety. According to a controlled trial, children with anxiety who were provided CCPT showed a statistically significant decrease in symptoms of worry and anxiety, while children in the control group experienced increases in levels of anxiety and worry (Stulmaker & Ray, 2015). The studies done show that children unable to speak in particular situations were able to speak in those same situations after having been treated with cognitive-behavioral therapy (Mendlowitz & Monga, 2007). The literature suggests that integrating play-based interventions with a cognitive-behavioral approach is effective (Bergman et al., 2013; Busse & Downey, 2011; Oerbeck et al., 2014).

Conclusion

SM can be a complex and difficult disorder to treat, but a prescriptive play therapy approach offers the therapist a broader selection of intervention options that can match up with the individual needs of each child tied to the severity of symptoms presented at every stage of the treatment process. Parent participation and inclusion in the treatment process are very important to ensure that the parents, therapist, and child are working as a team and are on track with the goals of treatment and the practices and strategies.

REFERENCES

American Psychiatric Association. (2013). *Diagnostic and statistical manual of mental disorders* (5th ed.). Arlington, VA: Author.

Beidel, D. C., & Alfano, C. A. (2011). *Child anxiety disorders: A guide to research and treatment* (2nd ed.). New York: Taylor & Francis.

Bergman, R. L., Gonzalez, A., Piacentini, J., & Keller, M. L. (2013). Integrated behavior therapy for selective mutism: A randomized controlled pilot study. *Behaviour Research and Therapy, 51,* 680–689.

Busse, R. T., & Downey, J. (2011). Selective mutism: A three-tiered approach to prevention and intervention. *Contemporary School Psychology, 15,* 53–63.

Camposano, L. (2011). Silent suffering: Children with selective mutism. *The Professional Counselor, 1*(1), 46–56.

Cohan, S. L., Chavira, D. A., & Stein, M. B. (2006). Practitioner review: Psychosocial interventions for children with selective mutism: A critical evaluation of the literature from 1990–2005. *Journal of Child Psychology and Psychiatry, 47*(11), 1085–1097.

Crosby Budinger, M., Drazdowski, T. K., & Ginsburg, G. S. (2013). Anxiety-promoting parenting behaviors: A comparison of anxious parents with and without social anxiety disorder. *Child Psychiatry and Human Development, 44*(3), 412–418.

Klein, E., Armstrong, S., Skira, K., & Gordin, J. (2017). Social communication anxiety treatment (S-CAT) for children and families with selective mutism: A pilot study. *Clinical Child Psychology and Psychiatry, 22*(1), 90–108.

Knell, S. M. (1993). *Cognitive-behavioral play therapy.* Northvale, NJ: Jason Aronson.

Kristensen, H. (2000). Selective mutism and comorbidity with developmental disorder/delay, anxiety disorder, and elimination disorder. *Journal of the American Academy of Child and Adolescent Psychiatry, 39,* 249–256.

Landreth, G. L. (1991). *Play therapy: The art of the relationship.* Muncie, IN: Accelerated Development.

Letamendi, A. M., Chavira, D. A., Hitchcock, C. A., Roesch, S. C., Shipon-Blum, E., & Stein, M. B. (2008). Selective Mutism Questionnaire: Measurement structure and validity. *Journal of the American Academy of Child and Adolescent Psychiatry, 47*(10), 1197–1204.

Lin, Y., & Bratton, S. C. (2015). A meta-analytic review of child-centered play therapy approaches. *Journal of Counseling and Development, 93*(1), 45–58.

Mendlowitz, S. L., & Monga, S. (2007). Unlocking speech where there is none: Practical approaches to the treatment of selective mutism. *The Behavior Therapist, 30*(1), 11–15.

Mendoza, L. (2013). Social superheroes. Retrieved from *www.schoolcounseling-files.com/social-superheroes.html.*

Muris, P., & Ollendick. H. (2015). Children who are anxious in silence: A review on selective mutism, the new anxiety disorder in DSM-5. *Clinical Child and Family Psychology Review, 18*(2), 151–169.

Nock, M., Kazdin, A., & Kazdin, P. (2001). Parent expectancies for child therapy: Assessment and relation to participation in treatment. *Journal of Child and Family Studies, 10*(2), 155–180.

O'Connor, K. J. (2000). *The play therapy primer.* New York: Wiley.

Oerbeck, B., Stein, M., Wentzel-Larsen, T., Langsrud, O., & Kristensen, H. (2014). A randomized controlled trial of a home and school-based intervention for selective mutism: Defocused communication and behavioural techniques. *Child and Adolescent Mental Health, 19*(3), 192–198.

Perednik, R. (2016). *The selective mutism treatment guide: Manuals for parents, teachers and therapists* (2nd ed.). Jerusalem: Oaklands.

Schottelkorb, A. A., Swan, K. L., Jahn, L., Haas, S., & Hacker, J. (2015). Effectiveness of play therapy on problematic behaviors of preschool children with somatization. *Journal of Child and Adolescent Counseling, 1*(1), 3–16.

Shipon-Blum, E. (2010). Social communication bridge for selective mutism. Retrieved January 11, 2011, from *www. selectivemutismcenter.org/cms/BRIDGE2010ALL.pdf.*

Shipon-Blum, E. (2012). *Selective mutism: Stages of social communication comfort scale.* Jenkintown, PA: Selective Mutism Anxiety Research and Treatment Center. Retrieved from *www.selectivemutismcenter.org/Media_Library/Stages.SM.pdf.*

Shipon-Blum, E. (2015). A brief guide to understanding and treating selective mutism via social communication anxiety treatment (S-CAT)®. Retrieved from *www.selectivemutismcenter.org/aboutus/SelectiveMutism.*

Shipon-Blum, E., & Stein, M. B. (2008). Selective Mutism Questionnaire: Measurement structure and validity. *Journal of the American Academy of Child and Adolescent Psychiatry, 47*, 1197–1204.

Spence, S. H., Donovan, C., & Brechman-Toussaint, M. (2000). The treatment of childhood social phobia: The effectiveness of a social skills training-based, cognitive-behavioural intervention, with and without parental involvement. *Journal of Child Psychology and Psychiatry, 41*(6), 713–726.

Stallard, P. (2013). Adapting cognitive behaviour therapy for children and adolescents. In P. Graham & S. Reynolds (Eds.), *Cognitive behaviour therapy for children and families* (pp. 22–33). Cambridge, UK: Cambridge University Press.

Stulmaker, H. L., & Ray, D. C. (2015). Child-centered play therapy with young children who are anxious: A controlled trial. *Children and Youth Services Review, 57,* 127–133.

Su, S. H., & Tsai, M. H. (2016). Group play therapy with children of new immigrants in Taiwan who are exhibiting relationship difficulties. *International Journal of Play Therapy, 25*(2), 91–101.

Vladair, H. B., Feyijinmi, G. O., & Feindler, E. L. (2017). Termination in cognitive-behavioral therapy with children, adolescents, and parents. *Psychotherapy, 54*(1), 15–21.

Wilson, B. J., & Ray, D. (2018). Child-centered play therapy: Aggression, empathy, and self-regulation. *Journal of Counseling and Development, 96*(4), 399–409.

Young, B. J., Bunnell, B. E., & Beidel, D. C. (2012). Evaluation of children with selective mutism and social phobia: A comparison of psychological and psychophysiological arousal. *Behavior Modification, 36,* 525–544.

PART III

Clinical Applications
of Prescriptive Play Therapy
for Stress/Trauma Reactions

CHAPTER 7

Play Interventions for Young Survivors of Disaster, Terrorism, and Other Tragic Events

Janine Shelby
Audrey D. Smith

Description of the Need for Intervention Following Disastrous Events

Tragic events befall children somewhere on earth every minute of every day. Over the past two decades, 8,154 natural disasters have affected millions of children globally (Ritchie & Roser, 2018). During the past 10 years, human conflict has resulted in the deaths of 2 million children, the homelessness of 6 million youth, and the injuries of 12 million young survivors (Danziger, 2015). Today, more than 250 million children live in areas impacted by violence (UNICEF, 2018). As a result, 40 million children and adults have become internally displaced, and over 25 million have become refugees (UNHCR, 2018). Additionally, many children in stable living conditions are also at risk of harm. In 2017, 11,000 terrorist-related attacks, including 65 in the United States, resulted in 26,445 fatalities (Roser, Nagdy, & Ritchie, 2018).

When disaster or terrorism impacts their communities, play therapists may find themselves suddenly called upon to assist young survivors. Early intervention protocols for disaster relief/humanitarian aid with children commonly encourage the use of play. Yet, there is surprisingly little agreement as to the purpose of the play (e.g., diversion method, amusement source, communication tool, or psychological intervention) or the best-practice standards when using play in early intervention settings. Furthermore, there is little guidance in acute intervention protocols to help interventionists distinguish helpful from unhelpful play. This chapter addresses these underexplored areas to assist play therapists as they intervene with children during the immediate aftermath of disastrous events. First, historical approaches to postdisaster intervention are reviewed. Then, we propose guidelines and practical strategies to aid interventionists as they provide developmentally and evidence-informed play-based interventions to young survivors immediately following disaster, terrorism, and other tragic events. We conclude by summarizing research in this area as well as the prevailing wisdom about how to avoid potentially harmful interventions. This chapter is an outgrowth of the authors' collective work with thousands of child survivors on five continents following a varied range of tragic events. Even so, we meekly acknowledge that scientific understanding evolves, best-practice standards change, and within each child we find a teacher who adds to our repository of knowledge.

Rationale for Using Play in Early Interventions

History of Early Psychological Intervention

For decades after mental health treatment programs became commonplace in community and hospital settings, psychological intervention efforts were largely absent from sites where disaster and terrorism survivors received assistance. However, in the 1980s and 1990s, psychological intervention programs sprang from numerous organizations and agencies. These acute intervention protocols were designed not only for individuals directly exposed to disaster or terrorism but also for the staff who assisted them and/or for emergency services personnel (e.g., first responders). At that time, psychological interventions reflected the widely held belief among mental health professionals that expression of experiences, thoughts, and feelings was beneficial or even curative, irrespective of the setting or the recency of the distressing event. One popular intervention, critical incident stress management (Mitchell, 1983) and the subsequent critical incident stress debriefing (CISD; Mitchell & Everly, 2001), was originally developed for first responders but later used with other trauma-exposed individuals. The intervention was believed to benefit participants by their detailed recounting of the event in a group comprised of others who experienced the same event. The intervention was typically held soon after the event and was thought to reduce or prevent psychological trauma symptoms while increasing a sense of group cohesion.

This era's initial assumptions about expression-based, early intervention fit well with play therapy's long tradition as a developmentally sensitive means for children to communicate and process their experiences. Concurrently, awareness of children's postdisaster play was increasing, with published accounts of kidnapped and then rescued children playing scenes of the crime they survived (Terr, 1979) and children using broccoli to depict the trees of Hurricane Hugo (Saylor, Swenson, & Powell, 1992). The expanded recognition of children's posttraumatic play manifested itself in humanitarian aid organizations, where children were often provided play space as well as art and play activities during the wake of disastrous events. Within these programs, interventionists with various levels of education, training, and experience in child development and play therapy offered acute interventions. With more than a dozen theoretically distinct forms of play therapy, interventions were delivered in vastly different ways with varying goals and outcomes. At the time, the research guiding these intervention practices was primarily anecdotal or quasi-experimental. Thus, some interventionists in acute intervention settings used approaches similar to those they might use in longer-term psychotherapies, where children were encouraged to symbolically express their postdisaster experiences and/or emotional responses through play with as little therapist direction as possible. In contrast, directive play activities were offered by other interventionists, who tended to focus on adaptive functioning and coping instead of expression- or retelling-oriented interventions.

Following a period of widespread dissemination and use of expressive- or debriefing-type interventions, research findings caused disaster mental health practices to shift away from the use of debriefing-oriented approaches. Despite generally high satisfaction levels with participation in debriefings, most studies found no effect on or increases in trauma symptoms (Rose & Bisson, 1998) among adult debriefing participants. Although little research had been conducted on debriefing interventions for children, CISD's research findings led to the widespread conclusion that early ventilation of feelings and emotions may be harmful and retraumatizing. Also, several anecdotal accounts raised questions about the possible iatrogenic effects of some expressive arts and play-based early interventions (e.g., Bisson & Cohen, 2006; Kim, 2011; Pfefferbaum & Shaw, 2013). Concerns were related to the indiscriminate application of interventions to all children (i.e., including highly distressed and asymptomatic youth), the focus on emotional expression rather than coping or soothing, and the timing of the interventions. For example, some children who received play or art interventions during the immediate aftermath of disastrous events were reported to show signs of increased physiological arousal or distress and/or insufficient coping resources to counter the stress associated with their participation in the intervention. Furthermore, follow-up mental health resources were not always readily available for young survivors. So, upsetting content expressed immediately following tragic events may have been left unresolved at a time in the postdisaster recovery period when individu-als' psychological resources were required to address basic needs and cope with the changed circumstances of their lives. Equally important, children who faced ongoing danger, deprivation, chaos, or tumult may have found expression-based interventions less helpful than coping-based interven-tions. As Bisson and Cohen (2006, p. 587) summarized, "The problem with some acute psychological interventions is that children are asked to talk about what happened . . . when there is no evidence that either screen-ing for [high] distress or risk factors has occurred."

During the same era when postdisaster intervention practice was evolving, Kaduson, Cangelosi, and Schaefer (1997) proposed the prescrip-tive eclectic approach to recommend that play therapists match therapeutic interventions, elements, and techniques with the individual needs of young therapy clients. This chapter is an offshoot of their approach, as we seek to tailor interventions to each child's unique characteristics and concerns, as well as to the acute intervention environment.

Contemporary Approaches to Postdisaster Psychological Assistance

In time, *early* interventions came to be regarded as distinct from *thera-peutic* interventions. Initial interventions are typically designed to focus on practical, immediate-term issues and may be provided by paraprofes-sionals. Also, early interventions may be single- or extremely short-term encounters, and therefore should not rely on intervention techniques that take several weeks or months to benefit survivors.

In response to the need for an effective, safe initial postdisaster psy-chological protocol, the *Psychological First Aid: Field Operations Guide* (PFA; Brymer et al., 2006) was developed and is now widely regarded as "the first, and most favored, early intervention approach" (Shultz & Forbes, 2014, p. 1). Based on expert consensus and principles extracted from existing research evidence, the PFA is an evidence-informed, but not yet evidence-based, intervention. Developed for use with both adults and children, eight core intervention modules are identified, with brief notes summarizing how to apply these components to children and adoles-cents. The eight core actions are as follows: (1) contact and engagement; (2) safety and comfort; (3) stabilization; (4) information gathering related to survivors' needs and concerns; (5) practical assistance; (6) social sup-port; (7) coping; and (8) linkage to collaborative services. Despite the lim-ited amount of research that has directly assessed the PFA's effectiveness (Dieltjens, Moonens, Van Praet, De Buck, & Vandekerckhove, 2014; Fox et al., 2012; Shultz & Forbes, 2014), the PFA has been actively propagated, is used in many parts of the world, and holds distinction as the most widely accepted protocol of its kind.

In the PFA and similar protocols, play is assigned a role in intervention with children, but the precise role, function, and parameters of play have yet to be articulated. Fittingly, the PFA has been described as a set of principles with variants rather than a detailed manual. The descriptions of these principles leave gaps in technical guidance, and a number of issues that commonly occur in postdisaster settings remain unaddressed (e.g., how to notify children of the disastrous event when caregivers are unavailable or seek assistance to do so, or how to assist overwhelmed caregivers meet the needs of their distressed children rather than merely advise them to do so). This chapter addresses these and other areas by proposing practical strategies for implementing some of the PFA's core actions with children during the immediate aftermath of disastrous events. In contrast to the PFA's set of principles with variants, here the focus is on a set of *variants with principles*, derived from both the PFA and the prescriptive play therapy approach.

Proposed Play-Based Early Intervention Strategies

Overview

The intervention recommendations presented here align with three of Schaefer's (1993) therapeutic factors of play (stress inoculation, stress management, and the enhancement of positive emotions). Therapeutic factors, called *powers of play,* have been described as the "specific targeted aspects within treatment in which play initiates, facilitates, or strengthens the therapeutic effect" (Drewes & Schaefer, 2016, p. 36). Later, Schaefer's 20 hypothesized powers of play are grouped into four fundamental categories, and the three factors used in this chapter are placed together in the category called *fostering emotional wellness* (Drewes & Schaefer, 2016).

This chapter is not intended as a comprehensive guide to early intervention; rather, it addresses selected issues common in postdisaster psychological intervention settings. Play therapists providing postdisaster interventions should refer to Baggerly's (2006) recommendations to adhere to incident command structures, maintain one's own affect regulation, develop hardiness and flexibility, emphasize survivors' normalcy and resilience rather than pathology, and provide a "safe space" for children. It is also essential to ensure that children are as physically safe and comfortable as possible. Medical issues should be treated, and biological needs should be addressed to the fullest extent possible. Finally, it is important for interventionists to be mindful of the fact that survivors receive many types of resources and services during the aftermath of disastrous events; psychological interventions may not be prioritized as the most important.

Specific Intervention Strategies

Death or Tragedy Notification

The information a child receives about a tragic event, as well as the informant's demeanor, commingle to shape children's understanding about what has occurred and the recovery trajectory. Yet, caregivers sometimes show reluctance to disclose tragic events to their children, or they provide misleading and/or confusing explanations (e.g., a deceased relative may be described as being on a long work trip or a mass shooting may be described as a loud party). This reluctance usually stems from the caregiver's desire to spare his or her child emotional pain, the caregiver's own use of avoidance-based coping, and/or the caregiver's sense of guilt that the child was not/could not be protected from suffering. In these cases, it is important to bear the family's cultural norms and practices in mind, and then, to gently acknowledge to the caregiver that large-scale disastrous events or intense parental distress almost always seep into children's awareness. With some caregivers, interventionists can inquire about the pros and cons of open communication with children and provide guidance about how disclosure is a powerful opportunity to teach children that they can face and survive adversity. Interventionists can offer caregivers guidance, psychological support, or the opportunity to rehearse the notification. Some caregivers prefer to have the interventionist notify the child, either in the caregiver's presence or without the caregiver. In cases where a caregiver wishes the interventionist to disclose the event, it is useful to explore the caregiver's concerns to determine whether the issue can be resolved so that the caregiver can remain present during the notification (e.g., making a plan with the caregiver for how to answer a child's question or what to do if the caregiver becomes overwhelmed with emotion). However, in our experience, there are many equally compassionate ways to disclose tragic events to children, and it is rarely productive to press emotionally drained caregivers to disclose when they strongly prefer not to do so. In these cases, interventionists can outline the content of the intended notification to the caregiver prior to meeting with the child and then refocus caregivers on how they can assist the child following the notification. Figure 7.1 provides a sample script of a notification to a child.

As presented in Figure 7.1, the notification has four primary components. The first component, *the four Rs*, involves the following subsections: rare, reveal, reassure, and reason. To begin, provide a framework for understanding the event so that children understand that the event is *rare*, almost

---

I. Rare, Reveal, Reassure, Reason

Rarity
Today, something happened that does not usually happen. Briefly (i.e., in one or two sentences) describe event.

Reassurance
You are safe now/in as safe a place as I/we could find. [If true] *Your family/ friends are safe.* [Alternate] *A lot of people are working hard to try to keep you/ as many people as possible safe.*

Attribution
The [event] *is not your fault at all. It happened because* [brief, developmentally appropriate explanation].

Pause to allow the child time to absorb the information and/or spontaneously ask questions.

II. Immediate Effect on Child, Others, Community

Now, [anticipated effects—for example, *You/your family will stay here until you have a safe place to live; You may feel confused/sad/scared/upset/nervous; Your parents might feel sad/scared/upset/nervous; People might talk or cry about this a lot*].

III. Questions and Clarification: Ask, Repeat, and Correct

Ask: *Do you have any questions about this?*
Respond honestly but age appropriately (i.e., simply for younger children and more elaborately for older children).

Repeat: When helpful but not if contraindicated (i.e., the child is overwhelmed, extremely upset, cognitively disorganized, or does not want to speak), ask children to repeat what they heard you say and/or what they had already heard from others.

Correct: Confirm children's accurate depictions and correct any misunderstandings.

IV. Coping and Normalization

Coping
After sufficient time has lapsed, assess whether it is appropriate to provide a brief discussion of soothing/coping techniques. For example, *No one can undo what happened, but doing* [ ] *might make you feel better* and/or *You can help* [caregivers, siblings, direct survivors] *by* [ ].

Normalization
Remember, it is okay/normal to have strong feelings right now.

FIGURE 7.1. Tragic event child notification script.

never occurs, or is not expected to happen to the child regularly. Then, briefly disclose, or *reveal*, the event using developmentally appropriate terminology while providing an accurate but understandable attribution, or *reason*, for the event (e.g., "Something didn't work well in his mind, and he didn't understand that he was hurting people" or "Deep under the ground, some parts of the earth moved, and that made your house fall down"). Next, offer realistic *reassurance* of safety or relative safety, but avoid offering unrealistic or untrue reassurance. For example, children can be told by an adult, "I will do everything possible to keep you safe," but safety can never be assured with absolute certainty. Afterward, briefly explain the impact of the incident on the child, family, friends, and/or community (e.g., "You may miss the way things used to be, many buildings fell down," or "Many people will cry about the people who died"). Of course, interventionists should modify the script based on the individual circumstances of the tragedy, environmental context, family, and child. After providing the four Rs and discussing the immediate effects of the event, interventionists should provide an opportunity for the child to ask questions. When possible, the interventionist should leave the child with practical methods of coping tailored to the event and its aftermath. Throughout the conversation, avoid extreme, negative language (e.g., "awful," "horrific," or "hopeless") and maintain the perspective that hardships, even particularly painful ones, can be survived.

Caregiver Reassurance Strategies

In the PFA, caregivers are encouraged to provide comfort and reassurance to their children, but not all caregivers have the psychological resources or preexisting parenting skills to adequately meet their children's heightened needs during the immediate aftermath of tragic events. In these cases, it may be more practical to identify high-likelihood/high-impact caregiver strategies (i.e., comforting strategies already included in caregivers' repertoires) that can be easily employed to reassure children. To structure this intervention, overwhelmed caregivers can be asked about their use of the following strategies: (1) verbal reassurance; (2) physical affection or close physical proximity; (3) provision of comforting materials (e.g., a comforting blanket or toy); (4) privileges (e.g., temporarily sleeping near caregivers, or spending extra time with people who comfort the child); (5) verbalization of a hope-based trajectory (e.g., "We will get through this and find a way to feel better in the future"); and (6) adherence to daily routines. From among these or other types of reassurance, caregivers can identify two or three strategies they are likely to use and their children find helpful. Other ways caregivers can promote their children's adjustment include explicitly pointing out steps adults have taken to enhance safety, modeling effective coping, and noting aloud their own use of helpful coping strategies (e.g., "I felt really sad today and that is okay/normal. After a while, I decided I wanted to think about something happier, so I thought about how lucky we are to have each other."). Finally, encourage caregivers to play with their children, explain children's ability to process their experiences through play, prepare caregivers for the possibility that disaster-related themes may appear in their children's play, and help them recognize signs that indicate a need for more intensive psychological assistance.

Play-Based Strategies to Foster Emotional Wellness

In the remainder of this chapter, we present several play-based, early interventions to foster emotional wellness. Our interventions are presented as three types. The first type, voiceless interventions, involves the use of highly visible activities or materials readily available to survivors and designed to promote helpful cognitions, adaptive coping, and hopefulness without the explicit aid of an interventionist. These interventions may be particularly helpful in the immediate aftermath of tragic events, when both children and adults often have difficulty verbalizing their needs and reactions. These interventions are also useful in cases where survivors might feel uncomfortable being directly approached by an interventionist. The second type, interventionist-directed techniques, calls for young survivors to engage in structured activities with interventionists. The final category, spontaneous play, is presented with specific suggestions for a prescriptive, tailored response to children's play in acute intervention settings.

Voiceless Interventions

HOPE WALL

In this activity, the label "reasons I can/have to get through this" is affixed to a chalk board, wall, or other identified space. A written notice should invite both children and adults to participate by writing or drawing the people, pets, spiritual or philosophical beliefs, or personal skills/experiences that provide a reason to keep going, despite the hardships they face (e.g., "because my sister needs me"; "because my Dad would want me to"; "to care for my pet"; or "because I am strong in many ways"). Materials (e.g., writing implements, sticky notes) should be readily available for survivors to contribute their own statements to the wall. Participation is voluntary, but even those who do not participate are likely to benefit from exposure to the varied sources of courage others have posted on the hope wall. The wall also provides a natural entry point for conversation between survivors and interventionists.

KNOWING TREE

In this psychoeducational intervention, a drawing or picture of a tree is placed atop and attached to a blank sheet of paper the same size. The foreground page with the picture of the tree contains "window" squares drawn at various points in the tree branches. Each window is cut on three of its four sides, such that it opens (i.e., it is attached by the fourth side of the square). On the forward-facing side of each window, a question or statement is written to reflect a concern children often have following disastrous events. Responses to these questions are written (i.e., prior to the intervention activity) on the sheet of paper in the background, behind the window, so that when the window is opened, the answer is revealed. Tying a piece of thread to each window not only makes it easier to pull open, but also generates additional enticement for children to explore the knowing tree's psychoeducational content. Windows might contain questions such as "Will I always feel this scared?"; "Is it my fault?"; or "Is it normal to feel this way?" Answers revealed when the windows are opened might include "There are many things you can try to feel better"; "It is not your fault"; and "It is normal to feel the way you do."

COPING BOX

This activity can be created from a wide array of materials, ranging from a simple cardboard box to an elaborately decorated wooden treasure chest. When opened, the coping box reveals a variety of coping/sensory-based materials, such as kinetic sand, squishy balls, cotton balls, play dough, items with fragrant smells, bubbles, music boxes, and other content likely to provide instant soothing and distraction. Multiple coping boxes, each containing different types of materials, can be placed in different locations in the intervention area for easy access by those in need of soothing activities.

COPING PUPPET SHOWS

Puppetry can be an effective tool for helping children develop and enhance coping skills. Using puppets, interventionists can portray a story about a character who seeks advice about his or her posttraumatic reactions. Other puppets are introduced into the narrative, sequentially explaining how to use various but specific coping skills and tips (e.g., how to use positive imagery, relaxation techniques, social support, and helpful cognitions/behaviors). When the circumstances are conducive to an interactive puppet show, puppets can encourage children to practice the coping skills at the same time the main character learns each technique.

Interventionist-Directed Activities

COPING ROAD

Following disastrous events, survivors often feel powerless and ruminate on how they wish the past could be altered. In this cognitive intervention strategy, survivors have the opportunity to refocus their efforts on their sense of agency (i.e., what they can change or do). First, a "road" can be created with chalk or construction paper used as stepping stones. A special symbol or piece of paper represents the tragedy, which is identified along the road but is not discussed in detail. Shortly thereafter, the road divides into two paths. The interventionist prepares the survivor for the intervention by saying that this pathway is like time. It moves in only the forward direction. Next, the interventionist and survivor stand on a "step" or point on the road past the place where the tragedy is symbolically depicted, and the interventionist points out that the disaster has already happened, so it cannot be changed. What remains in the survivor's power, however, is the choice to act and think in ways that lead to feeling better or worse. The paper "steps" of the "better" path can be completed with pictures or labels of methods in which the young person can engage in adaptive coping behaviors. When it is encouraging to do so, survivors can be invited to imagine a time much further ahead on the road when recovery efforts have progressed. Of note, this intervention is designed for those likely to benefit from a cognitive restructuring strategy, and it may not be suitable during the first hours or days following tragic events.

COPING MENU

From a selection of sticky notes or index cards with pictures and/or labels, young survivors can select strategies that they believe would help them. After selecting a strategy/behavior for each category of the coping menu (see Figure 7.2), they affix it to the corresponding section of the coping chart. Young survivors can practice using the selected strategy with the interventionist, teach their caregivers the techniques they have selected, and take the coping menu with them for future use.

PHYSIOLOGICAL SOOTHING SESSIONS

With increased physiological arousal common in the initial postdisaster period, interventions that provide opportunities for soothing are critically important to young children. For youth whose caregivers are available, frequently scheduled "soothing sessions" can be helpful in restoring a sense of calm. For example, children's favorite soothing experiences (e.g., being rocked, sung to, having a story read, or swaddled) can be provided. Follow-

Feeling Better		
Things I Can Do By Myself To Feel Better 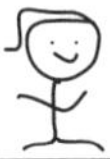		
Things I Can Do With Someone Else To Feel Better 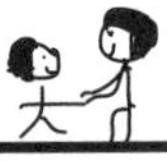		
Fun Things I Can Imagine I Am Doing 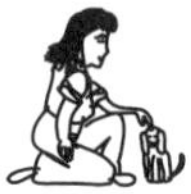		
Something I Can Tell Myself To Feel Better 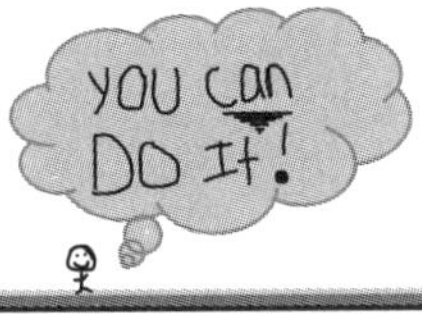		

FIGURE 7.2. Coping menu. Created by Samara Shelby-Nishita.

ing tragic events, children may wish for soothing methods commonly used by younger children. When caregivers are not available, interventionists can assist children select and use blankets, subdued lighting, soft music, large boxes in which to sit quietly, or other materials that might provide a comforting experience. Scheduling these soothing sessions several times each day gives children frequent opportunities to experience a calm state, despite the hardships surrounding them.

Spontaneous Play

Although posttraumatic play is more widely discussed as a maladaptive phenomenon, it is common, developmentally typical, and can be a helpful tool in children's processing of adverse experiences. In one study, a majority of traumatized children were found to spontaneously use play in an attempt to process the event (Cohen, Chazan, Lerner, & Maimon, 2010). In helpful posttraumatic play, children use symbolic materials to titrate and self-regulate their depictions of events, affect, and cognitions. Adaptive posttraumatic play feels gratifying to children. In contrast, unhelpful posttraumatic play is repetitive, static, and/or compulsive, and is usually experienced as unfulfilling (see Gil, 2017, for a thorough discussion of healthy vs. toxic play). When children play themes of the tragic event in acute intervention settings, interventionists must make choices about whether to allow, interrupt, redirect, or facilitate coping/problem solving/ hope within the play. Commonly used protocols recommend that adults recognize, tolerate, normalize, voice the feelings expressed during the play, and/or redirect the posttraumatic play (e.g., PFA for Children II [Øllgaard, 2017]; and PFA, [Brymer et al., 2006]). For example, the interventionist or caregiver is advised to explain to the child, "You're drawing a lot of pictures of what happened. Did you know that many children do that?" and/or "It might help to draw how you would like your school to be rebuilt to make it safer" (Øllgaard, 2017, p. 122). However, there is no guidance for differentiating helpful from unhelpful play of the adverse event, and the manualized instructions are not tailored to these distinct types of play. Table 7.1 summarizes and adapts the work of several authors to present key distinguishing factors for each type of posttraumatic play. This is written specifically for application in acute intervention settings where posttraumatic play during the first hours and days following disastrous events is likely to involve elements that may seem more pathological in clinical settings. These include frequent thematic references to the event, morbid content, a relatively restricted range affect or numbness, and less sophisticated, organized, or integrated play narratives. In early intervention settings, these features of posttraumatic play are typical, expected, and not necessarily indicative of unhelpful posttraumatic play.

TABLE 7.1. Helpful and Unhelpful Posttraumatic Play

	Characteristics of helpful posttraumatic play
Content	• Tragedy-related or non-tragedy-related themes
Pattern/narrative development	• Children externalize their memories, selecting what and when to remember • Meaning is developed from chaos • Adaptive outcomes emerge • Flexibility is present (e.g., new characters, play narratives begin or end differently)
Affect	• Variable and consistent with the themes depicted • General sense of relief or gratification from outcomes or symbolic expression of experiences expressed in the play narrative, even if they are difficult experiences • Reenactments or problems depicted in play narratives involve a sense of gratification, soothing, or relief.
Physiological	• No excessive physiological arousal
	Characteristics of unhelpful posttraumatic play
Content	• Persistently morbid at a level that supersedes the child's experience of the event (though play narratives that involve themes of recent traumatic events are common and often helpful).
Pattern/narrative development	• Repetitive and/or literal • Inflexible, static, rigid, mechanistic, absent new solutions or outcomes, and compulsive or driven in nature • Extremely disorganized or chaotic • Unproductive, lacking in resolution, reenactment without soothing, or reenactment with overwhelming reexperiencing
Affect	• Ungratifying, devoid of pleasure, • Does not decrease anxiety • Affect involving anxiety, inflexible sadness, or desperation • Abrupt shifts and/or sudden avoidance
Physiological	• Intense or shallow breath • Yawning • Exaggerated startle response

Note. Data from Cohen, Chazan, Lerner, and Maimon (2010); Findling, Bratton, and Henson (2006); Gil (2017); Schaefer (1994); and Terr (1981).

When the type of play is identified, an intervention response can then be formulated. Figure 7.3 provides an algorithm for suggested intervention decisions based on the characteristics of the child's play. First, interventionists should identify whether play is developmentally typical (e.g., enjoyable, no themes of the traumatic event), atypical (e.g., developmentally delayed), or posttraumatic. Developmentally typical play without trauma themes requires no intervention, but joining or inviting caregivers to participate in child-directed play can provide comfort and enhance adult–child relationships. Developmentally atypical play without trauma themes may be manifested when numbness or fear are the predominant influences steering children's play but may also indicate a neurodevelopmental disorder or mental health issue. In cases where a child's history, behaviors, quality of play, and parental interactions raise questions about possible neurodevelopmental, maltreatment, or mental health issues, a referral for follow-up contact with the appropriate agency and/or mental health care may be appropriate. Many children in disaster relief settings have histories of adverse events, diagnosed or undiagnosed mental disorders, and environmental stressors. At times, the interventionist may be the first person to recognize and link survivors to agencies where assistance and/or assessment can be provided to child and/or family.

When a child's play is developmentally typical but themes of the adverse event are present, the interventionist should differentiate whether the posttraumatic play is helpful, potentially helpful, or unhelpful. Those engaging in unhelpful play can be encouraged to participate in soothing, grounding, or coping activities instead. For youth whose posttraumatic play possesses both adaptive and unhelpful qualities, techniques proposed by Gil (2017) may be beneficial. These suggestions include verbalizing descriptive statements that may cause a shift in posttraumatic play, asking children to give characters a voice to deepen their expression of thoughts and feelings, or changing the sequence of the play by asking children to start at a midpoint to break the pattern of the narrative. As another set of strategies, we suggest several "What can be done?" interventions. For example, a child engaging in posttraumatic play can be asked, "Can anything be done to make this [scene/play narrative/world] better/safer today?" After this question is asked, many children explore potential solutions to the scenario they are depicting in their play. If the child responds that nothing can be done, we then ask whether anything can be done to make the characters in the play more comfortable, even if nothing can be done to make things better/safer today. Often, children offer soothing elements to the characters in their play and derive vicarious comfort from their ability to soothe the characters. Again, if the child responds that nothing can be done, he or she can be asked whether "we [the interventionists and child] can tell them [the characters] we know they are sad/scared/confused but that they [the

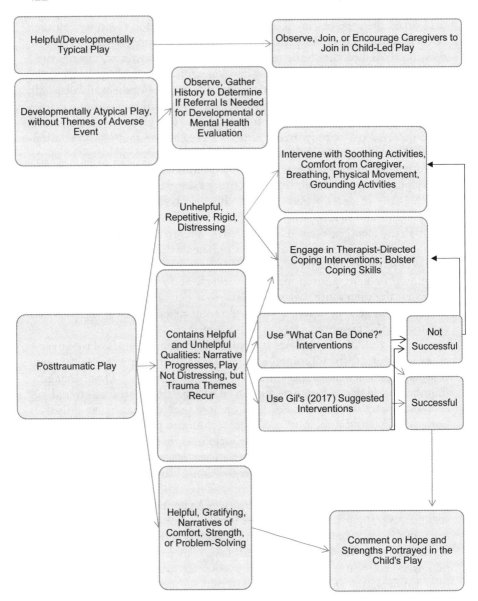

FIGURE 7.3. Posttraumatic play decision tree.

characters] are not alone. Even if the child once more indicates that the characters cannot receive this reassurance, the interventionist can speak directly to the characters, saying "Okay, not much can be done today, but I will remember you and I won't give up hope. I have seen a lot of things get better and I believe that you will get through this." When unhelpful play persists, children should be encouraged to engage in soothing, grounding, or coping activities instead. The interventionist should also consider making a referral for follow-up mental health care. On the other hand, when children engage in adaptive posttraumatic play, interventionists can highlight the characters' or child's ability to find solutions, survive hardships, demonstrate strengths, or cope well with adversity.

Caregiver Involvement

It is generally agreed that when children receive individual interventions, parallel attention to parental concerns and psychoeducation can be beneficial (Pfefferbaum & Shaw, 2013). Similarly, it is usually beneficial to provide coping-based and hope-enhancing interventions to caregivers as well as children. As described throughout this chapter, practical play-based strategies that help caregivers communicate about the event, provide realistic reassurance, facilitate coping, and instill hope can be easily implemented in early intervention settings.

Empirical Support for the Intervention

The research on disaster interventions for children has made considerably less progress than the research on disaster interventions for adults. In a comprehensive review of child disaster mental health interventions, Pfefferbaum et al. (2014) found that a variety of approaches (e.g., debriefings, exposure, humanistic therapy, and eye movement desensitization) have been used to address children's disaster-related reactions, but the most commonly used intervention techniques were cognitive behavioral in nature, including relaxation, coping, social support, and psychoeducation. Pfefferbaum and colleagues found insufficient data to assign superiority to any approach, and several programs used more than a single method of intervention. The absence of clear findings from extant research on early interventions for children highlights how little is known about effective early intervention strategies.

Few rigorously designed studies exist of play-based, disaster-related, immediate-term interventions of children. Among those that involved randomized controlled trials (RCTs), the play-based intervention was often used as the control condition and was rarely explicitly described. Yet, multiple quasi-experimental studies and clinical descriptions of postdisaster play-based interventions for children appear in the literature (e.g., Aiello, 2012; Cohen et al., 2010; Cohen, Pat-Horenczyk, & Haar-Shamir, 2014; Das & Mohanty, 2018; Ohnogi, 2010; Shen, 2002; Wolmer, Laor, & Yazgan, 2003), and play-based interventions are widely practiced in the field.

In the absence of strong research support, other sources of information must serve as the basis for conclusions about best practices for postdisaster intervention with young survivors. From these sources (e.g., clinical wisdom, common practice data, research extrapolated from somewhat similar populations, and expert consensus) some themes emerge. First, there is widespread agreement that early interventions should foster resilience, coping, and adaptive functioning. Second, there is also strong consensus that interventionists should avoid retraumatizing children by exposing them to information and emotions they may not be able to process or integrate. Thus, play-based interventions with children should not *require* them to draw or play the traumatic event during the initial postdisaster period (Pfefferbaum & Shaw, 2013). Third, there is general acceptance that nontrauma-specific interventions, such as relaxation and stabilizing activities (e.g., singing, art, storytelling, and playing), have a prominent role in early intervention (Bisson & Cohen, 2006). Fourth, recommendations to use play appear in most widely disseminated intervention protocols. In addition to being engaging and comforting to children, play also provides a developmentally sensitive vehicle for teaching and learning coping skills. Unhelpful posttraumatic play should be addressed or diverted, but self-initiated, adaptive play may facilitate the processing of disaster-related experiences.

Conclusion

In every disaster or terrorism intervention setting where children have access to toys, they play. Despite its ubiquity, the full potential of children's play in disaster relief settings has not been harnessed. Intervention protocols remain undetailed or ambiguous about the specific uses of play, and there is little research to guide practice. With this chapter, we hope to contribute to the play-based intervention literature by promoting greater consonance between common practice standards and real-world realities. Early interventions are typically brief, but they are not necessarily fleeting. Using the prescriptive approach to play-based interventions, we have safely and effectively reduced countless children's initial distress, bolstered their coping skills, and facilitated or intervened in their play in ways that empowered and galvanized them to begin their postdisaster recovery.

REFERENCES

Aiello, T. (2012). What the children said: Children's narrative constructions of the events of 9/11 in psychotherapy. *Journal of Infant, Child, and Adolescent Psychotherapy, 11*(1), 32–38.

Baggerly, J. N. (2006). Preparing play therapists for disaster response: Principles and practices. *International Journal of Play Therapy, 15*(2), 59–81.

Bisson, J. I., & Cohen, J. A. (2006). Disseminating early interventions following trauma. *Journal of Traumatic Stress, 19*, 583–595.

Brymer, M., Jacobs, A., Layne, C., Pynoos, R., Ruze, J., Steinberg, A., et al. (2006). *Psychological first aid: Field operations guide* (2nd ed.). Los Angeles: National Child Traumatic Stress Network and National Center for PTSD.

Cohen, E., Chazan, S., Lerner, M., & Maimon, E. (2010). Posttrauamtic play in young children exposed to terrorism: An empirical study. *Infant Mental Health Journal, 31*(2), 159–181.

Cohen, E., Pat-Horenczyk, R., & Haar-Shamir, D. (2014). Making room for play: An innovative intervention for toddlers and families under rocket fire. *Clinical Social Work Journal, 42*(4), 336–345.

Danziger, N. (2015). Children and war. Retrieved from *www.redcross.int/EN/mag/magazine2003_3/4-9.html.*

Das, M., & Mohanty, N. (2018). Physical activity and play as a medium of psychological first aid (PFA) leading to psychosocial care for building resiliency and helps to overcome trauma in emergency situations. *Clinical and Experimental Psychology, 4*, 184.

Dieltjens, T., Moonens, I., Van Praet, K., De Buck, E., & Vandekerckhove, P. (2014). A systematic literature search on psychological first aid: Lack of evidence to develop guidelines. *PLOS ONE, 9*(12), e114714.

Drewes, A., & Schaefer, C. E. (2016). Therapeutic powers of play. In K. J. O'Connor, C. E. Schaefer, & L. D. Braverman (Eds.), *Handbook of play therapy* (2nd ed., pp. 35–60). Hoboken, NJ: Wiley.

Findling, J. F., Bratton S. C., & Henson, R. K. (2006). Development of the trauma play scale: An observation based assessment of the impact of trauma on the play therapy behaviors of young children. *International Journal of Play Therapy, 15*, 7–36.

Fox, J. H., Burkle, F. M., Jr., Bass, J., Pia, F. A., Epstein, J. L., & Markenson, D. (2012). The effectiveness of psychological first aid as a disaster intervention tool: Research analysis of peer-reviewed literature from 1990–2010. *Disaster Medicine and Public Health Preparedness, 6*, 247–252.

Gil, E. (2017). *Posttraumatic play in children: What clinicians need to know.* New York: Guilford Press.

Kaduson, H. G., Cangelosi, D., & Schaefer, C. E. (1997). *The playing cure.* Lanham, MD: Rowman & Littlefield.

Kim, Y. (2011). Editorial: Great East Japan earthquake and early mental-health-care response. *Psychiatry and Clinical Neurosciences, 65*, 539–548.

Mitchell, J. T. (1983). When disaster strikes . . . The critical incident stress debriefing process. *Journal of Emergency Medical Services, 13*(11), 49–52.

Mitchell, J. T., & Everly, G. S., Jr. (2001). *Critical incident stress debriefing: An operations manual for CISD, defusing and other group crisis intervention services* (3rd ed.). Ellicott City, MD: Chevron.

Ohnogi, A. J. (2010). Using play to support children traumatized by natural disasters: Chuetsu earthquake series in Japan. In A. Kalayjian & D. Eugene (Eds.), *Mass trauma and emotional healing around the world: Rituals and practices for resilience and meaning-making* (pp. 37–54). Santa Barbara, CA: Praeger/ABC-CLIO.

Øllgaard, R. (2017). Psychological first aid for children: II. Retrieved from *http://resourcecentre.savethechildren.se*.

Pfefferbaum, B., & Shaw, J. A. (2013). Practice parameter on disaster preparedness. *Journal of the American Academy of Child and Adolescent Psychiatry, 52*(11), 1224–1238.

Ritchie, H., & Roser, M. (2018). Natural catastrophes. Retrieved from *https://ourworldindata.org/natural-catastrophes*.

Rose, S., & Bisson, J. (1998). Brief early psychological interventions following trauma: A systematic review of the literature. *Journal of Traumatic Stress, 11*(4), 697–710.

Roser, M., Nagdy, M., & Ritchie, H. (2018). Terrorism. Retrieved from *https://ourworldindata.org/terrorism*.

Saylor, C. F., Swenson, C. C., & Powell, P. (1992). Hurricane Hugo blows down the broccoli: Preschoolers' post-disaster play and adjustment. *Child Psychiatry and Human Development, 22*(3), 139–149.

Schaefer, C. E. (1993). *The therapeutic powers of play*. Northvale, NJ: Jason Aronson.

Schaefer, C. E. (1994). Play therapy for psychic trauma I children. In K. J. O'Connor & C. E. Schaefer (Eds.), *Handbook of play therapy: Advances and innovations* (Vol. 2, pp. 297–318). Hoboken, NJ: Wiley.

Shen, Y. (2002). Short-term group play therapy with Chinese earthquake victims: Effects on anxiety, depression and adjustment. *International Journal of Play Therapy, 11*(1), 43–63.

Shultz, J. M., & Forbes, D. (2014). Psychological first aid. *Disaster Health, 2*(1), 3–12.

Terr, L. C. (1979). The children of Chowchilla. *Psychoanalytic Study of the Child, 34*, 547–623.

Terr, L. C. (1981). "Forbidden games": Posttraumatic child's play. *Journal of the American Academy of Child Psychiatry, 20*, 741–760.

UNHCR. (2018). Figures at a glance: Statistical yearbook. Retrieved from *www.unhcr.org/figures-at-a-glance.html*.

UNICEF. (2018). Children in war and conflict. *UNICEF USA*. Retrieved from *www.unicefusa.org/mission/emergencies/conflict*.

Wolmer, L., Laor, N., & Yazgan, Y. (2003). School reactivation programs after disaster: Could teachers serve as clinical mediators? *Child and Adolescent Psychiatry Clinics of North America, 12*, 363–381.

CHAPTER 8

Play Therapy for Children of Divorce

Donna Cangelosi

Introduction and Presenting Problems

"My 6-year-old son is clingy and has been wetting the bed"; "My 8-year-old daughter is having difficulty sleeping"; "My 12-year-old son is doing terribly in school." These are just a few presenting problems commonly seen among children referred for play therapy during or after parental divorce. The breakup of the family can bring about regressive behaviors, hinder mastery of developmental tasks, and increase the risk of numerous social, emotional, cognitive, and behavioral difficulties.

Experiencing parental divorce often sets in motion enormous changes in children's lives. These changes can include the absence of one parent while living with the other, adjustment to moving between two households, the permanent or semipermanent loss of one parent, witnessing of parental anger or distress, ongoing parental conflict, added responsibilities, and increased emotional, social, and financial stressors in the home. Further complicating children's attempts to cope with these changes is the fact that they are also frequently faced with economic challenges, repartnering/remarriage, and relocation, which can result in loss of friendships and other significant relationships. Because children lack the cognitive and emotional skills needed to understand and negotiate these changes, they often struggle to make sense of them alone, resulting in a sense of loneliness, isolation, and confusion.

Researchers agree that children's reactions to parental divorce begin when one parent physically leaves the home. However, despite the difference between the legal date of divorce and the breakup of the family, the terms are commonly used interchangeably in the literature. This chapter also uses the terms *divorce, family rupture,* and *breakup of the family* interchangeably.

Historical Overview

Before the late 19th century, the incidence of divorce in the United States was rare and could only be based on adultery and desertion. However, after the suffragettes earned the right to divorce, women ended marriages for financial and emotional reasons as well, and so the number of broken marriages slowly rose until the 1950s, when it declined for the first time. With the women's movement in the 1960s, people were less compelled to stay in unhappy marriages in order to protect children from emotional turmoil. Divorce was seen as an opportunity for personal growth for parents as well as their children. This thinking was encouraged in the media and among scholars who argued that children were resilient and would be better off if their parents left unhappy marriages. In addition, "no fault divorce" bills allowed one spouse to end a marriage for any reason. In the decade that followed, approximately 50% of children born in the 1970s experienced parental divorce as compared to approximately 11% of children born in the 1950s (Wilcox, 2009). While statistics now vary depending on geographic location, ethnic background, and socioeconomic status, it is estimated that approximately 46% of children in this country experience parental divorce before the age of 17. Because a large number of divorced parents remarry, and 40% of these remarriages also end in divorce, this population of children may experience multiple losses and struggles (Anderson, 2014).

Effects of Divorce on Children

Researchers have found that while most children adjust well to divorce without intervention, others experience social, emotional, academic, and/ or behavioral difficulties following the family breakup (Amato, 2002; Emery, 1999; Kelly, 2012). Divorce has been associated with declines in reading and math scores, social skills, self-control, and increased internalizing and externalizing difficulties, such as anger, delinquent behaviors, anxiety, depression, self-blame, and separation/abandonment fears (Amato & Anthony, 2014; Fagan & Churchill, 2012; Hetherington & Kelly, 2002). In addition, it has also been found that children of divorce have difficulties with intimate relationships in adulthood (Hetherington, 1999).

Psychotherapists who work with children from divorced families have noted specific themes and struggles with this population. These include shame and worry about being different from peers; confusion about what to tell others; loyalty to one parent and fear of potential rejection; frustration and anger related to moving between two homes; discomfort with the nonprimary parent; fear the nonprimary parent will not provide adequate care; a perception of one parent as caring and competent and the other as not; becoming responsible for his or her own well-being and that of a fragile parent; loneliness; and concern for one or both parents, which may contribute to the child hiding his or her own feelings (Jordan, 2016).

Adjustment Factors

Children's adjustment to parental divorce is quite variable due to the countless influences inherent in this major change. To understand each child's unique needs, it is important to consider each individual child's age and stage of development, family dynamics, economic and social issues, and functioning prior to the breakup.

Age and Developmental Considerations

Age at the time of parental separation has a significant influence on children's abilities to understand and master the challenges brought about by divorce. Some researchers have found that preschoolers are at greater risk for difficulties because their limited cognitive abilities makes it difficult to understand the complexities of the family breakup (Wallerstein & Kelly, 1980). Children's thinking prior to the age of 7 is influenced by perceptions rather than reality, magical thinking, and egocentrism. They believe they can control their world and feel responsible when things wrong. Therefore, divorce commonly results in a sense of guilt and confusion as well as withdrawal or acting-out behaviors. In addition, young children rely on wishful thinking to cope with the losses associated with divorce and hold on to hope for a reunion much longer than do older children. Erik Erikson (1963) explained that preschoolers struggle with mastering a sense of initiative or, conversely, develop a sense of guilt, depending on the influences of the environment. Instead of exploring the world and pursuing age-appropriate activities, children of divorce may become clingy, experience separation anxiety, and have difficulties transitioning from one parent to another. The disruption of divorce during this age may cause these children to revert to an earlier, more dependent stage of development associated with a sense of security. Common presenting problems include separation anxiety, crying at bedtime, sleep problems, bedwetting, soiling, whining, tantrums, and thumb sucking.

By the age of 7, children begin to reason logically and their understanding of the world is less egocentric. However, their thinking is concrete and literal, and they are not yet able to reason abstractly. This can cause them to draw incorrect conclusions and not fully understand answers given to their questions. School-age children of divorce frequently worry about the unknown, wonder who will take care of them, and fear their parents who have stopped loving each other will stop loving them as well. Because their ability to name and express feelings and thoughts is still quite limited, they may internalize or externalize their grief and confusion. According to Erikson, it is at this stage that peer relationships and academic achievement become an important source of the child's self-esteem. If children gain a sense of pride in their accomplishments and are encouraged and acknowledged for their initiative, they begin to feel competent and confident in their abilities. However, if this initiative is not encouraged or is thwarted by the divorce, the child will feel inferior and experience self-doubt. School-age children who become preoccupied with loss and family concerns often show signs of depression and anxiety as well as behavioral difficulties. They fall behind or withdraw from age-appropriate academic and social activities, feel disempowered, and suffer from low self esteem.

Whereas parental divorce tends to intensify young children's dependence and regressive tendencies, the opposite tends to occur with older children and adolescents. The more independent-minded adolescent may react with anger, depression, anxiety, guilt, and a loss of trust. The latter may result in a premature flight toward adulthood, rebellion, and counterdependent behaviors stemming from an attitude that they are on their own. In addition, some adolescents attempt to take control of their lives by behaving distantly and defiantly (Dong et al., 2004; Oliver, Kuhns, & Pomeranz, 2006).

Family Dynamics

In her review of research, Kelly (2012) found that family processes following divorce are strong predictors of risk versus resilience. Important aspects of family dynamics include quality of parenting, parent–child relationships, level of conflict between parents, economic resources, and social support (Amato, 1994; Kelly, 2012; Lamb, 2012). Lamb's meta-analysis of research showed that children benefit when parents adjust to the divorce well enough to provide loving, emotionally responsive parenting with reasonable age-appropriate discipline. However, when parents become preoccupied with their own losses and emotions, engage in ongoing conflict, or are unable to manage single parenting with social and work demands, the child is left without affection and the support needed to negotiate the many changes associated with divorce (Hetherington, 1999).

Children also benefit from positive relationships with both parents and knowing that their parents have found a way to get along. However, when parents are embroiled in anger toward their former spouse, ask children to deliver hostile messages, or talk badly about the other parent in front of the child, profound stress and loyalty conflicts, and long-term ramifications occur. In one study, young adults whose parents had low conflict after divorce were less depressed and had fewer emotional symptoms than those who experienced high levels of parental conflict (Zill, Morrison, & Coiro, 1993).

Economic and Social Issues

Divorce often contributes to financial struggles or intensifies challenges that already existed in the family. Custodial parents may have to work longer hours, resulting in less contact, increased stress, and greater responsibilities for children at home. In addition, financial restraints may make it impossible for children to participate in sports, lessons, and organizations that give pleasure. In some cases, families may be forced to move, creating a series of additional changes and disruptions. Relocation may interfere with relationships between children and the noncustodial parent and extended family, and may take them away from friendships. At a time when children need supportive relationships most, they are forced to adjust to a new neighborhood, new school, and numerous changes and losses. Still another loss/adjustment occurs when parents date, cohabitate, and remarry. Children may experience confusion, loneliness and isolation, and anger. This situation commonly stirs family conflict, which can further complicate children's adjustment.

Functioning Prior to Divorce

Children's functioning prior to parental separation, the quality of parenting they received before the breakup, and the amount of conflict and violence they witnessed during the marriage play a significant role in adjustment (Kelly & Emery, 2003). Risk factors including developmental, social, emotional, cognitive, learning, and psychiatric challenges that were present before the breakup will affect the child's adjustment. To best understand the effects of divorce, a thorough assessment must be conducted. Important factors to consider include the child's temperament, pattern of coping with challenges, affect and behavioral regulation, self-perception/esteem, relationships with family and friends, social skills, academic achievement, psychiatric vulnerabilities, and prior history of losses and trauma.

Parent–child relationships prior to the divorce are also important factors to consider. Attachment theory has shown that children who are provided a strong bond with a loving, responsive caretaker develop a secure base, enabling them to cope with losses and separations. Children with a solid sense of self and a feeling of security in their relationships with parents are better able to negotiate the family breakup. It is also important for children to see that the divorce benefits the family, especially with regard to the level of parental conflict. Divorce makes sense, and children benefit most when conflict diminishes and parents become more emotionally available after the breakup.

Rationale for Psychodynamic Play Therapy

A psychodynamic approach to treating children of divorce incorporates psychoanalytic theories of child development, including the work of Erik Erikson, Anna Freud, Margaret Mahler, John Bowlby, and Mary Ainsworth. Like other forms of therapy, the immediate goal of treatment is to alleviate emotional, behavioral, and adjustment-related issues and to help children return to their former level of functioning. However, psychodynamic psychotherapy also aims to address deeper issues, including strengthening ego resources to improve coping, reducing a harsh superego/conscience, mastering developmental challenges, fostering spontaneity and joy, promoting resiliency and resourcefulness, and containing anger, rage, and impulsivity.

In her seminal 25-year longitudinal study, Wallerstein (1983) found that children's adjustment to parental divorce was dependent on their mastery of five essential psychological tasks: understanding the significance of the divorce; disengaging from the crisis and resuming usual activities; coping with related loss, dealing with anger and resolving guilt and self-blame; accepting the permanence of the divorce; and achieving hope regarding future relationships. Given this broad range of issues, treatment requires an in-depth understanding of the whole child and how the circumstances, changes, and challenges of divorce affect their relationships, sense of self, functioning, and adjustment. Play therapists are faced with several simultaneous goals when working with children of divorce. These include helping them understand and resolve feelings, thoughts, and conflicts; helping them return to their developmental track; and providing psychoeducational guidance to parents to help them minimize stressors. This chapter demonstrates the effectiveness of psychodynamically oriented play therapy, along with psychoeducational parent counseling, for meeting these needs.

Step-by-Step Details of the Intervention

The model of psychodynamic play therapy discussed in this chapter entails three overlapping phases of treatment: assessment, treatment, and termination.

Assessment

Treatment begins with an initial intake with parents, without the child present. This session is designed to take a developmental history; gain an understanding of family and social dynamics before and after the divorce; and gain a preliminary understanding of the child's social, emotional, behavioral, and academic functioning, as well as his or her needs, readiness for play therapy, and any possible factors that may impede treatment. In addition, the therapist uses this session to establish an alliance with parents and to assess factors that contribute to the child's presenting problem, such as level of parental conflict.

Following the parent session, the therapist meets with the child for several play assessment sessions. Two are commonly sufficient, but in some cases, additional sessions may be needed. During this time, a therapeutic alliance is established, the needs of the child are further assessed, and a treatment plan is developed. Useful techniques for assessing the inner world of children include D. W. Winnicott's squiggle game (Berger, 1980), the Color-Your-Life technique (O'Connor, 1983), Pounding Away Bad Feelings (Cangelosi, 1997a), the Before and After Drawing technique (Cangelosi, 1997c), as well as use of the sandtray and other drawing or play activities that foster free expression.

A second meeting with parents is then scheduled to discuss recommendations for treatment. Because each child is unique, each treatment will be different, depending on factors such as presenting problems, when the divorce occurred, the amount of change and turmoil brought about by the divorce, and the amount of parental conflict present. In general, children are seen for individual play therapy once a week, and psychoeducational parent counseling sessions are scheduled one to two times per month.

Treatment

Everything that happens in the lives of children of divorce is beyond their control—the decision for parents to break up, the living and custody arrangement, ongoing parental conflict, moving, changing schools, and the many other forced adjustments brought about by the family breakup. In the midst of this whirlwind of change and readjustment, psychodynamic play therapy offers an opportunity for children to play out their feelings in a safe, accepting atmosphere, centered around his or her needs. In this treatment model, children are encouraged to use the session however they wish— building a world in the sandtray, creating with art materials, choosing a game. By following the child's lead, the therapist gains an understanding of the child's feelings, thoughts, conflicts, and needs, as well as his or her coping skills and way of relating. The therapist joins the child by engaging in a play dialogue, asking what he or she should do or say. In this way, the therapist establishes him- or herself as someone who is genuinely interested in the child—someone who is safe and emotionally attuned to the child's inner world. This process enables the therapist to gradually and sensitively intervene in ways that help the child replace problematic defenses, symptoms, thoughts, perceptions, and behaviors with healthy, age-appropriate coping skills. This is achieved by introducing play materials and, when necessary, providing information and/or ego-enhancing ideas or suggestions to improve the child's understanding of his or her feelings, thoughts, or problematic situations. For example, if a child's play reveals anger about having to leave one parent to be with the other, the therapist would point out that the doll is angry about only being with one parent at a time. The therapist would also validate the child's feelings by noting that many kids feel that way. These kinds of ego-supportive interventions support healthy adjustment, strengthen coping skills, and help the child achieve a sense of competence, hopefulness, and mastery.

Termination

Termination is an integral part of psychodynamic play therapy and can affect children's feelings about the entire therapeutic relationship. The sensitive handling of this phase of treatment is particularly important for children of divorce because they endure many losses and separations, which they do not have a say in. Therefore, it is crucial that they have a distinctly different experience when saying goodbye to the therapist. In contrast to being a passive recipient of change and loss, termination provides an opportunity for children to choose how and when therapy ends. A period of several weeks are set aside to prepare for the ending of treatment in a new, emotionally corrective way. During this final phase of treatment, the therapist helps the child integrate and consolidate the lessons and coping skills they learned in treatment and works to empower the child to cope with difficulties that may come up in the future.

Some child analysts adhere to the adult philosophy for termination, where a final break is made at an agreed-upon date. However, this author follows the viewpoint proposed by Anna Freud in which treatment is ended but not the therapeutic relationship (Cangelosi, 1997b). Anna Freud believed that development is a process that determines children's needs, and therefore, children may need to return for treatment at a later date. For this reason, she argued that it is important not to sever the tie to the therapist. She wrote:

> To make an absolute break from a certain date onward merely sets up another separation, and an unnecessary one. If normal progress is achieved, the child will detach himself anyway, in the course of time, just

as children outgrow their nursery school teachers. The analyst can allow this detaching process to occur by reducing the frequency of visits, and often this is suggested by the child. The analyst then becomes a benign figure in the background for the child. The analyst can thereafter be visited and remembered on certain occasions, and should be available for this kind of contact. (in Sandler, Kennedy, & Tyson, 1980, p. 243)

Parent Involvement

After decades of study, researchers have highlighted that divorce is not simply a single event, but rather a process extending over time that involves myriad changes and challenges for children. Decades of empirical research have shown that several specific stressors of the divorce process can increase the risk of psychological difficulties over time. These stressors include inadequate preparation for the initial separation, ongoing parental conflict, loss of the noncustodial parent and/or other important relationships, loss of social and economic opportunities, and changes related to remarriages (Kelly & Emery, 2003). Researchers have further found that reducing these stressors may lessen the risks and struggles associated with parental divorce. With regard to divorce, Amato's (1994) review of research showed that children's adjustment to divorce depends on several key factors: the amount of parental conflict following the divorce, the quality of the child's relationship with the noncustodial parent, the custodial parent's emotional adjustment and parenting skills, and the extent of financial and social stressors affecting the family. For these reasons, involvement with parents is an essential component of psychodynamic psychotherapy.

Case Vignette: Sam

Sam was 8 years old when his mother brought him for counseling. His parents had separated 4 months earlier, after which he had become increasingly anxious, insecure, and clingy. In the weeks prior to the initial intake, he complained of frequent stomachaches and would work himself up so much when separating from his mother that he would hyperventilate. The separation was a contentious one, so Sam's parents chose to meet separately for the initial parent sessions.

Assessment

The therapist first met with Sam's mother, who was very concerned about her son's anxiety. She shared that Sam was an only child who had always been quiet and insightful. He tended to have a hard time talking about feelings but expressed relief when his parents separated because he did not like the fighting. Mom shared that although periodic disagreements with Sam's father had continued since the breakup, they only occurred via phone messages and emails and Sam was not aware of them. She was keenly aware of not wanting the breakup to affect Sam.

Sam's symptoms developed gradually over the months prior to the intake. He had more and more difficulties with transitions when leaving for school, going to after-school activities, and leaving for bimonthly weekend visits with his father. His teacher was informed of his difficulties and was having great success distracting him when he arrived for school, which decreased his anxiety. However, this was not the case with his after-school activities or visits with his father. In these situations, Sam's anxiety would intensify. On several occasions, just before the intake, he refused to go to after-school activities and had to leave his father's apartment just a few hours after arriving for a scheduled visit.

Sam's mother described him as an easygoing child who presented with no behavioral difficulties. He was an excellent student and curious learner, and he preferred quiet activities such as reading, puzzles, and building toys rather than sports. While this kept him apart from more athletic boys at school, he got along with everyone and always managed to find ways to enjoy his free time. Sam lived with his mother in the home where he had grown up. She reported that they had a close relationship, but that Sam had never experienced separation anxiety prior to the marital breakup. Her parents and siblings lived in the same town and visited often. Sam's father also lived locally with his brother, Sam's uncle.

Before meeting with Sam, the therapist also met with his father, Mr. K, who was also concerned about Sam's anxiety. However, he felt that Sam needed to simply adjust to the divorce and cope with being away from his mother. Mr. K shared that his parents had divorced when he was 6 years old and that he did not have any difficulties with the change. He did not understand why Sam was having such a hard time. Nonetheless, he was concerned that Sam's symptoms were interfering with their visits, and he wanted to help his son overcome his difficulties. Although open to therapy, he was not able to reflect about Sam's internal experience of the family breakup.

During the initial session, Sam separated easily from his mother. He presented as a very appealing, though anxious, child who was comfortable meeting with the therapist and eager to receive help. He willingly spoke about his feelings of panic and shared that he gets so upset he stops breathing. The therapist felt that Sam was asking for help and his suffering was so extreme that an intervention was needed to help him regulate and self-soothe. Therefore, she introduced a picture book about stress and anxiety and practiced bubble breathing with him. Sam caught on quickly but remained very serious throughout this fun activity. There was a sadness in his eyes, which became increasingly apparent when he chose to create a sandtray later in this session. He assembled a battlefield of soldiers versus significantly larger aliens. Themes of aggression and extreme pain unfolded. Soldiers were buried and screamed for help. Similar themes were seen in Sam's sandtrays in the following session. This time, Sam shoved an army figure in the sand and shouted that he was drowning and could not breathe. The desperation in Sam's voice was very disturbing to witness and showed the intensity of his panic and sense of powerlessness.

Feedback Session and Recommendations

Sam was immersed in his play during both assessment sessions but was able to shift easily when the session was over. The organization of his play, together with his awareness of his problems, his ability to express his worries, and his responses to interventions were strong indications that he had good ego strength. His initial presentation revealed he felt powerless, was flooded with anxiety, and struggled for a sense of mastery. Sam's interest in play and in creating worlds in the sandtray were strong indications that play therapy was an ideal treatment to help him overcome his difficulties.

During the parent feedback sessions, the therapist recommended weekly play therapy for Sam and bimonthly meetings for each of his parents to help them foster his adjustment. She also recommended that Sam see his pediatrician to rule out any medical reason for his symptoms, particularly his stomachaches, which had become worse over time. The treatment goals set out for Sam were to continue establishing rapport and trust with Sam and his parents; to provide a safe place for Sam to express, understand, and master his sense of powerlessness; to help Sam self-soothe and manage his anxiety; to help Sam's father understand and empathize with Sam's feelings; and to better understand Sam's relationship with his mother and help him cope with separating from her.

Treatment

Throughout the beginning phase of treatment, Sam continued to create battle scenes in the sandtray. Initially, his play was replete with themes of drowning, sinking in quicksand, and being buried. He consistently identified with the figure being defeated and was flooded with a sense of powerlessness and despair. During this phase of therapy, Sam also continued to have difficulty during weekend visits with his father. His panic when separating from his mother had become so intense that he was unable to stay over at his father's house at all. In Session 6, two large monster figures stomped on a soldier, and Sam shouted, "I can't take this! There's no hope now!" As his level of anguish peaked, the therapist pointed to the other miniatures and asked if the soldier needed a backup. Sam rummaged through a pile of figures and eventually found a rather small, but "mighty," robot who proceeded to zap the monsters with his radar capabilities.

In the following sessions, Sam brought several action figures to his sessions and used them, along with the mighty robot, to construct new battles. However, now the encounters were more balanced and fair because each superhero was about the same size and had different, but equal, powers and vulnerabilities. Because of this equality, both sides won and lost, and there was less anguish when defeat occurred. Around this time, Sam had completed a series of medical tests which showed that his stomachaches were not due to a physical problem. With this knowledge, he seemed relieved and more open to discussing why his anxiety about staying at his father's house continued. Using the feeling chart, Sam identified several emotions, including, nervous, angry, and worried. He reported that he had not spent a lot of time with his father prior to the divorce and felt their visits were awkward. His father wanted to go fishing and watch sports on TV, which were activities that did not interest Sam. Eventually, Sam also expressed annoyance that his father did not already know this about him. In an attempt to empower Sam, the therapist asked if he ever made suggestions for fun things to do with his father. He responded that he was afraid to do so because he did not want to hurt his father's feelings or make him mad. Apparently, Mr. K scheduled weekend visits with so many preplanned activities that there was no room for Sam to have a voice about how to spend their time together. Sam's uncle often accompanied them, which made Sam feel outnumbered and uncomfortable expressing his needs. By this point in treatment, Sam often shared these feelings spontaneously. He had become more open to discussing his emotions and experiences and he now looked forward to using therapy to get things off his shoulders. However, despite identifying anger as an emotion associated with visiting dad, he was not yet able to discuss this emotion openly.

In the weeks that followed, battles in the sandtray had come to a halt. Sam brought new toys to his sessions, and themes of competence and mastery followed. He brought Pokémon cards to several sessions and discussed each character's powers as well as things that disempowered them. He brought a maze game and demonstrated an uncanny ability to anticipate moves. Finally, Sam brought elaborate Lego constructions which he had assembled, and the therapist highlighted his patience and problem-solving ability. Sam's overall anxiety, insecurity, and clinginess with his mother had subsided by this time. However, he refused to participate in after-school activities and continued to have stomachaches during weekend visits with his father, which made it impossible for him to sleep over.

At this point in treatment, it was unclear whether Sam actually experienced stomachaches or if he was using them to avoid anxiety-provoking situations. In one session, he told the therapist he did not mind spending days with his father but didn't understand why he had to stay entire weekends. He complained that his father's apartment, which was shared with Sam's uncle, was loud and uncomfortable. Sam felt that weekend visits pulled him away from his life, and he became anxious each time he described his overnight visits. He noted that being in the apartment made him miss his home, and he worried his father would think he was being a baby if he asked to call his mother. Sam further felt that his father didn't understand him and frequently told him to be strong.

It was no surprise why Sam's feelings resulted in so much anxiety, despite his attempts to use the deep breathing and mindfulness activities the play therapist had taught him. Furthermore, it was clear that more work was needed to help Mr. K adjust his parenting style. Sam's stomachaches provided a temporary solution around the unbending nature of their visits, which gave him a reason not to stay over and provided a break from his sense of helplessness. While this was clearly not the most desirable coping mechanism, it significantly reduced Sam's internal suffering and level of anxiety. Using the defense of avoidance was helping his ego to cope better, and he became lighter and more interested in age-appropriate activities. In his discussions with the therapist, Sam became aware that this was just a temporary solution. Treatment focused on helping him recognize when this defense surfaced in order to prevent it from being overused and to replace it with more proactive behaviors. Stress was placed on exploring healthy ways to deal with problems and uncomfortable feelings. Simultaneously, parent counseling with Mr. K focused on listening to Sam's desire for shorter visits in order to decrease his sense of powerlessness and improve the father–son relationship.

Six months into treatment, Sam's interests and confidence increased, and he was more open to trying new things. Among these was his willingness to try swimming lessons and to join a board game club after school. He made a friend who shared his interest in building, and together they attended an after-school Lego class together. Sam continued to use his sessions to get things off his shoulders, but there was significantly less anxiety and turmoil in his play and conversation. He walked and talked more confidently and typically chose competitive games such as checkers and chess. Interestingly, Sam was comfortable not only teaching the therapist new strategies but winning, which he often did by a landslide. However, this was done in a lighthearted, nonboasting way.

When summer approached, Sam decided to attend a Lego camp with his friend, and his mother reported that he wanted to come to sessions every other week. The therapist used this opportunity to let Sam know that therapy was his place where he could express anything he needed. She hoped this would provide an emotionally correcting experience given Sam's history of not feeling heard by his father. The therapist also hoped to reinforce Sam's use of assertiveness rather than retreat and avoidance. Sam continued bimonthly sessions for an additional 7 months. During this time, less and less anxiety was noted. He had settled into a comfortable visiting pattern with his dad, which included a short dinner during the week and one long day together every weekend. In addition, Sam's father had purchased a video game system that became a mutually enjoyable activity for them to share. As the months passed, Sam became so busy and symptom free that he decided to stop treatment. However, he did not want to stop forever and requested to return if needed.

During the termination phase, the therapist encouraged Sam to make a list of the many things he accomplished during treatment. In each of the three last sessions, Sam added to the list, which ultimately included 33 items. The therapist's favorite was number 8, "I can breathe!" She gave Sam a bottle filled with sand from the sandtray as a goodbye gift (an idea that she heard about from her colleague, Robin Bottino) to remember the work he had done in therapy and, more importantly, his personal power. Approximately 18 months after treatment ended, Sam returned for several sessions to process his father's upcoming wedding. He showed no signs of anxiety, had a closer relationship with his father, and had internalized a sense of competence and confidence. Sam was involved in several after-school activities and made several like-minded friends.

Work with Parents

The therapist initially met with Sam's mother two times per month to help her empower Sam to separate more easily. She was very responsive and consistently went out of her way to help him branch out and gain a sense of comfort, confidence, and autonomy. After several months, these meetings took place less often and were used mainly to exchange information and help her understand her son's needs.

The therapist's work with Sam's father involved two monthly consultations throughout the treatment. Despite having an authoritarian parenting style, he was very motivated to be close to his son. Over time, he was able to see that they had different personalities, interests, and ways of coping. Although he did not fully understand Sam's feelings, he was able to see that not making adjustments with the visitation plan would ultimately distance them further. It took many sessions, but this awareness enabled him to change to an arrangement consisting of shorter, more frequent visits with Sam, which ultimately gave them more quality time together. Sam's mother saw the benefits of this arrangement and willingly cooperated. Over time,

Sam spent more time with his father because their relationship had become more comfortable. Although he did spend entire weekends at his father's apartment, Sam and his father, as well as his mother, were happy with the agreed-upon arrangement.

Empirical Support for Psychodynamic Psychotherapy

Empirical research shows increasing evidence that demonstrates the effectiveness of psychodynamic psychotherapy for treating both adult and child populations. Shedler's (2010) landmark publication entitled "The Efficacy of Psychodynamic Psychotherapy" showed evidence from a variety of randomized controlled studies that effect sizes for psychodynamic therapy are as large as those reported for other forms of therapy that have been endorsed as "empirically supported" and "evidence based." In addition, Shedler found that patients who receive psychodynamic therapy not only maintain therapeutic gains but often continue to improve after treatment ends.

In her review of 59 studies, Gaskin (2012) found strong support for the use of psychodynamic psychotherapy for treating a wide variety of presenting problems, including depressive disorders, somatic symptoms and some anxiety, and somatoform and personality disorders. In addition, a smaller number of studies showed that psychodynamic psychotherapy is an effective approach for treating eating disorders, posttraumatic stress disorder, and some substance-related disorders. Gaskin noted that meta-analysts and researchers have reported medium, large, and very large (exceeding two standard deviations) effect sizes for improvement on primary outcome measures and that these improvements remain beyond the termination of therapy.

A number of studies have demonstrated that psychodynamic therapy is an effective treatment for children as well. Fonagy and Target (1996) systematically reviewed 763 records at the Hampstead Clinic and found significant improvement in children's levels of anxiety and depression. Children treated for conduct problems with once or twice per week psychodynamic psychotherapy responded less well but improved with greater frequency of sessions. Furthermore, in their review of a vast number of research studies, Midgley and Kennedy (2011) found that when direct comparisons were made, psychodynamic treatment of children and adolescents appeared to be equally effective as comparison treatments. Children with a variety of emotional and behavioral difficulties showed significant improvement with both internalizing and externalizing problems when provided with psychodynamic play therapy. Most impressively, they found that psychodynamic treatment may have a different pattern of effect compared to other treatments. For instance, depressed children who received family therapy improved more quickly, while improvements for those receiving individual psychodynamic therapy were slower but more sustained, with some children continuing to improve beyond the termination of treatment. Thus, in contrast to therapies that bring about quicker changes, psychodynamic psychotherapy has been found to have a "sleeper effect," benefiting children after treatment has ended. In addition, Midgley and Kennedy's review showed that when age groups are compared, younger children benefit more than older ones. In general, children with emotional or internalizing disorders seem to respond better than individuals with behavioral/externalizing disorders.

Conclusion

Parental divorce brings about countless changes and losses in children's lives. Effective treatment must address a wide variety of social, emotional, and developmental issues, while simultaneously focusing on family dynamics that can hinder adjustment. Given the unique, multifaceted needs of these children, psychodynamic play therapy combined with parent counseling is an ideal modality of treatment.

This approach addresses psychological functioning beyond observable behavior, which is crucial when working with children of divorce who often conceal or disguise their internal pain to avoid worrying (or burdening) their parents. For some children of divorce, the therapy session is the only time when their needs come first and their deepest emotions are acknowledged. Most importantly, the psychodynamic play therapist does not tell them how to think, feel, or readjust, but instead shows patience and respect and empowers them to gain a sense of mastery.

Psychodynamic play therapy allows children to express their emotional struggles and perceptions of the family breakup in a disguised, nonthreatening way. Using the metaphor of play allows the therapist to respond in a sensitive, ego-enhancing manner so that a sense of empowerment can be achieved and healing can take place. In addition, the therapist's understanding of the child's inner world and background in child development can be extremely helpful when counseling parents. Psychodynamic play therapists are in an ideal position to translate the child's inner struggles and developmental needs to parents to help them understand how to foster their child's adjustment.

Empirical studies have shown that adults and children who receive psychodynamic psychotherapy not only maintain therapeutic gains, but also continue to improve after treatment ends. This is of great importance for children of divorce who, in many cases, are faced with long-term stressors stemming from the breakup of the family unit. Integrating psychodynamic principles with play therapy further serves to restore hope, joy, and a sense of personal well-being.

REFERENCES

Amato, P. R. (1994). Life-span adjustment of children to their parents' divorce. *The Future of Children, 4*(1), 143–164.

Amato, P. R., & Anthony, C. J. (2014). Estimating the effects of divorce and death with fixed effects models. *Journal of Marriage and Family, 76*(2), 370–384.

Anderson, J. (2014). The impact of family structure on the health of children: Effects of divorce. *The Linacre Quarterly, 81*(4), 378–387.

Berger, L. R. (1980). The Winnicott squiggle game: A vehicle for communicating with school-aged children. *Pediatrics, 66*(6), 921–924.

Cangelosi, D. (1997a). Pounding away bad feelings. In H. G. Kaduson & C. E. Schaefer (Eds.), *101 favorite play therapy techniques* (pp. 142–144). Northvale, NJ: Jason Aronson.

Cangelosi, D. (1997b). *Saying goodbye in child psychotherapy: Planned, unplanned and premature endings.* Northvale, NJ: Jason Aronson.

Cangelosi, D. (1997c). The Before and After Drawing technique. In H. G. Kaduson & C. E. Schaefer (Eds.), *101 favorite play therapy techniques* (pp. 55–58). Northvale, NJ: Jason Aronson.

Dong, M., Anda, R. F., Felitti, V. J., Dube, S. R., Williamson, D. F., Thompson, T. J., et al. (2004). The interrelatedness of multiple forms of childhood abuse, neglect, and household dysfunction. *Child Abuse and Neglect, 28*(7), 771–784.

Emery, R. E. (1999). *Marriage, divorce, and children's adjustment* (Vol. 14). Thousand Oaks, CA: SAGE.

Erikson, E. H. (1963). *Childhood and society.* New York: Norton.

Fagan, P. F., & Churchill, A. (2012). The effects of divorce on children. *Marriage and Religion Institute, 12,* 1–48.

Fonagy, P., & Target, M. (1996). Prediction of outcome in child psychoanalysis: A retrospective study of 763 cases at the Anna Freud Centre. *Journal of the American Psychoanalytic Association, 44*(1), 27–77.

Gaskin, C. (2012). *The effectiveness of psychodynamic psychotherapy: A systematic review of recent international and Australian research.* Melbourne: Psychotherapy and Counseling Federation of Australia.

Hetherington, E. M., & Kelly, J. (2002). *For better or worse: Divorce reconsidered.* New York: Norton.

Hetherington, E. M., & Stanley-Hagan, M. (1999). The adjustment of children with divorced parents: A risk and resiliency perspective. *Journal of Child Psychology and Psychiatry and Allied Disciplines, 40*(1), 129–140.

Jordan, P. H. (2016). Individual therapy with a child of divorced parents. *Journal of Clinical Psychology, 72*(5), 430–443.

Kelly, J. B. (2012). Risk and protective factors associated with child adolescent adjustment following separation and divorce. In K. Kuehule & E. L. Drozd (Eds.), *Parenting plan evaluations: Applied research for the family court* (pp. 49–84). New York: Oxford University Press.

Kelly, J. B., & Emery, R. E. (2003). Children's adjustment following divorce: Risk and resilience perspectives. *Family Relations, 52*(4), 352–362.

Lamb, M. E. (2012). Mothers, fathers, families, and circumstances: Factors affecting children's adjustment. *Applied Developmental Science, 16*(2), 98–111.

Midgley, N., & Kennedy, E. (2011). Psychodynamic psychotherapy for children and adolescents: A critical review of evidence base. *Journal of Child Psychotherapy, 37*(3), 232–260.

O'Connor, K. (1983). Color-your-life technique. In C. Schaefer & K. O'Connor (Eds.), *Handbook of play therapy* (pp. 251–258). New York: Wiley.

Oliver, W. J., Kuhns, L. R., & Pomeranz, E. S. (2006). Family structure and child abuse. *Clinical Pediatrics, 45*(2), 111–118.

Sandler, J., Kennedy, H., & Tyson, R. L. (1980). *The technique of child psychoanalysis: Discussions with Anna Freud.* Cambridge, MA: Harvard University Press.

Shedler, J. (2010). The efficacy of psychodynamic psychotherapy. *American Psychologist, 65*(2), 98.

Wallerstein, J. S. (1983). Children of divorce: The psychological tasks of the child. *American Journal of Orthopsychiatry, 53*(2), 230–243.

Wallerstein, J. S., & Kelly, J. B. (1980). *Surviving the breakup: How children and parents cope with divorce.* New York: Basic Books.

Wilcox, W. B. (2009). The evolution of divorce. Retrieved from *http://ohiofamilyrights.com/Reports/Reports/Special-Reports-Page-4/The-Evolution-of-Divorce.pdf.*

Zill, N., Morrison, D. R., & Coiro, M. J. (1993). Long-term effects of parental divorce on parent–child relationships, adjustment, and achievement in young adulthood. *Journal of Family Psychology, 7*(1), 91–103.

CHAPTER 9

Play Therapy for Children Who Have Been Sexually Abused

Eliana Gil
Quinn Koelfgen Smelser

Description of the Problem

In the last two decades, a great deal of research and clinical work has focused on children who are sexually abused by family members or other caretakers as well as older children or people in positions of authority in children's lives. There appears to be a consensus on the major effects of childhood sexual abuse and the long-term consequences of untreated early trauma. In fact, the Adverse Childhood Experiences (ACE) study has revolutionized the way many people think about the dangers inherent in allowing sexual abuse to go unrecognized, unreported, or untreated in children's lives (Felitti et al., 1998). The findings consistently point to what the National Child Traumatic Stress Network (NCTSN) proposes as typical target areas that are most affected by these adverse childhood experiences (NCTSN, 2012). Those target areas include behavioral and emotional dysregulation; depression; dissociation; biological and cognitive issues; attachment; and self-esteem. Of course, these are merely symptoms of a variety of emotional conditions manifested in many ways (NCTSN, 2012). Studies find that most abused children have varying degrees of fear and anxiety, anger, sadness, and identity confusion or lowered self-esteem. In addition, many sexually abused children experience the events as traumatic, that is, non-normative events that produce an overwhelming sense of helplessness and loss of control, and they may struggle with long-term somatic, psychological, sensory, neurological, psychiatric, and medical challenges (van der Kolk, 2014). van der Kolk (2005) states that dissociating is the greatest predictor of the development of posttraumatic stress disorder (PTSD) symptoms in young children. He purports that this diagnosis does not fully function for abused/traumatized children and suggests developmental trauma disorder in its place.

There is little consensus among researchers and clinicians, however, about how to treat the issues associated with child sexual abuse. Lanktree and Briere (2016) may have a powerful and innovative proposal based on their work with high-risk children in the past decade. They suggest that clinical focus be placed on assessment and that subsequent assessment findings guide the treatment approach. Lanktree and Briere (2016) go on to suggest a robust prescriptive approach in which the symptoms are lined up with what the research indicates is the appropriate treatment of choice. Thus, clinicians must be well versed in a variety of approaches and techniques, relying on their clinical judgment as well as some hard assessment data to reach conclusions about how to present and promote treatment.

Another layer of significant work includes clinical attention to the work of Bruce Perry (2006) and his neurosequential model of therapy (NMT). He suggests that many techniques are inherently effective treatment tools; however, they must be offered based on what part of the child's brain is over- or underdeveloped and in need of stimulation (Perry, 2006; Perry & Dobson, 2013). So, most clinicians favor individualized treatment plans, based on the needs of specific children and their families instead of manualized protocols that are delivered to all children whose families seek out treatment.

In the play therapy field, a schism emerged between the child-centered and more "directive" therapists. However, most child therapists who specialize in play therapy seem to be moving toward delivering services along a continuum of therapist-led and child-led activities, attending to the theories that underlie those approaches.

Schaefer (2001) has pioneered the use of prescriptive therapy with children and continues to advocate for this approach as consistent with quality service delivery. Instead of privileging the theories or techniques, he suggests that clinicians be conversant enough with the scientific literature to discern which treatment approaches have been found effective with specific problems (Schaefer, 2001). Schaefer and Drewes (2013) wrote a seminal book that requires all clinicians to dig a little deeper and know what play therapy has to offer what children, under what circumstances, and how and why it works, always informed by a good assessment and target problem areas.

Rationale for Prescriptive Play Therapy

Sexually abused children are as diverse as can be and have never really fit into a "profile." Thus, a singular approach to treating all sexually abused children will not follow. Each child and family will have unique experiences, needs, strengths, and vulnerabilities that can never fit into a "one-size-fits-all" approach. Target areas help us to assess for specific clusters of problems, systemic and contextual issues, family strengths and vulnerabilities, and children's individual learning styles, internal and external resources, or what is commonly understood as resiliency.

A prescriptive approach allows for this matching of child/family and specific vulnerabilities to treatment approaches based on goal-setting. Thus, this particular problem with all its layers of complexity requires a tapestry of carefully selected interventions.

Step-by-Step Details of the Intervention

As mentioned above, because sexual abuse occurs in a family system (whether or not the abuse itself occurs by a family member), the whole family is often traumatized, and individual reactions can be initially self-serving and less than useful to children. Parents, for example, may feel guilty, be ashamed and angry at their child's disclosure, and may express disbelief or disappointment that they were not informed sooner. Although this response is understandable, it often ends up creating more difficulties for children who need as much comfort and support as they can get, especially when they get up the nerve to tell a trusted family member.

After an initial intake with parents or caregivers, in order to both learn about the situation and how it came to light, parents are given specific coaching on what to say or do with the child who has disclosed abuse, as well as how to handle the situation with other children and extended family members. When cases involve extended family members, more confusion and uncertainty can come into play. When the abusers are trusted family friends, who were befriended or entrusted with their children's care, the level of responses becomes multilayered. Parents will need very specific coaching and will require additional services for their own processing of the abuse.

Sexually abused children are initially seen alone. At the Gil Institute for Trauma Recovery and Education (GITRE), children are often self-conscious in the presence of parents or siblings and may check them constantly for their own emotional reactions. There have been many children who try to cheer up their parents or try to recant their stories once they see their parents unhappy or scared.

The initial sessions with children are assessment-based, trust-building, and supportive. A combination of child-centered approaches along with parental information-sharing is very important at the outset, so that children know that it's okay to "show or tell" their thoughts and feelings about the abuse and the abuser. This is often done by clinicians verbalizing to child clients what they know from what the parent shared and telling the child that the clinician works with children who have been inappropriately touched or with children who have had something happen to them that was confusing or difficult. This genuineness with the child aids in beginning a therapeutic relationship built on unconditional positive regard, congruence, and trust. Building trust is part of all good therapy. When working with abused children, building trust is imperative, as broken trust is inherent in child maltreatment and building it with the therapist sets the foundation for all things to follow. Building trust requires the therapist to be attuned, patient, and emotionally present, willing to be tested and challenged at every turn, or able to tolerate being ignored or painfully avoided.

Over time, clinicians watch as children either play out their abuse or find a way to "show" what they are unable to speak. They may also blurt out their truths without apparent provocation or suggestion. They may tease the clinician with feigned interest in specific topics, or they may ask the therapist to help them do some of the work they know is needed in the forms of talking, expressive arts, or play activities. In any case, the clinical posture is to let the child lead the way and/or find a way to gradually introduce difficult material.

Just as there are consensus areas in terms of target treatment areas, there is agreement that sexual abuse treatment always includes attention to three major areas: building trust and establishing safety, addressing the traumatic memories directly, and helping the child with coping strategies so that children can continue to manage whatever trauma-associated problems surface as they get older. Most clinicians who specialize in this area recognize that children process the traumatic memories at their own developmental level and may return to reorganizing and integrating material differently as they mature. Thus, a 4-year-old who is sexually abused may feel confused or scared and may have sensory experiences of pain and/or pleasure. However, when this child turns 11 or 12, there may be a cognitive reevaluation of what that early experience was. The child may now realize that what happened was unique, and he or she might feel concurrent embarrassment or shame. He or she may also realize that what occurred was something sexual and not simply an innocent game. The child might recognize that he or she did not have control and was manipulated. All these insights can occur because the child's perceptual and cognitive abilities have grown according to their developmental level.

Parent Involvement

Levels of parental involvement vary greatly among professionals who work with sexually abused children, but at a minimum, psychoeducation seems to remain in the forefront. Most of the time, clinicians must provide information to parents about what to expect in their child, how to respond to them, how to manage the feelings/thoughts they are having, and what resources are available. There are tons of nagging questions about why children didn't tell sooner, why parents couldn't somehow detect there was a problem, concerns about children's behaviors, their adult sexuality, and so on. The clinician must meet these questions with great compassion, for they often come from a place of intense fear and/or guilt that the parent might now hold.

While therapists encourage psychoeducation, they are also keenly aware that often parents have their own histories of physical and sexual abuse and idiosyncratic ways of coping with difficult emotions; family bonds may be tested during these challenging situations. Thus, we encourage parents to participate in group therapy with other parents of abused children, and we suggest individual therapy to address the impact of abuse on themselves and other members of the family. Nonabused children are often neglected and must be included in some form of psychoeducation or treatment.

Case Vignette: Tony

Tony was brought to therapy by highly anxious parents who noticed a variety of changes in their 7-year-old immediately after he started school. They said that Tony used to be their "happy, outgoing, obedient" child, quite the contrast to his 4-year-old sister, Ana, who seemed demanding and cranky all the time. Tony's father, Mark, stated that he was with his son in the hammock reading him a book when Mark asked if it was okay for someone to "kiss his pee pee." Mark was quite startled by his son's question and sat up abruptly, asking "What are you talking about Tony?" Mark regretted that he reacted so poorly because he thinks that his reaction might have caused Tony to shut down and not want to talk to him anymore. Mark then said that he took Tony inside by the hand and told him to repeat what he had asked to his mother. At that point, Tony clung to his mother and cried.

Tony's mother, Linda, said that she comforted him and sat him on her lap on the rocking chair, as they had a habit to do before he went to sleep each night. She explained that Daddy wasn't angry, just worried. Tony kept repeating that Dad was "mad" and that he was "in trouble." By then, his father had whispered what Tony had said to him, and his mother gently began to reassure her son. Eventually, Tony was able to say that "someone" had touched his penis and had kissed it. Tony said that he didn't like it and told him to stop, but he wouldn't. He would not say who had done this, but he seemed very distressed and embarrassed to talk to his mother. In addition, he was worried about his father being angry at him. So, before Linda went to sleep, she encouraged Mark to go in and talk to his son and let him know that rather than being mad at him, he was proud that he had talked to his parents.

Following this disclosure, they noticed that Tony was clingy, unable to sleep through the night, and had developed the habit of biting his nails and pulling his hair—so much so, his mother confided, that he had started a small bald spot on his head. And there was one last disturbing fact: Mark had walked into the bathroom to find Tony putting a rubber band around his penis. Mark said that it looked "tight and painful," and he took it off, telling Tony not to do that again. This time, he hugged Tony first before correcting his behavior.

The play therapist talked to the parents about meeting with Tony individually to get to know him a little and to see if the play therapist could figure out what was on his mind. They told the play therapist that Tony was usually pretty self-confident and should be able to meet and come into the session alone. The play therapist told them that they could come in if that arrangement was more comfortable for Tony, but they should find a way to leave when Tony looked okay to them. The therapist also told his parents to tell Tony that he would be meeting with a play therapist who works with children, and that many of the children the therapist works with have had problems with being touched in their private parts. Linda and Mark shared with Tony what a therapist was, but they neglected to say that this therapist worked with sexually abused children. When the play therapist asked Tony, he seemed to know about counseling. The play therapist added that therapists at this office worked with many children who had been touched on their private parts. Tony seemed stunned when the play therapist said that. The therapist added that at some point, he could say or show whatever he wished about what had happened to him, since his parents know that it was on his mind. However, the play therapist emphasized that the therapist's first job was to get to know him a little and make sure he felt comfortable.

As the play therapist showed Tony around the play therapy office, Tony seemed cautious but curious. He asked if he could draw or paint with the paints set up at the easel. He drew the shape of a tear drop and painted the inside with various dark colors that eventually turned into a muddy brown. The play therapist noted how carefully he stayed within the shape he had drawn and how central it was on the page. The play therapist didn't interrupt his painting, and Tony seemed quite invested in what he was doing. At times, he would stop and look around the office without moving from his position in front of the easel. The play therapist sat to one side and was in his peripheral view. Tony asked a few questions, one of which seemed particularly important: "Do you ever see boys like me?" The play therapist responded that she sees "lots of boys your age." "Yeah, but, are they like me?" The play therapist said, "I'm not sure what you're asking. Like you in that someone has touched your private parts, or like you in that you like to paint, or like you in that you speak Spanish and English?" He responded, "the touching part." The play therapist reassured him that many boys his age who had someone touch them on their private parts came to this office. The play therapist added: "You can say or show as much or as little as you want about how you think or feel about the touching, any time you want." When he left the office he said quietly, "maybe next time." The play therapist said "Sure."

Tony wanted to leave his painting in the office, and he seemed to melt into his mother's arms when he returned to her in the waiting room. As he was leaving with his mom, the play therapist told them both that Tony had done a good job finding something he liked to do and that the play therapist worked with lots of other children who have had someone touch their private parts. Mom thanked her and they left. Tony's mom called midweek to say that Tony was asking daily when he could come to the play therapy office again.

Working with sexually abused children is unpredictable. There are so many defensive strategies that can be at play: Some children find it necessary to blurt things out almost immediately, and other children avoid the topic fiercely. In treating the children who blurt things out (and this includes telling stories, playing out themes, drawing pictures, etc.), it's best to follow their lead as they seem to make a gradual release of the secrets they have carried. With those who avoid, we eventually start "tickling the defenses" and encourage their willingness to face the difficult feelings and/ or thoughts that they find unbearable (Gil, 2010). Still others find that play is their first language, the language of trauma release, and they are able to show what has happened to them using miniatures. The task of the assessment is to understand each child's unique defensive strategies and to understand the kind of impact the abusive experiences have had, starting with how the events were perceived, what meaning the child has made of them, and how the child is coping with what's occurred. Many sexually abused children carry some guilt about doing or not doing something. In addition to assessing the negative impact of abuse, clinicians are encouraged to look for positive and resilient signs of how children have coped and how they have tried to help themselves.

Over the next 10 sessions, Tony developed comfort and trust. As his parents shared, he seemed eager to come to see the play therapist. In therapy, he had developed predictable routines. The one issue that seemed constant in Tony's behaviors in the clinical setting and in interactions with others as reported by his parents was his fear and anxiety. It appeared that Tony was frightened that something bad was going to come of his telling that he had been touched. So, he held on to the abuser's identity carefully. One of the ways Tony manifested anxiety was an increased sense of needing control in his various settings. Thus, in his new school, he had asked to sit in the front row, next to his friend Daman. He also pushed his mom to get him to school early, and on every dropoff he reminded his mom to be on time picking him up. In the play therapy office, he always started with drawing, moved to a board game, and then spent some time in the sandtray. He always asked how many minutes he had left and seemed to organize his time very well. At the same time, he never appeared relaxed. He was always a little on edge. In fact, he had a heightened startle response, and, as workmen hammered next door, he started to count the number of hammer hits or the seconds between hammering noises.

Because of his high anxiety, the play therapist developed a plan that included introducing cognitive-behavioral techniques, long recognized as an effective method for reducing anxiety (Sawyer & Nunez, 2014). The first step was to meet with Tony and his parents to share the assessment and what the treatment plan would be. Tony listened quietly as the play therapist told his parents that it was a joy getting to know Tony better. The play therapist shared that Tony was a worrier and that worrying all the time could begin to feel heavy and uncomfortable. The play therapist shared a book with them called *The Huge Bag of Worries* about a little girl who has a worry and it keeps getting bigger and bigger, so big in fact, that the girl found it impossible to carry it all by herself. The play therapist told the parents that she and Tony would be working on "shrinking his worry" and that she would be asking him to share what he learned with them, and to practice some of the worry-busting ideas they learned in therapy at home. Tony asked if he and the therapist would still get to play, and the play therapist told him, "Yes, half the time you can decide what you want to do, and half the time I will bring an idea or activity designed to work on the worry problem." "Half and half?" he asked. The play therapist reassured him and told him he could decide each time whether to do the play time or the worry work time first. He seemed satisfied, and so did his parents.

Tony's treatment goals for his worry problem included helping him to become less uneasy when he went to bed at night, to increase the number of hours he slept, and to express his specific worries as a way of beginning to shrink them. The play therapist mentioned to the parents that from time to time they would be asked to join the session for family therapy as well since they would need to know specific ways to help Tony with his worries. In this first session, as homework the play therapist asked Tony and his family to mark down the size of the worry problem each day after school and each day as he went to sleep. The sheet of paper had worry faces that started very small and got very large (see Figure 9.1). Tony and his parents were given their own sheets so that they could circle how big the worry problem was, and they were not to show each other what they had circled. When the play therapist first reviewed the sheets, it was clear that the parents seemed to be reading Tony's cues accurately and that the three of them seemed happy that most of their sheets matched.

This task was specific to affect identification and affect modulation. Later, the play therapist would follow up on the concept, so that if they marked a worry feeling at level 5, they would try some interventions to see if the feeling could shrink to level 4½. The parents quickly learned to rock Tony in the chair, give him a massage on his back, or have him draw a picture of his worry feeling, as ways to shrink it a little. They especially loved using Biodots (2001) and seeing what color the worry problem was when it was a 5 and how they could change the color by relaxing, breathing, or reading a book.

During one of the worry problem work times, the play therapist asked Tony to do a family play genogram (Gil, 2016). The play therapist encouraged him to think of "all the important people in his life, both at home and outside." Once the play therapist was sure all the important people who spent time in his life were included, he was asked to pick miniatures to show his thoughts and feelings about everyone, including himself (see Figure 9.2). Tony took this task seriously. He was very purposeful in his choices, often taking quite a bit of time to pick miniatures and sometimes replacing them in favor of something else. In his mind, he was limited to one object (which is not necessarily in the directive for the activity but demonstrated his control issues).

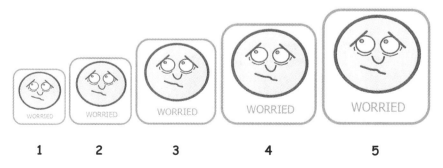

FIGURE 9.1. Affective Scaling Worksheet—Worried. Created by Jennifer Shaw.

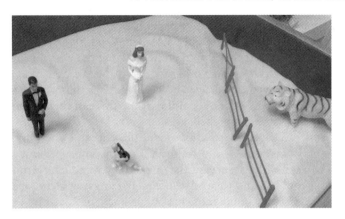

FIGURE 9.2. Family play genogram.

As can be seen in Figure 9.2, there is only one wild animal selected, and an aggressive one at that. It's pointing in the direction of the family. It's also interesting to note that Tony opted to put a fence encapsulating the animal, which suggested his need to keep this figure separate from the others. When the play therapist told him to "say a little about the miniatures he had chosen," he spoke about all of them, except that animal. When the play therapist pointed that out to him, he simply shrugged his shoulders and only said, "That one's name is Miguel." This remained a curiosity, so the play therapist asked the parents about this person and his relationship to Tony. His parents initially described a close and friendly relationship, noting that this was Tony's 10-year-old cousin who had lived nearby "forever" and that they spent many holidays and vacations together. The boys shared a love for soccer and video games, and they spent much time playing and laughing. Tony's father noted, as a postscript, that "now that I think about it, Miguel doesn't come around as much right now and when I've suggested to Tony that he go play at his cousin's house, he's refused . . . nothing big, he just does something else."

It's important to remember that as clinicians, we are not detectives, nor are we investigators of crimes. Especially in cases where a potential abuser has not been named, we as clinicians can sometimes find ourselves suddenly pressured to assume a detective role because we want to protect children from harm, respond to parental anxiety, figure out who harmed them, and bring justice to the situation. Seeking supervision and/or consultation with colleagues can help identify and relieve this countertransference. It's imperative to assert the clinical role and to keep from compromising the therapeutic relationship by taking on the investigative posture. Needless to say, once clinicians do develop a suspicion of child abuse, reporting to Child Protective Services is necessary and required.

Empirical Support for the Intervention

The treatment of choice for anxiety, as well as anxiety related to child sexual abuse, is cognitive-behavioral therapy and trauma-focused cognitive-behavioral therapy (Cohen & Mannarino, 2015). Because of that, the play therapist selected a number of playful cognitive-behavioral techniques that invited Tony to reveal more about the sources of his anxiety. Eventually, Tony was able to state that he was holding a secret about Miguel, on a scale of 11+++++ that he didn't feel comfortable telling anyone. The play therapist told Tony that was fine, that it happened to lots of people, and that in their "work time," they would look a little at secrets. Tony and the play therapist read a book called *Woody and Willy,* a book about a bear and a boy spending time together and getting to know each other. The boy eventually confides that he has been touched inappropriately on his private parts and talks about the difficult feelings he has had as a result. Tony listened very attentively.

After the book reading, the play therapist brought out some art materials and talked about secrets as "layers." On the first piece of construction paper, the play therapist wrote "Secret" and then had Tony select colors, explaining that each one was a wall that kept the secret from getting out. He seemed to enjoy working on a color scheme with the darker colors closer to the secret and the top color as yellow. "Wow, the top color is yellow," the play therapist said, and Tony replied, "Yeah, sunshiny day." Given that they were now engaged in cognitive-behavioral play therapy, the play therapist said, "Seems like the closer to the secret, the darker the colors, and the farther away from the secret, the more sunshiny. Sounds like leaving the secret behind might make for a sunshiny day." Tony was pretty smart and remarked, "Or keeping it buried makes you feel more sunshiny."

The play therapist then told him that they should take a look at all the walls that were keeping this secret buried, and she started to write headings on each page. The headings included: "Things I say to myself about the secret," "How I feel about the secret being buried/brought to the light," "Who might help me move some of these heavy walls," "Ways I can make the walls lighter," and "How many walls do I actually need." Tony added the headings: "Things my friends would say" and "Trouble that would happen if I told." They had laid out their work: to explore his defensive strategies, to try to provide options to his rigid thinking, and finally, to prepare a "construction plan" for removing the heavy walls.

Tony was able to follow this metaphor easily and with great enthusiasm. He brought some new pieces of paper to add that were transparent. The heading was, "If someone could see the secret, what would they see," and finally, "The person most upset if the secret comes out is. . . ." His answer was "Miguel," written in the faintest pencil, barely visible to the eye. The play therapist's clinical intuition had been that Miguel was involved in some way, and finally, Tony felt brave and safe enough to tell his mother that Miguel was the one who had kissed his penis and that it happened "lots of times." The play therapist made a child abuse report to the police, since the abuse had occurred in Miguel's house. Fortunately, this report went to a very experienced and well-trained juvenile officer, who recognized that Tony was in treatment, that his parents had done the right thing to believe him and get help, and that Miguel was still in fact a child, who likely needed help himself. Thus, this case could be viewed from a clinical rather than a criminal lens. Miguel's parents were devastated, but they were willing to get their son help (see Gil & Smelser, Chapter 11, this volume).

Conclusion

Sexual abuse of children is a serious national concern with many long-term consequences (Dube et al., 2005). Children need treatment in order to ameliorate the impact of these experiences, many of which are quite traumatic. In the last few decades, a consensus has emerged on impact areas as well as treatment goals and interventions (van der Kolk, 2005; Perry, 2006; Schaefer & Drewes, 2013). Those interventions are delivered in a variety of ways depending on the clinician's theoretical orientation. However, prescriptive play therapy relies on the research to determine the efficiency and desirability of specific approaches to target symptoms, many of which have been isolated and studied. At the same time, any consideration of treatment of young children must be provided in a reasonable way, taking into consideration their strengths and vulnerabilities in the areas of cognitive and linguistic factors. In addition, the neuroscientific community has provided another lens in which to consider the child's current brain functioning, in order to consider what sequence to provide interventions (Perry, 2006).

The case example in this chapter references an assessment process that allows for the establishment of safety and development of trust, followed by the identification of the target problem area. Once that target area is identified, the research literature is consulted in order to design play therapy interventions that deliver an evidence-based approach. Since the child's symptoms clustered around anxiety in this case example, a trauma-informed cognitive-behavioral approach was selected and provided utilizing play therapy techniques.

Parents and caregivers play a significant role in the health and recovery of their children. As a result, conjoint sessions and homework assignments are selected to share information to all family members and to include non-offending parents/caregivers in the healing process. Parents' follow-through is critical to provide repetition of clinical lessons.

REFERENCES

Biodot International. (2001). *Teacher's guide*. Bedford, IN: Biodot of Indiana.

Cohen, J. A., & Mannarino, A. P. (2015). Trauma-focused cognitive behavioral therapy for traumatized children and families. *Child and Adolescent Psychiatry Clinics of North America, 24*(3), 557–570.

Dube, S. R., Anda, R. F., Whitfield, C. L., Brown, D. W., Felitti, V. J., Dong, M., et al. (2005). Long-term consequences of childhood sexual abuse by gender of victim. *American Journal of Preventive Medicine, 28*(5), 430–438.

Felitti, V. J., Anda, R. F., Nordenberg, D., Williamson, D. F., Spitz, A. M., Edwards, V., et al. (1998). Relationship of childhood abuse and household dysfunction to many of the leading causes of death in adults: The Adverse Childhood Experiences (ACE) Study. *American Journal of Preventive Medicine, 14*(4), 245–258.

Gil, E. (2010). *Working with children to heal interpersonal trauma: The power of play*. New York: Guilford Press.

Gil, E. (2016). *Play in family therapy* (2nd ed.). New York: Guilford Press.

Ironside, V. (1996). *The huge bag of worries*. London: Hodder Children's Books.

Lanktree, C. B., & Briere, J. N. (2016). *Treating complex trauma in children and their families: An integrative approach*. Thousand Oaks, CA: SAGE.

National Child Traumatic Stress Network. (2012). Trauma affect regulation: Guide for education and therapy. Retrieved September 10, 2018, from *www.nctsn.org/interventions/trauma-affect-regulation-guide-education-and-therapy*.

Perry, B. D. (2006) The neurosequential model of therapeutics: Applying principles of neuroscience to clinical work with traumatized and maltreated children. In N. B. Webb (Ed.), *Working with traumatized youth in child welfare* (pp. 27–52). New York: Guilford Press.

Perry, B. D., & Dobson, C. (2013). Application of the neurosequential model (NMT) in maltreated children. In J. Ford & C. Courtois (Eds.), *Treating complex traumatic stress disorders in children and adolescents* (pp. 249–260). New York: Guilford Press.

Sawyer, M. C., & Nunez, D. E. (2014). Cognitive behavioral therapy for anxious children: From evidence to practice. *World Views on Evidence-Based Nursing, 11*(1), 65–71.

Schaefer, C. E. (2001). Prescriptive play therapy. *International Journal of Play Therapy, 10*(2), 57–73.

Schaefer, C. E., & Drewes, A. A. (2013). *The therapeutic powers of play: 20 Core agents of change* (2nd ed.). Hoboken, NJ: Wiley.

van der Kolk, B. A. (2005). Developmental trauma disorder: Toward a rational diagnosis for children with complex trauma histories. *Psychiatric Annals, 35*(5), 401–408.

van der Kolk, B. A. (2014). *The body keeps the score: Brain, mind, and body in the healing of trauma*. New York: Viking Press.

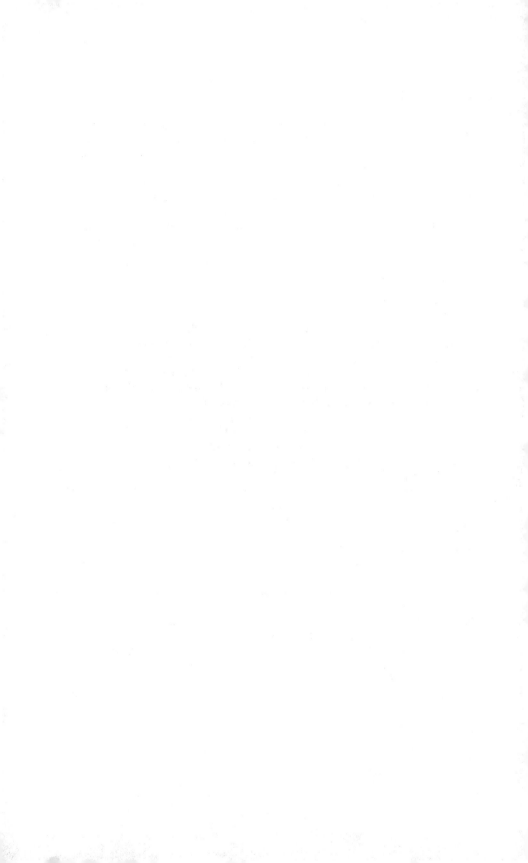

PART IV

Clinical Applications of Prescriptive Play Therapy for Externalizing Disorders

CHAPTER 10

Play Therapy for Children with Attention-Deficit/Hyperactivity Disorder

Heidi Gerard Kaduson

Description of the Disorder

Attention-deficit/hyperactivity disorder (ADHD), one of the most commonly diagnosed neurobehavioral disorders in children, consists of developmental delays or deficiencies in at least two types of neuropsychological abilities. These two dimensions are inattention and hyperactive–impulsive symptoms. The disorder is also classified as neurodevelopmental because the scientific evidence for the substantial role of neurological and genetic causes in ADHD is now overwhelming and irrefutable (Barkley, 2016). ADHD is considered to be neurodevelopmental because it is primarily the result of a delay or lag in specific mental abilities. The deficits are largely due to delays and/or dysfunction in the maturation of the brain areas that underlie those abilities. Barkley (2016, p. 1) states that "such brain maldevelopment seems to arise largely from genetics but can also occur as a consequence of damage or other disruptive influences experienced by the child or teen at any time during development but most often during prenatal brain formation."

Controversy surrounding ADHD, as well as our understanding of the disorder, continues to evolve. Although ADHD was once characterized primarily in terms of overactive and inattentive behavior, and later by marked impulsivity, it can also be described by deficits in executive function (Barkley, 2012) and motivation (Sonuga-Barke, 2005). Challenges with activity level, attention, and impulsivity are viewed as behavioral manifestations of problems in the capacity for self-regulation and corresponding deficits in planning and successfully completing goal-directed activities.

ADHD is one of the most prevalent mental disorders diagnosed in children, affecting about 3–5% of children globally (Frank-Briggs, 2013). A study by the Centers for Disease Control and Prevention (2011) reported that approximately 11% of U.S. children ages 4–17 (6.4 million) have received a medical diagnosis of ADHD. This constitutes an increase from 7.8% in 2003 and has raised concerns about the overdiagnosis and overmedication of children by some medical practitioners (Schwarz & Cohen, 2013). Although psychostimulants continue to be the most dominant treatment implemented, the use of medication for ADHD actually decreased from 15% of visits (to the pediatrician or psychiatrist) in 2003 to 6% in 2010, and the management of ADHD in the community has shifted away from pediatricians to psychiatrists.

Behaviorally, the symptoms of ADHD are dimensional because they reflect the extreme end of a continuum of normal or typical human ability in inattention and hyperactive–impulsive symptoms. The fifth edition of the American Psychiatric Association's (2013) *Diagnostic and Statistical Manual of Mental Disorders* (DSM-5) provides a consistent set of criteria used to confer a diagnosis of ADHD. The diagnosis requires that the symptoms must occur often for over 6 months and to a degree that is excessive for their age. It includes six or more of the following summarized symptoms in inattention and/or hyperactivity and impulsivity to be present.

Inattention can include failure to give close attention to details, leading to careless mistakes; difficulty sustaining attention in tasks or play activities; frequent failure to listen when spoken to directly, to follow through on instructions, and to finish schoolwork, chores, etc.; difficulty in organizing tasks and activities (e.g., difficulty in managing sequential tasks and in keeping materials in order; being messy and disorganized); avoidance, dislike, or reluctance to engage in tasks that require sustained mental effort; repeated loss of things necessary for tasks or activities; tendency to be easily distracted by extraneous stimuli; and, often, forgetfulness in daily activities.

Hyperactivity and impulsivity can include the child's frequent tendency to fidget with or tap hands or feet or squirm in his or her seat; leave his or her seat in situations when remaining seated is expected; run about or climb in situations at inappropriate times; be unable to play or engage in leisure activities quietly; be "on the go," acting as if "driven by a motor"; talk excessively; blurt out an answer before a question has been completed; find it difficult to wait his or her turn; and interrupt or intrude on others. Additionally, symptoms need to have been present prior to age 12; are present in two or more settings; and interfere with or reduce the quality of functioning.

As can be seen, the constellation of symptoms that make up ADHD is quite varied, and the presentation can change over time, making it one of the most complex disorders with which to work. Based on the nature of the symptoms, three types of ADHD can be diagnosed applying the DSM-5 criteria: combined presentation, predominantly inattentive presentation, and predominantly hyperactive–impulsive presentation. The symptoms of ADHD affect children's interactions in all areas of their environment and result in an inability to meet situational demands in an age-appropriate way (Imeraj et al., 2013).

Other Treatment Approaches

Treatment for ADHD exists in many different types of approaches. The most common treatments are medication therapy, behavior modification, cognitive training, cognitive-behavioral therapy, and family systems therapy. In addition, over the last 20 years, play therapy has become a viable treatment alternative.

Medication Therapy

Psychostimulant medication, the most common treatment for children with ADHD, is given to more than 600,000 children annually. Numerous studies clearly demonstrate medication-induced, short-term enhancement of the behavioral, academic, and social functioning of the majority of children being treated (Barkley, 2012). Many families, however, report behavior problems resulting in negative interactions during unmedicated after-school hours, as well as side effects (insomnia, loss of appetite, increased anxiety, and exacerbation of tics (Barkley, 2012). Because children may still experience low self-esteem, poor social skills, and depression, other approaches are necessary to supplement the medication. Many researchers now agree that the combination of two treatments is superior to either given in isolation (Pelham & Murphy, 1986; Abdollahian, Mokhber, Balaghi, & Moharrari, 2013).

Behavior Therapy

Cumulative evidence now attests to the effectiveness of behavior therapy treatment for a variety of problematic and nonfunctional behaviors, such as talking out of turn, getting out of one's seat, and off-task behavior (Mash & Barkley, 2003). Common interventions include (1) positive reinforcement and stimulus control (Mischel, 1974); (2) reinforcement of competing responses (Kazdin, 1975); (3) time-out (Forehand & Baumeister, 1976); (4) prompting and fading (Craighead, Kazdin, & Mahoney, 1981); and modeling (Cohen & Przbycien, 1974). The methods of behavior modifi-cation are particularly well suited to achieving these behavioral deficits. Many techniques for this form of treatment can be applied to children with ADHD-related deficits (Barkley, 2016).

Compared with pharmacological approaches, behavior therapy has a number of advantages as a single treatment for children with ADHD (Hersen & Barlow, 1976; O'Leary & O'Leary, 1972). It does not produce the negative side effects often found with pharmaceutical treatment. It also focuses on antecedent and consequence events, which could result in greater understanding of the elicitation and maintenance of problem behav-ior. However, many studies have shown that behavior changes observed during treatment have tended not to persist or do not generalize beyond conditions under which the contingencies have been operative (Kazdin, 1975). Barkley (2016) reiterates that concern, but he recognizes (1) inter-nalized, self-generated behavior; (2) externalized sources of motivation, often artificial, which must be arranged within the context at the point of performance; and (3) compensatory, prosthetic forms of motivation, which must be sustained for long periods. If the external motivation is removed, the behavior will not be further sustained, and the individual will regress to more erratic goal-directed behavior with less ability to sustain actions toward tasks and goals.

Cognitive Approaches

The lack of generalization and maintenance evidenced by the behavioral approach prompted the development of alternative and more cognitively based treatment options. Much of the research was focused on problems associated with children with ADHD (Camp, Bloom, Herbert, & van Doorninck, 1977; Kendall & Finch, 1978; Meichenbaum & Goodman, 1971). Cognitively based techniques, such as self-instruction training and problem-solving skills training, constitute special procedures that may also be useful in maintaining and generalizing behaviors.

There is a growing body of research that is exploring the efficacy of self-instructional programs with children (Wulfert, Block, Santa Ana, Rodriguez, & Colsman, 2002; Meichenbaum, 1977). However, children with ADHD have behaviors, which, to an important extent, are the result of cognitive deficiencies. In the treatment of children with ADHD, cognitive training has more face validity than perhaps any other therapeutic modality.

Cognitive-Behavioral Approaches

With many successful specific treatment approaches in both the cognitive and behavioral therapies, an effort was made to investigate the efficacy of cognitive and behavioral interventions together. Again, the goal was to reduce or eliminate maladaptive, inappropriate behaviors and to establish a more efficient, adaptive mode of response. To accomplish this goal, children need to develop self-control skills and reflective problem-solving strategies. It was thought that this would help in the acquisition and internalization of skills and would provide the child with the means for self-regulation of behavior (Reid, Trout, & Schartz, 2005; Meichenbaum & Asarnow, 1979).

Some researchers have found that traditional cognitive-behavioral programs may be less effective with children who exhibit severe behavior problems (Bugental, Whalen, & Henker, 1977; Sprafkin & Rubenstein, 1982). It is quite common for children with ADHD to not listen, fail to comply with instructions, or be unable to maintain instruction compliance over time (Barkley, 1990). As a therapist attempts to train children to use the methods, ADHD children may become bored and refuse to engage in the treatment. Therefore, to overcome these difficulties, presenting the training in a playful, nonthreatening environment would increase children's participation.

Rationale for Prescriptive Play Therapy

Play therapy has grown over the last 20 years and is used most often as the treatment of choice for children. Play is their language, and within a play therapy session, children are free and open to learning more. Cognitive-behavioral play therapy can incorporate the cognitive and behavioral techniques used but in a fun, nonthreatening format. Because the interventions are interesting and playful, children with ADHD comply and engage in their own treatment.

Over the last 20 years, the efficacy of play therapy with children with ADHD has been reported clinically and empirically, and play therapy is increasingly being recognized as a helpful tool to use for this population (Barzegary & Zamini, 2011; Bratton et al., 2013; Kaduson, 1993; Ray, Schottelkorb, & Tsai, 2007). The therapeutic powers of play, such as facilitating communication, self-regulation, and direct and indirect teaching (Schaefer & Drewes, 2014), can help children with ADHD identify and communicate their problems through play and to participate more fully in treatment. A vital aspect of using play therapy is that the child is *actively engaged, practicing, and developing needed skills* in treatment. Play therapy treatment for children with ADHD focuses on remediation of skill deficits and also allows children to work through any related psychological issues, such as anxiety and poor self-esteem. The play therapist facilitates this psychological work by keeping the child focused on his or her own play, simultaneously working on important issues and skills, without distraction. Another vital aspect of successful intervention is parent education and consultation. This collaborative effort permits more therapeutic engagement to occur directly with the child.

In addition, play therapy allows the therapeutic powers of play to assist in healing psychological difficulties in the context of a caring relationship. Many children who experience years of negative feedback, negative reinforcement, and an inability to meet the reasonable demands of family, friends, and teachers because of such skill deficits, will certainly be affected. Play therapists must be aware not only of the core symptoms of this disorder, but also of the significant secondary impact they have on both the child and family members (Barkley, 2012; Kaduson, 2000). Play therapy gives children a safe place where they are accepted as they are, and it allows them the freedom to learn coping mechanisms and to feel the self-confidence they need.

It has been documented that cognitive-behavioral treatment can result in positive outcomes for children with ADHD (Antshel, Faraone, & Gordon, 2014; Raggi & Chronis, 2006; Harris, Friedlander, Saddler, Frizzelle, & Graham, 2005; Kaduson, 1997b). However, cognitive-behavioral play therapy adds the important aspect of play to the tasks or techniques (Abdollahian et al., 2013; Kaduson, 1997a). Since play has been emphasized as being a necessity in the lives of children in general (Yogman, Garner, Hutchinson, Hirsch-Pasek, & Michnick Golinkoff, 2018; Ginsburg, 2007), it clearly follows that incorporating it into the treatment of children would enhance the outcome.

Play is intrinsically motivating, so that external motivation may not be needed. Children with ADHD have many impulsive behaviors, and they need help to attend and stay on task. Pleasure is inherent in any activity that is playful, which sustains children's attention and can satisfy the inner desire of children (Schaefer, 1993). Additionally, play is about the process and not the goal. With ADHD children focusing on the process, they are open to learn, to problem-solve, and to experience. The pleasure and positive feelings of play allow children with ADHD to experience more positive feelings to counter the negative environment impact of teachers, parents, siblings, and peers telling them to stop, pay attention, and behave (Kaduson, 1997b). Furthermore, play allows children with ADHD to be actively involved in their own treatment through play. Children with ADHD tend not to complete tasks and may go from one activity to another, but during a play period, children are able to stick to a task with the help of the play therapist and to experience a sense of accomplishment. Lastly, play has an "as-if" quality, which means that children's play is carried out as if it was real life. This is extremely beneficial to children with ADHD because they can work through problems, make mistakes, try out solutions, all without the critical eye of others. Play incorporates specific factors (causal agents of change specific to a particular therapeutic approach). These factors are also known as the therapeutic powers of play, and they transcend culture, language, age, and gender (Schaefer, 2004). So it is important for the play therapist to know what theoretical approach would increase the clinical effectiveness of treatment (Prochaska & Marcus, 1995). In addition, the more therapeutic powers of play in one's repertoire, the better able the play therapist will be to eclectically select the one(s) with the best empirical support for treating a particular disorder (Schaefer, 2014). For children with ADHD, the following therapeutic powers are especially important in strengthening the impact of the play interventions.

Step-by-Step Details of the Intervention

Facilitating Communication

Play is the natural language of the child, and it is often the easiest way for children to express difficult thoughts and feelings from either the conscious or unconscious. Perhaps it is for this reason that play enables children with ADHD to communicate thoughts and feelings that they are aware of but cannot express in words directly. In addition, children's play helps to uncover unconscious wishes and conflicts, which may be the underlying reasons for the inappropriate behavior patterns (Kaduson, 1997b). Because the play is "as if" it were real, children with ADHD express themselves freely and open up in any games or techniques created that are fun.

Feeling Word Game (Kaduson, 1997a)

Materials: Eight pieces of copy paper, marker, and a bag of bingo chips. This game is used easily either at the intake session of children with ADHD or after the occurrence of some situation that has not yet been talked about.

   The play therapist can introduce this new game to play with the child. Ask the child for feelings that a 9-year old child would have (if the client is 9 years old; always use the age of the child). As the child lists feelings, the therapist writes them down on separate pieces of paper. The therapist must get the feelings happy, sad, mad, and scared. If the child doesn't spontaneously give, then the therapist must push to get them. It is very rare to have a child supply the word *scared,* so the therapist usually brings up that word so that it is on the table for the game. Generally, feeling words listed by a 9-year-old might be confused, frustrated, worried, or tired, as well as many others. If one of the feeling words is very specific (e.g., excluded), then the therapist can make the second or third story about that. While 4- to 6-year-olds can only play with the four basic feelings (happy, sad, mad, and scared), children 9 years of age and above can work with eight feelings. When all eight feelings are written, the therapist begins the introduction:

   "Suppose I said a story like this: I go to the mall to buy a new toy, park my car, go in and buy the toy, and when I come out, my car is missing. Then I would feel happy to have my toy [putting chips down on that paper], feel mad that I didn't know where my car was parked [putting a larger number of chips to represent intensity on that paper], and maybe I would be happier because I do have the toy (adding chips to the *happy* paper again), and maybe confused [if the child used that as a feeling word] because I didn't know where I parked it. I think that is how I would feel."

As the therapist is placing the chips on the paper, he or she should look at the child to see if both therapist and child are agreeing with the feeling choices before moving on to the next feeling. Most children will nod or tell you another feeling you can have. The therapist then introduces another story for the child about something that has opposite feelings involved, such as "You are playing soccer. You kick three goals, but your team loses." Then the child puts down his or her feelings about that story. The play therapist does not ask why when the child places the chips, but may lead the child and ask "because?" . . . so that the child lets the therapist know what he or she is thinking.

Next it is the child's turn to make up the story, and the child projects his or her issues into the story. The play therapist must put the feelings he or she would suspect the child would have under those conditions (once again making sure to look at the child to make sure there is agreement on what the play therapist is expressing).

Lastly, the play therapist does another story, but this one is almost exactly like an issue that the child is having or had earlier. The story must be somewhat different from what really happened, so that it is not personally recognizable. If the child asks, "Is this story about me?" the play therapist should say, "No, I am making up a story."

In addition to enhancing verbalization of feelings (both conscious and unconscious), direct teaching can be done through other game formats to allow children with ADHD to experience success in maintaining on-task behavior as seen by the next intervention.

Beat the Clock (Kaduson, 1997a)

Materials: Kitchen timer, bingo chips, drawing materials, blocks, and some easy reading books. The child is introduced to the task at hand (building a tower out of blocks, drawing a picture, coloring in stencils, or reading a book). The play therapist begins this technique by saying:

"We are going to play the game Beat the Clock. First I will give you 10 poker chips. Now I am going to give you a piece of paper with a design on it. You must color the design and keep your eyes on the work the entire time. If you look up, distracted by anything around you, you will have to pay me one chip. Each time you get distracted or ask questions or do anything except color the picture, you will give me another chip. We will have three trials, and when you have accumulated 25 chips, then you may pick from the Treasure Box."

On the first trial, the therapist will find the child's baseline ability. Therefore, the therapist uses a second hand on his or her own watch to time the child. When the therapist has to take away the fourth chip, she will tell the child that time is up and that the child has beaten the clock. The length of time the child can attend before taking away the fourth chip is the baseline.

The therapist remains nonintrusive for the first and subsequent trials, except that the therapist does focus on giving a lot of positive reinforcement using words that are usually used against the child (concentrate, attention, focus) in a positive framework ("You are really concentrating," etc.). After several or more sessions of training (depending on the severity of the inattentiveness), the child will increase his or her attention span to 5 minutes per timing. At this point, the therapist will begin to create distractions to make sure that the child is trained enough to do this time span during homework or in a classroom.

Fostering Emotional Wellness

While various forms of therapeutic play help children develop better awareness of and control over distressing feelings, it is most helpful for children with ADHD because of the cathartic effect and positive emotions that they experience while in play therapy. Catharsis involves the release of pent-up negative affect such as anger, which then results in lessening the negative affect. Many children with ADHD have a lot of anger from frustration, feeling incompetent, and from the constant feelings of never doing it correctly. In order to release this anger, another technique that can be used frequently with school-age children and older is the "Splatz."

Splatz (Kaduson, 2015)

Materials: Whiteboard and Egg Splat Balls (Oriental Trading Company). This technique is easily introduced by the play therapist with school-age or older children in the second session of the treatment. The therapist tells the child that it is time to get his or her "mads" out—mad about school, about home, about anything. First, the therapist shows the Egg Splat Balls and describes that they look like eggs, but are rubber, with water inside and a rubber yolk. Then the therapist illustrates how to use the Splat Balls by making an anger statement (e.g., "I hate mean people") and then throwing the Splat Ball against the whiteboard. Children are then encouraged to take a Splat Ball and do the same thing—saying what they hate. Based on the children's throwing ability, the therapist will throw similarly but with slightly more force, illustrating how the ball looks when it hits the whiteboard (looking like a fried egg). Then the child does the same thing, but also must express what makes him or her angry during the throw. Because children with ADHD are corrected much of their daily lives, some will be hesitant to do this if they feel that something might not be correct. The therapist must become silly when throwing, reducing any anxiety the child might have about it. If a child gets stuck and says, "I don't know what I hate" or something similar, the therapist can prompt the child with "What do you hate that your mother [or any other person] does?" That usually opens up the child to feel the freedom of being able to say whatever he or she wants to say. The positive affect created by this release is seen almost immediately. If the Splat Ball breaks and the water goes all over the room, the therapist (while putting paper towels down on the water for safety to avoid slipping) reinforces how that anger is broken apart now, and the child can throw the ball (without the water in it) onto the ceiling so that the "mads" stay here in the playroom and the child can leave without that feeling (this is clearly the therapist's choice since it will stay on the ceiling and sometimes stain the corkboard).

Increasing Personal Strengths

Self-regulation is extremely difficult for children with ADHD. While much research has been done evaluating self-regulation (Reid et al., 2005; Mischel, Shoda, & Rodriguez, 1989), strategies have also been created to help teach self-regulation, usually in school curriculum of preschools (Bodrova & Leong, 2007). However, when it comes to school-age children, the impulsivity can still be a problem, and self-control is difficult for children to understand (Barkley, 1997) unless they can feel what it is like to have self-control. Techniques in play therapy can provide that experience for children. One such technique involves the game Rebound.

Rebound (Mattel)

The therapist can bring the game board to the floor and encourage the child to take some practice slides with the ball-bearing game pieces. It is easy for the therapist to see when children are able to have self-control in this game because they must slow themselves down significantly to get into the target area. During the practice, the therapist will comment and praise whenever self-control is exhibited. This reinforces the appropriate move for the game in order to score points. Every time the game is started, the therapist tells the child to practice so that reinforcement can be consistent, along with having the child feel what it is like to have self-control. The therapist must play this game very well in order to win or lose at will. Then the therapist can keep the game even with the child winning at the end most of the time. This will help the child to practice more and to feel more competent while playing.

Parent Involvement

To facilitate the healing of children, parents must be trained in how to understand and manage their children's behavior and how to be the advocate they need. A multimodal approach also includes education of the parents regarding the facts about the diagnosis and treatment of ADHD. Parent training is conducted on a weekly basis, incorporating medication referrals (when indicated), classroom interventions, teacher consultation, social skills training, as well as the individual play therapy.

Parents need to have the support as well, and with that comes the responsibility of the play therapist to educate parents about what is within the range of normal with regard to certain behaviors. Most healthy children exhibit many of the behaviors listed in DSM-5 at one time or another. Certainly, not all preschoolers have the ability to listen to a story from beginning to end or to finish a drawing they started. That is normal behavior for preschoolers. They have a short attention span and aren't able to stick to a task for long periods of time. Being different isn't ADHD. The same is true about hyperactivity. Young children are generally very energetic and can easily wear their parents out before they get tired themselves. And children can become much more active when they are tired, hungry, anxious, etc. Every child is unique with differences that should not be compared to others and then diagnosed based on what they see. Normalizing what their child can and cannot do will help lower the expectations of the parents, and many times the result is a more reasonable parenting style (Kaduson, 1997b). Therefore, the positive parenting program (Kaduson, 1997b), with modifications if necessary, helps keep the parents involved and enhances the relationship between parent and child.

Empirical Support
for Cognitive-Behavioral Play Therapy

It has been documented that cognitive-behavioral treatment can result in positive outcomes for children with ADHD (Antshel et al., 2014; Raggi & Chronis, 2006; Harris et al., 2005; Kaduson, 1997b). However, cognitive-behavioral play therapy adds the important aspect of play to the tasks or techniques (Abdollahian et al., 2013; Kaduson, 1997b). Since play has been emphasized as being a necessity in the lives of children in general (Yogman et al., 2018; Ginsburg, 2007), it clearly follows that incorporating it into the treatment of children would enhance treatment results.

Case Vignette: Bob

Bob, age 9, was referred for therapy after being diagnosed with ADHD (combined type). He had the core symptoms of ADHD: inattentiveness, hyperactivity, and impulsivity. Since he was athletic, he had been successfully involved with group sports (soccer and basketball), and it was only when he started fourth grade that his symptoms seemed to interfere with functioning.

Cognitive-behavioral therapy had been utilized for Bob's treatment over the last 2 years. However, his participation in it had become a problem. He no longer wanted to see his therapist and was no longer benefiting from treatment. Since Bob had made some progress in the beginning, cognitive-behavioral play therapy was the treatment of choice, for it allowed him to have fun and to practice skills that he had not mastered yet, namely, self-control and anger outbursts. This model provided a framework for Bob's active participation by addressing issues of control, mastery, and responsibility for his own behavior changes (Kaduson, 1997b; Knell, 1993). Using cognitive-behavioral play therapy to enhance verbalization of his feelings and to teach self-control were the goals of treatment based on information that had been gathered from parents and the prior therapist. Most important in the treatment goals was the effort to engage Bob in play to keep him feeling positive and enjoying his treatment. In fact, during his intake, he was amazed that a therapist could have such "cool" toys to play with. Bob began playing with transformers and racing cars as a way of grounding himself in the playroom. When he experienced difficulty attending to whatever he chose to play with, the therapist would contain his play by asking him something about the items he was playing with. When he was playing with the cars, the therapist used some interpretation through the cars as the metaphor, illustrating how some of the other cars could not keep up with the energy of his car (rather than saying the slower cars wanted to play with him but he was too fast). He fully enjoyed this portion of his sessions, and similar metaphors were discussed each week. In addition to his spontaneous play, cognitive-behavioral play therapy techniques were directly introduced. Even when this was done, it was in a game format, and he happily joined and participated.

The first technique presented was the Feeling Word game to teach Bob the interrelationship of thoughts, behaviors, and emotions. Bob was asked what feelings a 9-year-old would have, and it was clear that at first he was not sure. He said that 9-year-olds could feel *happy, mad, frustrated,* and *sad.* Bob was prompted to include *scared* since he did not identify that feeling, and then he added, *confused, bored, and tired.* Through this game, it became clear that Bob had a lot of irrational thinking about his world, including feelings about having to win at sports all the time in order to be considered a good player, doing whatever was asked of him or he would not be loved, and getting A's in school to show how smart he was. Rather than immediately working on his irrational thinking, metaphorical stories were used to illustrate for Bob that modifications in his emotional response and behaviors would be desirable. Bob could easily role-play his parents talking to him, as the play therapist played his role of being the child. Through several role-plays, Bob began to understand that his parents could have perceived some of his behavior differently than he had thought before. Since his parents were doing the parent training, the slow change of their reactions to his behavior could be seen in the play therapy sessions as well.

To enhance his expression of feelings and to allow for his anger to be released, *Splatz* was introduced in the third session. Bob took immediately to this technique and was freely expressing things that he hated (e.g., feeling stupid, never being good enough, feeling that people would wait for him to make mistakes, not understanding what was required of him, always feeling left out). After he broke the first Splatz and the water sprayed all over, he laughed much more and began to open up more each week. He was able to express his need for self-control, and that was illustrated when the game Rebound was brought out. He loved playing it but found it difficult in the beginning. Using the pieces as a metaphor, he was able to put silly comments on each piece as he and the therapist played (e.g., "There goes the slow poke," "Oh, oh, too fast for the scoring zone"). This helped him stay focused on doing what he had to do to win the game over several weeks, and he commented that he felt self-control when he was winning. The therapist used self-talk and self-monitoring (cognitive-behavioral techniques) during the game by saying aloud her own thought process about what she was planning, when she took her turn, and then praising herself for success (Gawrilow, Gollwitzer, & Oettingen, 2011). By the fifth week of treatment, Bob began using these techniques too.

In addition to self-control, Bob had mentioned that he could not stay focused on homework because it was so boring. The therapist introduced the Beat the Clock game and spoke about on-task behavior (Harris et al., 2005). While the game is usually started with a simple drawing to color, Bob wanted to try to do easy math problems while he kept his eyes on his work. By participating in the goal making, Bob was more engaged in making himself successful. Over several sessions, he had increased his on-task behavior baseline of 2 minutes to 6 minutes, and he brought in some of his real homework from school to play the game. This gave him a lot of confidence, and he even wanted his parents to time him at home. Including his parents in a positive feeling that he felt responsible for achieving, enhanced their relationship with him as well.

Each session would incorporate a technique to enhance verbalization of feelings (Color Your Heart, Stamp Stories; Kaduson, 1997a), as well as the self-control game (Rebound) and Splatz. Several of Bob's disclosures showed that he had a lot of trouble when stressed because he didn't know what to do to calm down. He had tried to count to 10 and take deep breaths, but nothing seemed to work. He was open to trying to do it with the play therapist, which made it more fun. Bob was beginning to take responsibility for some of his actions, and he was finally feeling that he could control some of his actions that he initially thought others were responsible for creating. This shifted his perception of his parents and teachers to a more positive one (Wiener et al., 2012).

Along with Bob's parents' shift in attending to the positive behaviors he exhibited and his own realization that he could have self-control and express himself, Bob's behavior began to become more positive, and the family was more willing to try other interventions that might assist Bob in school and at home. Bob was much more comfortable with himself, and he began to feel more confident in school. He continued to have to work within the limitations of ADHD, but now he would ask for help when needed and would take more personal responsibility for making himself successful.

Conclusion

ADHD continues to be one of the most frequently diagnosed disorders in children. While there are several ways to treat this disorder, a multimodal approach seems to be the most successful. Inherent in this approach is cognitive-behavioral play therapy, for it is rich with empirically proven techniques and enhances those techniques with the play that each and every child needs and wants. The therapeutic powers of play continually engage children in treatment, enhance their verbalization of feelings, and help them to self-regulate and foster positive relationships that can counter the world that is so critical of who they are.

REFERENCES

Abdollahian, E., Mokhber, N., Balaghi, A., & Moharrari, F. (2013). The effectiveness of cognitive-behavioral play therapy on the symptoms of attention-deficit/hyperactivity disorder in children aged 7–9 years. *ADHD Attention Deficit and Hyperactivity Disorders, 5*(1), 41–46.

American Psychiatric Association. (2013). *Diagnostic and statistical manual of mental disorders* (5th ed.). Arlington, VA: Author.

Antshel, K. M., Faraone, S. V., & Gordon, M. (2014). Cognitive behavioral treatment outcomes in adolescent ADHD. *Journal of Attention Disorders, 18*(6), 483–495.

Barkley, R. A. (1990). A critique of current diagnostic criteria for attention deficit hyperactivity disorder: Clinical, and research implications. *Journal of Developmental and Behavioral Pediatrics, 11*, 343–352.

Barkley, R. A. (1997). *ADHD and the nature of self-control*. New York: Guilford Press.

Barkley, R. A. (2012). *Executive functions: What they are, how they work, and why they evolved*. New York: Guilford Press.

Barkley, R. (2016). *Managing ADHD in schools: The best evidence-based methods for teachers*. Eau Clair, WI: PESI Publishing and Media.

Barzegary, L., & Zamini, S. (2011). The effect of play therapy on children with ADHD. *Procedia—Social and Behavioral Sciences, 30*, 2216–2218.

Bodrova, E., & Leong, D. J. (2007). *Tools of the mind: The Vygotskian approach to early childhood education*. Upper Saddle River, NJ: Pearson.

Bratton, S., Ceballos, P., Sheely-Moore, A., Meany-Walen, K., Pronchenko, Y., & Jones, L. (2013). Head Start early mental health intervention: Effects of child-centered play therapy on disruptive behaviors. *International Journal of Play Therapy, 22*(1), 28–42.

Bugental, D. B., Whalen, C. K., & Henker, B. (1977). Causal attributions of hyperactive children and motivational assumptions of two behavior change approaches: Evidence for interactionist position. *Child Development, 49*, 874–884.

Camp, B., Bloom, G., Herbert, F., & van Doorninck, W. (1977). "Think aloud": A program for developing self-control in young aggressive boys. *Journal of Abnormal Child Psychology, 5*, 157–169.

Cohen, S., & Przbycien, C. (1974). Some effects of sociometrically selected peer models on the cognitive styles of impulsive children. *Journal of Genetic Psychology, 124*, 213–220.

Centers for Disease Control and Prevention. (2011). *2011 DHHS Publication No. (PHS) 2013-1582*. Hyattsville, MD: U.S. Department of Health and Human Services, Centers for Disease Control and Prevention, National Center for Health Statistics.

Craighead, W., Kazdin, A., & Mahoney, M. (1981). *Behavior modification: Principles, issues and application* (2nd ed.). Boston: Houghton Mifflin.

Forehand, R., & Baumeister, A. (1976). Deceleration of aberrant behavior among retarded individuals. In M. Hersen, R. Eisler, & P. Miller (Eds.), *Progress in behavior modification* (2nd ed., pp. 112–123). New York: Academic Press.

Frank-Briggs, A. I. (2013). Attention deficit hyperactivity disorder (ADHD). *Journal of Pediatric Neurology, 9*, 291–298.

Gawrilow, C., Gollwitzer, P. M., & Oettingen, G. (2011, December). Self-regulation in children with ADHD: How if–then plans improve executive functions and delay of gratification in children with ADHD. *ADHD Report, 19*(6), 4–8.

Ginsburg, K. R. (2007). The importance of play promoting healthy child development and maintaining strong parent–child bonds. *Pediatrics, 119*, 182–191.

Harris, K. R., Friedlander, B. D., Saddler, B., Frizzelle R., & Graham, S. (2005).

Self-monitoring of attention versus self-monitoring of academic performance: Effects among students with ADHD in the general education classroom. *Journal of Special Education, 39*(3), 145–156.

Hersen, M., & Barlow, D. H. (1976). *Single case experimental designs: Strategies for studying behavior change.* New York: Pergamon Press.

Imeraj, L., Antrop, I., Sonuga-Barket, E., Deboutte, D., Deschepper, E., Bal, S., et al. (2013). The impact of instructional context on classroom on task-behavior. *Journal of School Psychology, 51,* 487–498.

Kaduson, H. G. (1993). Self control game interventions for attention-deficit hyperactivity disorder. *Dissertation Abstracts International, 54*(3-A), 868.

Kaduson, H. G. (1997a). *101 Favorite play therapy techniques.* Northvale, NJ: Jason Aronson.

Kaduson, H. G. (1997b). Play therapy for children with attention-deficit hyperactivity disorder. In H. G. Kaduson, D. Cangelosi, & C. Schaefer (Eds.), *The playing cure: Individualized play therapy for specific childhood problems* (pp. 197–227). New York: Rowman & Littlefield.

Kaduson, H. G. (2000). Structured short-term play therapy for children with attention-deficit hyperactivity disorder. In H. G. Kaduson & C. E. Schaefer (Eds.), *Short-term play therapy for children* (pp. 105–143). New York: Guilford Press.

Kaduson, H. G. (2015). Play therapy with children with attention-deficit hyperactivity disorder. In D. A. Crenshaw & A. L. Stewart (Eds.), *Play therapy: A comprehensive guide to theory and practice* (pp. 415–438). New York: Guilford Press.

Kazdin, A. E. (1975). Covert modeling, model similarity, and reduction of avoidance behavior. *Behavior Therapy, 5,* 325–340.

Kendall, P. C., & Finch, A. J. (1978). A cognitive-behavioral treatment for impulsivity: A group comparison study. *Journal of Consulting and Clinical Psychology, 46,* 110–118.

Knell, S. M. (1993). *Cognitive-behavioral play therapy.* Northvale, NJ: Jason Aronson.

Mash, E. J., & Barkley, R. A. (Eds.). (2003). *Child psychopathology* (2nd ed.). New York: Guilford Press.

Meichenbaum, D. H. (1977). *Cognitive behavior modification.* New York: Plenum Press.

Meichenbaum, D. H., & Asarnow, J. (1979). Cognitive-behavioral modification and metacognitive development: Implications for the classroom. In P. C. Kendall & S. D. Hollon (Eds.), *Cognitive behavioral interventions: Theory, research and procedures* (pp. 11–36). New York: Academic Press.

Meichenbaum, D. H., & Goodman, J. (1971). Training impulsive children to talk to themselves: A means of developing self-control. *Journal of Abnormal Psychology, 77,* 115–126.

Mischel, W. (1974). Processes in delay of gratification. In L. Berkowitz (Ed.), *Advances in experimental social psychology* (Vol. 7, pp. 34–50). New York: Academic Press.

Mischel, W., Shoda, Y., & Rodriguez, M. L. (1989). Delay of gratification in children. *Science, 244,* 933–938.

O'Leary, K. D., & O'Leary, S. G. (1972). *Classroom management: The successful use of behavior modification.* New York: Pergamon Press.

Pelham, W. E., & Murphy, H. A. (1986). Attention deficit and conduct disorders. In M. Hersen (Ed.), *Pharmacological and behavioral treatment: An integrative approach* (pp. 108–148). Hoboken, NJ: Wiley.

Prochaska, J. O., & Marcus, B. H. (1995). The transtheoretical model: Applications to exercise. In R. Dishman (Ed.), *Exercise adherence II* (pp. 164–170). Champaign, IL: Human Kinetics Press.

Raggi, V. L., & Chronis, A. M. (2006). Interventions to address the academic impairment of children and adolescents with ADHD. *Clinical Child and Family Psychology Review, 9* (2), 85–111.

Ray, D., Schottelkorb, A., & Tsai, M. (2007). Play therapy with children exhibiting symptoms of attention deficit hyperactivity disorder. *International Journal of Play Therapy, 16*(2), 95–111.

Reid, R., Trout, A. L., & Schartz, M. (2005). Self-regulation interventions for children with attention deficit/hyperactivity disorder. *Council for Exceptional Children, 71*(4), 361–377.

Schaefer, C. E. (1993). *The therapeutic powers of play.* Hoboken, NJ: Wiley.

Schaefer, C. E., & Drewes, A. A. (2014). *The therapeutic powers of play: 20 core agents of change* (2nd ed.). Hoboken, NJ: Wiley.

Schwarz, A., & Cohen, S. (2013). ADHD seen in 11% of U.S. children as diagnoses rise. Retrieved from *www.nytimes.com/2013/04/01/health/more-diagnoses-of-hyperactivity-causing-concern.html.*

Sonuga-Barke, E. J. S. (2005). Causal models of attention-deficit/hyperactivity disorder: From common simple deficits to multiple developmental pathways. *Biological Psychiatry, 57,* 1231–1238.

Sprafkin, J., & Rubenstein, E. A. (1982). Using television to improve the social behavior of institutionalized children. In J. Sprafkin, C. Swift, & R. H. Ross (Eds.), *Prevention in human services: Rx television: Enhancing the preventive impact of TV* (pp. 5–16). New York: Haworth Press.

Wiener, J., Malone, M., Varma, A., Markel, C., Biondic, D., Tannock, R., et al. (2012). Children's perceptions of their ADHD symptoms: Positive illusions, attributions, and stigma. *Canadian Journal of School Psychology, 27*(3), 217–242.

Wulfert, E., Block, J. A., Santa Ana, E., Rodriguez, M. L., & Colsman, M. (2002). Delay of gratification: Impulsive choices and problem behaviors in early and late adolescence. *Journal of Personality, 70*(4), 533–552.

Yogman, M., Garner, A., Hutchinson, J. K., Hirsch-Pasek, K., & Michnick Golinkoff, R. (2018). The power of play: A pediatric role in enhancing development in young children. *Pediatrics, 142*(3), 2018–2058.

CHAPTER 11

Play Therapy for Children with Problem Sexual Behaviors

Eliana Gil
Quinn Koelfgen Smelser

Description of the Problem

Children with sexual behavior problems have been referred for clinical interventions with great frequency and consistency in the last 20 years. Adolescent sex offenders have been widely recognized and treated in specialized programs for even longer. However, children with sexual behavior problems are treated without uniformity, and few treatment programs exist solely for young children, some as young as 3 years of age (Chaffin, Letourneau, & Silovsky, 2002; Friedrich, 2007). This age group appears to perplex professionals and the lay public alike. It is the most likely population to receive a continuum of responses, ranging from ignoring problem behaviors in the hopes they will resolve alone to punitive responses to viewing child sexual behavior problems as predictive of adolescent and adult sexual offending behaviors (Chaffin et al., 2006). Thus, these child clients receive the most indiscriminate interventions, and parental guidance can be misguided, personalized, and misinformed (Silovsky, Niec, Bard, & Hecht, 2007; Friedrich, 2007; Gil & Shaw, 2014). This area is worthy of rigorous attention by child and play therapists—those most likely to be consulted about any childhood behavior problems.

Most child-serving professionals who provide therapeutic services have likely received phone calls from parents, educators, or others regarding this particular problem area. Even those who specialize in childhood trauma and who work with victims of child sexual abuse may feel sty-mied regarding these particular sexual behavior problems and may view them as requiring specialized services, often separating victim from victim-izer therapies (Silovsky, Swisher, Widdifield, & Burris, 2012; Gil & Shaw, 2014). The problem is that specialization in this area has not grown in tan-dem with the actual need itself; thus, many communities are still uncertain about how to proceed with these inquiries for clinical attention. There is a paucity of services for parents who want to help their children or are being asked by others to get their children help.

This ambivalence about childhood sexual behavior problems may stem from the underlying topic area: childhood sexuality and the multi-tude of thoughts, feelings, and reactions that are elicited in professionals and parents alike (Friedrich, 2007). Interestingly, even the youngest child with problematic sexual behaviors can elicit fear and confusion in others—feelings that render parents and/or professionals confused about what direction to take.

Sexual behavior problems in children range from noncontact types of behaviors, such as focused attention on issues of sexuality (e.g., children who make explicit sexual drawings or use inappropriate or provocative language) to behaviors like public and/or excessive masturbation or insert-ing objects in the vagina or anus. There are few firm guidelines about what is and is not normative, so parents and others constantly worry that some-thing may or may not be appropriate or expectable (Gil, 1993; Friedrich, 2007; Hagan, Shaw, & Duncan, 2008). Rather than relying on external information that may or may not be accurate, it is more useful to think of things along a developmental continuum. For example, if a 4-year-old child touches himself in public, parents might remove his or her hand from the private parts, put something in his or her hands, or redirect the child's attention. These responses may be sufficient to decrease or eliminate the behaviors if they are repeated a few times. When children do not respond to limits, become angry and defiant, and persist in acting inappropriately, clinical assessments may be warranted (Gil, 1993; American Academy of Pediatrics, 2016). Since there is a typical general trajectory for childhood sexual development (a general rule of thumb is that interest increases with age and as physical changes occur), parents and others must always gauge the behavior in comparison to that of peers and try to provide guidance and/or limits when appropriate (Gil & Shaw, 2014; American Academy of Pediatrics, 2016). Parents will typically need guidance on how to address specific sexual behaviors, however, since they often report feeling uncer-tain and awkward about what to say or do. If children's behaviors are not responsive to redirection, limits, or alternatives, persistence could suggest a range of other possibilities: namely, exposure or experience. These might include the child's exposure to inappropriate images, TV shows, or witnessing sexual behaviors by others, and/or a child's direct experience with inappropriate sexual behaviors initiated by others, that is, the child's own sexual abuse (Gil, 1993; American Academy of Pediatrics, 2016). In addition, sometimes the family's boundaries about sexuality are too loose or too constricted. A well-trained clinician can assess this gamut of reasons for sexual behaviors. Good clinical assessments will also rule out medical needs. Urinary tract infections, for example, can cause intense itching, and thus, children will pay inordinate attention to their genitals, touching or rubbing themselves in private or public.

In summary, non-normative sexual behavior problems do not occur in a vacuum. A high percentage of children who exhibit inappropriate sexual behaviors are likely to have experiences with or exposure to some form of sexual information. These behaviors include explicit knowledge of sexual acts (those that are beyond their developmental knowledge base) and/or mimicking learned behaviors and/or using threatening or aggressive interactions in order to secure cooperation (Gil & Shaw, 2014). When these behaviors occur without parental guidance and/or with/without peer encouragement, this can add another layer of complexity. In addition, direct experience with child sexual abuse can cause children to develop trauma-based behaviors—distress signals that are in fact a call for help. Given that contemporary use of technology makes graphic images more accessible in children's environments, it becomes important to develop clinical clarity about contextual/familial issues in the child's environment that might be contributing to sexual acting out.

Rationale for Prescriptive Play Therapy

Treating sexual behavior problems in children requires knowledge of a diverse group of youngsters such that a "one-size-fits-all" approach would not be sufficient (Hackett, Masson, Balfe, & Phillips, 2013). This specific behavioral problem is fraught with challenges regarding identification and responsiveness. Often, parents who feel uncomfortable about how to respond, simply do not respond at all. In addition, these behaviors can elicit a range of responses from others, including those who have histories of sexual abuse. An adult mother with a history of her own victimization may view her young son as threatening or scary and may begin to perceive the behavior from the lens of victim/victimizers (Gil, 1993; Gil & Shaw, 2014). Parents may feel hesitant to let others know that their children are struggling with this type of behavioral issue and/or may experience varying degrees of guilt and shame (Gil, 1993; Gil & Shaw, 2014). These emotions can contribute to parental over- or underfunctioning (i.e., parental ability and willingness to provide careful supervision, monitoring, and concrete verbal and behavioral interventions).

In addition, clinicians who assess this specific problem behavior may also have a range of idiosyncratic thoughts and feelings about young children's sexuality and sexual behavior problems specifically. Based on those responses, the clinician may favor early intervention with the child, the child and his or her parents, the child and his siblings, as well as considering the different settings that the child may frequent: school, day care, neighborhood children, etc. Given the uncertainty about how to proceed, the scarce, but consistent, literature provides a foundation for selecting child and family interventions. The research on this topic area suggests that children do better with a cognitive-behavioral approach (whether or not it includes play-based techniques) and, in addition, that parental education is required to optimize the impact of services (Gil & Shaw, 2014). There is consensus among researchers in the arena of sexual behavior problems that treatment should cover three areas: attention to trauma, involvement of caregivers, and psychoeducation and cognitive-behavioral techniques to manage the sexual behavior problems (Gil & Shaw, 2014). A prescriptive approach allows clinicians to cover all of these treatment areas in ways that specifically meet the needs of the child and the child's family.

Step-by-Step Details of the Intervention

Likely taking the format from the rich history of sex offender treatment programs, most approaches to treating sexual behavior problems are group-based (Chaffin et al., 2006; Friedrich, 2007). Providing interventions within a group format offers destigmatization, gives children opportunities to share with peers (which might be less intimidating than individual therapy with an adult), and allows children to relate to others who have similar issues (Yalom, 2005; Gil & Shaw, 2014). The group approach somewhat normalizes the behavior and allows children to learn together.

Most group programs are time-limited and gender-specific, and work in gradually increasing age groups (Friedrich, 2007). In addition, all groups tend to focus on teaching children about boundaries, affect identification, and modulation; expressing difficult emotions; learning what is and is not appropriate in terms of physical boundaries and social skills; and recognizing triggers for the problem behavior as well as self-soothing and redirecting behaviors (i.e., "What do I say or do when I feel specific feelings, have specific thoughts, or get uncomfortable physical sensations?") (Pithers, Gray, Busconi, & Houchens, 1998; Bonner, Walker, & Berliner, 1999; Chaffin et al., 2006). These programs emphasize self-regulation, including the child keeping him- or herself out of potentially high-risk situations (unique to each child). Almost always, helpers and coping strategies are identified and practiced. When behavioral concerns arise, group members discuss how to keep a problem behavior from growing in the future (Gil &

Shaw, 2014). Thus, a certain modicum of self-control is encouraged, even in the youngest children. Also, play therapists work diligently to help even the youngest child understand what leads them to thoughts about touching others and what alternative behaviors can be employed to avoid problem behaviors (Gil & Shaw, 2014). Because children with sexual behavior problems can be as young as 3 years of age (up to 11 or 12), we recommend that the group process (with lessons to be addressed) be offered by integrating play therapy with cognitive-behavioral therapy (Cavett & Drewes, 2012; Malchiodi, 2014). More specifically, because these youngsters may have experienced their own victimization, an integrated play therapy approach will provide a continuum of directive and nondirective interventions (Gil, 2006; Malchiodi, 2014).

These authors suggest an assessment process that allows for child-centered play therapy so that children can gradually show or tell what might be on their minds and establish a sense of safety with the clinician and setting. This approach also facilitates children's use of a reparative process called posttraumatic play (Gil, 2017). However, many children experience shame about their problem behaviors and require some direct messages from the clinician as well as more directive ways of addressing behavioral alternatives, so that the problem behaviors can subside. Thus, cognitive-behavioral play therapy (Knell, 1995, 2015) is most desirable with this population during treatment.

Parent Involvement

As mentioned earlier, it is imperative that parents feel competent and adequate about their responses to young children with sexual behavior problems (Gil, 1993; Gil & Shaw, 2014). Most of the time, parents want very concrete help, including what language to use when talking to their children and the type of consequences to set for sexual behavior problems. Parents need to be confident that they are delivering interventions in a nonpunitive way, so that children are more likely to feel care and respect. Therapists are well advised to help parents recognize that their child has a behavioral problem like any other and to differentiate between the behavior and the person. Parents will also need help honestly facing whatever emotions or reactions are triggered by the child's behavior and finding a way to decrease negativity and increase positive interactions with their child (Gil, 1993; Gil & Shaw, 2014). Clinicians are well advised to help parent–child dyads establish or reinforce positive attachment behaviors, and some activities are designed to promote secure attachment.

Because childhood sexuality is a complex topic that requires a range of services depending on children's ages, developmental stages, or gender, it's important for parents to have opportunities to hold candid and problem-solving discussions that clarify what behaviors are appropriate or inappropriate (Gil, 1993; Chaffin et al., 2006; Gil & Shaw, 2014). Parents need to know how to be nonjudgmental with a child who engages in inappropriate behaviors. Kindness is a prerequisite for play therapists and parents when working with children with sexual behavior problems. The second prerequisite is clarity in setting limits, with the ability to teach alternative behaviors.

Case Vignette: Miguel

Ten-year-old Miguel was referred to one of us (Gil) as a result of his problem sexual behaviors[1] when his 7-year-old cousin, Tony, made a disclosure of child sexual abuse.[2] Miguel's parents, Cynthia and Matt, were initially skeptical about the possibility that Miguel would have been guilty of such wrongdoing, but after talking to Miguel numerous times, Miguel broke down and confessed that he had touched his cousin, "but only one time," and only after Tony asked him to do it.

Parents Cynthia and Matt attended the intake session and seemed somewhat embarrassed, but they were mostly concerned about their son. They described him as a "good boy, quiet and studious." They described cousin Miguel's relationship to Tony as "very close," and they were surprised that there had been any problems between them. Their early questions concentrated on Miguel: specifically, would he be in trouble with the law, would he be labeled a sex offender at his age, would he have to go to court, and did this mean that he was homosexual? Given the fact that Matt was Latino, this therapist (Gil) could see the look of grave concern when he asked that question. Mother added her own questions about this behavior being predictive of a life-long problem, and whether there was any reason to believe that someone had molested Miguel. These questions are typical of parents when they are confronted with their child's sexual behaviors.

Subsequently, the first clinical responses are quite important since they set the context for treatment going forward. After the questions were answered and basic psychoeducation was provided, a description of assessment and treatment was given.

---

[1] One of us (Gil) developed a program called Boundary Project (Gil, 1993; Gil & Shaw, 2014) to serve children with sexual behavior problems. The program includes a group therapy format for children and a collateral parental group. This family-based program can be delivered individually or in group, depending on group availability and the child's ability and/or willingness to fully participate in group therapy with peers and later within a multiparent group.

[2] Tony's case is described in a separate chapter (see Gil & Smelser, Chapter 9, this volume).

Assessment

Early in treatment, most young children with sexual behavior problems are loathe to admit their "touching problem." Therefore, the play therapist simply communicates that he or she knows about the problem behavior and adds that "lots of kids don't want to talk about this until, after we get to know each other," and moves on to some playful assessment techniques that don't rely on verbal question-and-answer sessions. The typical assessment process includes child-centered play therapy, as well as invitations to participate in expressive therapies. Play therapists allow children a range of expression and focus on getting to know each child and to develop trust with each child as best as they can. Thus, the assessment allows clinicians to observe children's play for thematic material or the emergence of post-trauma play (Gil, 2017), as well as responses to specific activities, such as drawing a Kinetic Family Drawing, a play genogram, or a sandtray (Gil, 2015). Once children participate in an assessment, play therapists have a better idea of how receptive they will be to group, how open they may or may not be about the sexual behavior problems, and what their strengths and vulnerabilities might be. Children are usually referred to an appropriate group; however, at times groups are not currently running or the wait time may be long. When this occurs, the play therapist can choose instead to deliver important "lessons" in individual therapy, with the parent joining the last 15 minutes of the session (Gil & Shaw, 2014).

Miguel's assessment revealed a youngster in distress. He was overwhelmed with feelings of guilt and shame, and keeping the secret about his inappropriate sexual behavior with Tony had taken its toll. Miguel participated easily in all expressive activities, and, although he did not reveal much verbally, his expressive images spoke clearly and consistently. In a family play genogram, he chose an alligator and a graduate for himself and a ladybug for Tony. In a Kinetic Family Drawing, he put himself playing soccer with Tony and letting him make a goal by stepping out of the way. In a story that he told with puppets, a monster lived in the forest, out of sight, attacking birds' nests to eat the baby eggs before they were born. In this way, Miguel began to reveal issues of helplessness, aggression, and predatory behavior, as well as kindness and an interest in school.

Individual Therapy

Typical sexual behavior problem services include teaching children a number of "lessons" designed to target the underlying areas that can contribute to sexual acting out (Gil, 1993; Gil & Shaw, 2014). In some cases, the assessment may also identify the child's sexual abuse, and individual therapy may be necessary for victimization issues. Children are referred to group therapy when it is determined that they will be successful in a group setting designed to review pertinent information about acting-out behaviors.

For Miguel, we had to delay participating in group for a few months, so I (Gil) began a series of playful activities designed to set a foundation for subsequent group work. I had Miguel and me sit in the room within hoola-hoops, and we talked about "private space" called physical boundaries. We then stood holding our hoola-hoops around our waists and practiced getting close without touching each other's boundaries. We also took this concept and shared a large space of easel paper in which Miguel drew whatever he wanted to in his half of the page, and I drew in my half of the page.

We also did collage work on self-image, and I asked him to place pictures of how he saw himself in school, at home, or with his extended family or specific friends. Initially, his images were mostly negative, although a later collage showed that he had managed to integrate the lesson that the inappropriate sexual touching was a behavior, and not something that defined who he was. For Miguel, it was important for him to learn that he had made bad decisions when he had approached Tony, but he was not a bad person. It was gratifying to clinician and client to see a drawing he made of his brain, with a key on the perimeter of the brain. He said, "I know what to do when I have a bad thought now. I have the key to 'move along' my thoughts, and choose a good behavior." During treatment, Miguel grew in confidence about self-control. He also came to understand how his own abuse had contributed to his acting-out behaviors—all important steps in his recovery. As a termination present, I gave Miguel a safe with a key and told him he could decide what to put inside it and how often to open or lock it up. He offered a big smile in recognition of this metaphor.

Group Therapy

Group therapy is universally accepted as a beneficial format when working with children with a common problem. The research indicates that a cognitive-behavioral framework is preferred for teaching children important concepts designed to help them self-regulate, identify and respond to triggers, and find alternative behaviors to sexual acting out. Lessons must be repeated numerous times and across settings to be successfully integrated by young children. The Boundary Project, for example, utilizes a minimum of 12 sessions, which can be repeated if it seems necessary to reinforce lessons or if children continue to act out (Gil & Shaw, 2014).

For the parent group sessions, psychoeducation is provided specific to sexual behavior problems. Most of the questions that Miguel's parents had at intake are reviewed. The goal of working with parents is to ensure that they feel confident enough to deliver clear, kind, and firm limits as well as to provide alternative behaviors to their children. In addition, play therapists challenge parental judgments that are negative, punitive, cruel, or misinformed. A secondary goal is to strengthen the parent–child relationship so that each child can view his or her parent as a resource and can turn to the parent(s) for help in an open and candid way (Gil & Shaw, 2014).

Family Therapy

In cases of familial sexual abuse, it is important to provide family therapy to address the countless conflicts that can arise among family members. Mark and Matt were brothers and parents, but their focus was and remained their children first. However, they were also uncles to Tony and Miguel, and spent family holidays together and planned to continue to do so. It became critical to have Tony and Miguel, who had been separated upon disclosure, have an opportunity to come together and eventually have an open conversation about the inappropriate sexual behavior that Miguel had initiated. It was also important, as it is with every sexual abuse situation, to ensure that secrecy was broken and that everyone was able to speak openly about what had occurred, in order to move forward.

Both families were asked to come in to plan how to reestablish contact between the children and how to support the reunification process. Each set of parents was to talk to their children about touching private parts, what to do if anyone asked them to participate in this type of touching, and who to tell what was going on. Parents were asked to name what was inappropriate about the behavior and likewise to state what was appropriate between children of the same or different ages. Once this was achieved, Tony and Miguel were invited to come into the office, and Miguel had a chance to be accountable to Tony for his behavior. Tony was allowed to say whatever was on his mind about the behavior. They were able to shake hands and understood that they would be supervised when they were playing together until everyone was sure that there would be no repeat of inappropriate sexual behaviors. Tony had been in his own therapy and was able to clearly state how scared he had felt, how confused, and how embarrassed. Miguel was able to provide empathy and apologize for making Tony experience those uncomfortable feelings. Miguel also shared what he had learned in group and how he would keep himself from engaging in inappropriate behaviors in the future.

Miguel's parents were very supportive of their son and nephew and were able to set aside their fears and worries to provide Miguel with some very clear limits about what was appropriate and not appropriate for a child his age. Miguel's father was impressive with his ability to talk openly to his boy about erections, ejaculation, "wet dreams," and masturbation. Although they were Roman Catholics and believed that masturbation was a sin, Miguel's father was able to tell Miguel that he should try other things before touching himself, but if he did, he should confess to the priest in church. Miguel also shared that it was important that he have "good fantasies" when he was touching himself and imagine himself loving someone, not just having sex. Cynthia was not actively involved in these conversations, but she was supportive of talking openly about how important consent was, and how respect and love were paramount to having any sexual relationship. Cynthia always talked about sex in the context of marriage; Matt's contribution was about sex accompanied by love and respect. These conversations often included Miguel's 13-year-old brother, Juan, who benefited greatly from these conversations since he was just becoming interested in dating.

Treatment Summary

Miguel was just as his parents had described him: a sweet and polite boy who seemed shy and embarrassed at first. He participated well in the assessment process, following directives for expressive activities such as "Draw a picture of yourself" (self-portrait) and "Draw a picture of you and your family doing something together" (Kinetic Family Drawing). In addition, he was able to build a scenario in the sandtray and was forthcoming about his acting-out behavior. By the end of the individual assessment process, he had confided that Tony "didn't really ask me to touch him" and that instead, it had been his idea. He shared that he had seen some pictures at school that got him curious about erections. He was able to state quietly that he was worried about getting the bed wet some nights because he touched himself "a lot." Over time, this child was able to provide a great deal of information about a school friend who showed them pornography on his iPhone, as well as a game that this boy played in the bathroom, in which the boys had to lick each other's penises. This was reported to the authorities since the initiator of the behavior was an older high school boy who sought out the younger ones at recess and after school. It's important to note that Miguel was able to communicate verbally once he participated in nonverbal, expressive activities that allowed him to "show" what was on his mind. After these activities, I (Gil) noted that he could "say as much or as little as he wanted," and often he would shrug his shoulders and yet remain very engaged as I talked about the metaphors he had used. Once he felt safe in his interactions with me, he began to share spontaneously about his private parts.

We had about eight individual therapy sessions in which several issues about boundaries and self-control were reviewed playfully. Miguel always responded well to active, playful, physical activities. Probably his favorite was when we went outside and threw water balloons against the wall, as he identified angry feelings about the boy who had shown him pornography and encouraged him to engage in sexual behaviors that were fraught with shame and guilt for him.

In group therapy, Miguel was a leader. He and another child were the oldest kids in the group, and they took the younger ones under their wings. With Miguel's help, the play therapist was able to deliver the lessons and obtain a high level of cooperation. Miguel became an asset and role model, encouraging children to participate fully in whatever game or activity was selected.

In family therapy, Miguel was forthcoming and sensitive to his cousin. Both Miguel and Tony were lucky in that their parents did not blame each other for what had happened and thus created a positive experience for their children.

One of the closing activities was to do a family sandtray in which everyone placed a miniature in the center of the tray, which represented what it was like when Tony first disclosed the sexual abuse. On the outside of the center, the family was asked to place miniatures that showed what they had learned, what resources they had now, and how they were conceptualizing moving forward. The miniatures chosen for the abuse were a fire, a lightning rod, a scream figure, an alligator, and a turtle with its head inside the shell. The miniatures chosen for the outside doubled these: a fire extinguisher, a priest and a church, a cage with a lock and key, a head with an open mouth, a family of elephants with their babies, and lots of little circles in the sand. When I asked the family to say as much or as little as they wanted about what they had done, they smiled. Both sets of parents hugged their boys and thanked them for being who they were. Miguel and Tony also hugged as they left the last session with a clear prevention plan and within a context of family warmth and guidance.

Empirical Support for the Intervention

In the realm of treating sexual behavior problems, the majority of existing research centers on adult sex offenders (Boyd, Hagan, & Cho, 2000). Most programs for treating children with sexual behavior problems rely on psychoeducation delivered in a group and/or individual format and from a cognitive-behavioral framework (Gil & Shaw, 2014). Few studies on the whole focus on outcomes research for treating sexual behavior problems in children. Cognitive-behavioral approaches are considered evidence-based for a variety of presenting problems. There is also much empirical support for play-based interventions, family-systems models, and trauma-informed treatments when it comes to treating sexual behavior problems (Gil & Shaw, 2014).

These authors promote a family-focused, trauma-informed, play-based, and phase-based (Gil & Shaw, 2014) treatment response for children with sexual behavior problems. We encourage a three-phase trauma-treatment model similar to that of Judith Herman's (1992) approach. In the first phase of treatment (assessment), safety and security are established in a therapeutic relationship and play therapy environment (Herman, 1992; Gil & Shaw, 2014). Then, the second phase of treatment includes attention to the specific trauma experience, whether it be victim or victimizer dynamics (Herman, 1992; Gil & Shaw, 2014). Finally, the child and parents are offered an opportunity to affiliate with others who experience similar struggles, thus providing them a future orientation to overcome these struggles (Herman, 1992; Yalom, 2005; Gil & Shaw, 2014).

The intervention presented in this case vignette includes directive and nondirective play therapy, collateral family work, cognitive-behavioral therapy, as well as expressive activities. It allows the play therapist to pick what is needed for treatment of each child, whether or not they might benefit from an individual or group format or both, and it provides a variety of techniques selected from differing theoretical orientations (Gil & Shaw, 2014). Additionally, it covers all the aforementioned areas that researchers agree are necessary for treatment of sexual behavior problems. Chaffin et al. (2006) suggested focusing on trauma-related symptoms if those are also present in the child's behavior prior to treating the sexual behavior problems. A well-trained, trauma-informed clinician can assess whether this treatment area is relevant on a case-by-case basis during the assessment phase. Silovsky et al. (2012) cited the importance of caregiver involvement in the treatment of sexual behavior problems of children. This treatment area is central to the Boundary Project. Psychoeducation and a cognitive-behavioral focus are the final treatment area researchers agree upon and should be included as necessary treatment approaches (Chaffin et al., 2006; Gil & Shaw, 2014).

Conclusion

Children with sexual behavior problems need kind, clear, and nonpunitive interventions designed to help them understand what is appropriate and inappropriate behavior in regards to the private parts of their bodies (Gil, 1993; Gil & Shaw, 2014). Most children who engage in inappropriate sexual behaviors are ashamed to discuss what they've done and may need support and patience in developing a trusting therapy relationship prior to fuller engagement in processing. A group play therapy experience helps destigmatize the issue of sexual behavior problems and may provide a less intimidating environment in which children can be more candid (Gil &

Shaw, 2014). In addition, parents of children with sexual behavior problems have an array of responses to their children's behaviors and may feel uncertain and/or misinformed about how to respond. Thus, a collateral psychoeducational treatment program is pivotal to success (Silovsky et al., 2012). Play therapists may also need to confront negative parental attitudes and/or other feelings or memories that might surface in the face of learning about children's sexual behavior problems.

There are limited specialized services for this population, and many professionals may harbor their own fears and negative subjective reactions about these behaviors. Play therapists are encouraged to seek supervision, consultation, and psychoeducation about sexual behavior problems, and to view these behavioral problems in the same way they might view general behavioral problems in their playrooms.

REFERENCES

American Academy of Pediatrics. (2016). Sexual behaviors in young children: What's normal, what's not? Retrieved from *www.healthychildren.org/English/ages-stages/preschool/Pages/Sexual-Behaviors-Young-Children.aspx*.

Bonner, B. L., Walker, C. E., & Berliner, L. (1999). *Children with sexual behavior problems: Assessment and treatment* (Final Report, Grant No. 90-CA-1469). Washington, DC: U.S. Department of Health and Human Services, National Clearinghouse on Child Abuse and Neglect.

Boyd, N. J. A., Hagan, M., & Cho, M. E. (2000). Characteristics of adolescent sex offenders: A review of the research. *Aggression and Violent Behavior, 5*(2), 137–146.

Cavett, A., & Drewes, A. (2012). Play applications and trauma specific components. In J. A. Cohen, A. P. Mannarino, & E. Deblinger (Eds.), *Trauma-focused CBT for children and adolescents: Treatment applications* (pp. 105–123). New York: Guilford Press.

Chaffin, M., Berliner, L., Block, R., Johnson, T. C., Friedrich, W., Louis, D. G., et al. (2006). Report of the Task Force on Children with Sexual Behavior Problems. Retrieved from *www.atsa.com/atsa-csb-task-force-report*.

Chaffin, M., Letourneau, E., & Silovsky, J. F. (2002). Adults, adolescents, and children who sexually abuse children: A developmental perspective. In J. E. B. Myers, L. Berliner, J. Briere, C. Jenny, T. Hendrix, & T. E. Reid (Eds.), *The APSAC handbook on child maltreatment* (2nd ed., pp. 205–232). Thousand Oaks, CA: SAGE.

Friedrich, W. N. (2007). *Children with sexual behavior problems: Family-based attachment-focused therapy.* New York: Norton.

Gil, E. (1993). Age-appropriate sex play versus problematic sexual behaviors. In E. Gil & T. C. Johnson (Eds.), *Sexualized children: Assessment and treatment of sexualized children and children who molest* (pp. 21–40). Royal Oak, MI: Self-Esteem Shop.

Gil, E. (2006). *Helping abused and traumatized children: Using directive and non-directive techniques.* New York: Guilford Press.

Gil, E. (2015). *Extended play-based developmental assessment.* Grand Rapids: MI: Self-Esteem Shop.

Gil, E. (2017). *Posttraumatic play: What clinicians should know.* New York: Guilford Press.

Gil, E., & Shaw, J. A. (2014). *Working with children with sexual behavior problems.* New York: Guilford Press.

Hackett, S., Masson, H., Balfe, M., & Phillips, J. (2013). Individual, family and abuse characteristics of 700 British child and adolescent sexual abusers. *Child Abuse Review, 22,* 232–245.

Hagan, J. F., Shaw, J. S., & Duncan, P. M. (Eds.). (2008). *Bright futures: Guidelines for health supervision of infants, children, and adolescents* (3rd ed.). Elk Grove Village, IL: American Academy of Pediatrics.

Herman, J. L. (1992). *Trauma and recovery.* New York: Basic Books.

Knell, S. (1995). *Cognitive-behavioral play therapy.* New York: Jason Aronson.

Knell, S. (2015). Cognitive-behavioral play therapy. In K. J. O'Connor, C. E. Schaefer, & L. D. Braverman (Eds.), *Handbook of play therapy* (2nd ed., pp. 119–133). New York: Jason Aronson.

Malchiodi, C. (2014.). *Creative interventions with traumatized children* (2nd ed.). New York: Guilford Press.

Pithers, W. D., Gray, A., Busconi, A., & Houchens, P. (1998). Children with sexual behavior problems: Identification of five distinct child types and related treatment considerations. *Child Maltreatment, 3*(4), 384–406.

Silovskyk, J. F., Niec, L., Bard, D., & Hecht, D. B. (2007). Treatment for preschool children with interpersonal sexual behavior problems: A pilot study. *Journal of Clincial Adolescent Psychology, 36*(3), 378–391.

Silovsky, J. F., Swisher, L. M., Widdifield, J., Jr., & Burris, L. (2012). Clinical considerations when children have problematic sexual behavior. In P. Goodyear-Brown (Ed.), *Handbook of child sexual abuse: Identification, assessment, and treatment* (pp. 401–428). Hoboken, NJ: Wiley.

Yalom, I. D. (2005). *Theory and practice of group psychotherapy.* New York: Basic Books.

CHAPTER 12

Play Therapy for Children Exhibiting Aggressive Behaviors

David A. Crenshaw
Alyssa Swan

Description of the Problem

Aggressive behaviors manifest as children's external, nonverbal communication of a range, and sometimes an intersection, of internal emotional, physical, social, and relational experiences. Play therapy delivered prior to or at early identification of childhood aggressive behaviors can serve as prevention for continuation and heightening of aggressive behaviors. When assessing childhood aggression, clinicians take care to avoid misattribution of intentionality to children for exhibiting aggressive behaviors. Play therapists can consider aggression and behavior as symptomology of emotional, relational, cultural, and social difficulties experienced by children and externalized as behavior. In this way, aggressive behavior can be conceptualized as a means for communication of pain or loss that is more difficult to articulate verbally, particularly for children. It is fair to validate that often children's aggressive behaviors can feel hurtful or manipulative to caregivers and teachers on the receiving end; aggressive behavior is a way that children attempt, consciously and unconsciously, to get their needs met. Typically, however, the emotional or relational needs (e.g., relational safety, care/attention, respect) they are attempting to meet through aggression go unmet due to the disruptive nature of their behaviors. Intentional assessment of children's aggressive behaviors can help pinpoint the underlying needs motivating their aggression.

Holistic assessment of the origins of observed aggressive behavior is essential. Wilson and Ray (2018) described the typical development of childhood aggression, normalizing that all children express aggressive behavior more or less during different periods of child development. Considering the developmental context and being able to articulate the externalization of aggression at different stages of development can help play therapists identify typical and atypical aggression in child clients. Play therapists can then account for the developmental appropriateness in consideration of children's unique presenting concerns, experiences, and cultural contexts. Some children will exhibit heightened behavior problems due to disruptions in daily life, such as nutrition (Jansen et al., 2017) and sleep (Mazurek & Sohl, 2016; Rubens et al., 2017). For such problems, counselors can recommend diet and sleep changes in conjunction with psychological intervention.

Beginning in early childhood, children who live in poverty and low-income neighborhoods are identified as exhibiting higher levels of aggressive behavior. African American children are more likely to be identified as aggressive or as exhibiting disruptive behavior, compared to their counterparts (Sacco, Bright, Jun, & Stapleton, 2015). Experiencing racial discrimination is related to valid feelings of anger and, subsequently, is correlated with increased levels of aggression (Chng & Tan, 2017). Researchers also describe gender differences in expression of aggressive behavior, specifically higher levels of physical aggression among male children and higher levels of relational aggression among female children (Card, Stucky, Sawalani, & Little, 2008; Cullerton-Sen et al., 2008; Ostrov & Crick, 2007). Thoroughly considering the cultural impacts of aggression can reduce the risk of pathologizing reactions to oppression, increase the accuracy of identifying the roots of children's aggression, and allow play therapists to most accurately tailor play therapy intervention and advocacy efforts.

In conjunction with the intentional gathering of accurate and thorough background information on children's development of aggressive behaviors, across various settings (e.g., home, school) and from multiple informants (e.g., caregivers, teachers, self-report), play therapists can utilize observations and instruments to assess childhood aggression. Informal observations of children in their normal environments during daily activity and/or during particularly stressful, aggression-precipitating times are particularly useful in identifying environmental and relational experiences that may trigger an aggressive response. Some formal assessments of aggressive behaviors include the Child Behavior Checklist (CBCL; Achenbach, 1994), the Children's Aggression Scale (CAS; Halperin & McKay, 2012), and the Social Emotional Assets and Resilience Scales (SEARS; Merrell, 2011).

Rationale for Play Therapy

Risk factors for higher levels of aggressive behaviors during childhood include, but are not limited to, child maltreatment (Augsburger, Dohrmann, Schauer, & Elbert, 2016), residential placement (Boxer, 2007), parental physical punishment (Piché, Huỳnh, Clément, & Durrant, 2016), insecure caregiver–child attachment (Finzi, Ram, Har-Even, Shnit, & Weizman, 2001), community violence (Houston & Grych, 2016), depressive symptomology (Barnes, Howell, Thurston, & Cohen, 2017), and peer rejection (Prinstein & La Greca, 2004). The long-term impacts of childhood aggression begin as early as adolescence, during which children who demonstrated elevated levels of aggression during early childhood may be more likely to experience lower academic achievement (Scott, Lapre, Marsee, & Weems, 2014), school adjustment (Kokko & Pulkkinen, 2000), and mental health diagnosis (Harrison, Genders, Davies, Treasure, & Tchanturia, 2011) as adolescents. Although not the sole determiner or a direct factor, youth aggression has been correlated with higher rates of adulthood domestic violence (Gabriel et al., 2017), sensation seeking and risk taking (Cui, Colasante, Malti, Ribeaud, & Eisner, 2015), mood and substance use disorders (Reef, Diamantpoulou, van Meurs, Verhulst, & van der Ende, 2011), incarceration (Neller, Denney, Pietz, & Thomlinson, 2006), and unemployment (Kokko & Pulkkinen, 2000).

The connection between childhood aggression and adolescent/adult maladjustment may not be surprising; however, the connection is nonetheless troubling and nonlinear. For play therapists working with teens and adolescents, early identification of concerns connected to early childhood aggression can streamline treatment. Play therapists target mediating factors shown to help disrupt the development and continuation of childhood aggression to reduce the risk of persistence of aggression into adulthood. The goals of play therapy align with these mediating factors, situating play therapy as both prevention and intervention treatment to reduce children's risk factors for developing aggressive behaviors and/or reduce aggressive behaviors to mitigate long-term impact. See Figure 12.1 for a visual depiction of the role of play therapy as prevention of aggression development by targeting risk factors and intervention of aggression by bolstering positive mediating factors for youth.

Play therapy provides a relationship in which children, even children who exhibit the most aggressive behaviors, can experience unconditional acceptance and genuine empathy, which serve as platforms upon which children can begin to experience themselves as worthy of such acceptance. In play therapy, hopefully and eventually, children begin to experience themselves as someone worthy of the play therapist's consistent and unwavering relationship. In this relationship, children can experiment

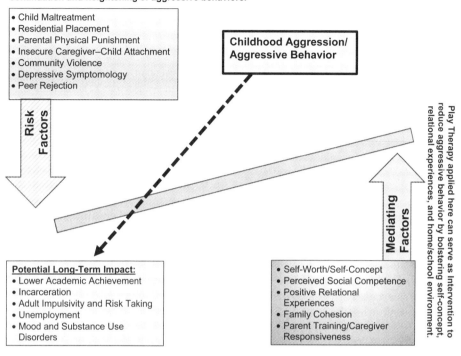

Play Therapy applied here can serve as Prevention for continuation and heightening of aggressive behaviors.

- Child Maltreatment
- Residential Placement
- Parental Physical Punishment
- Insecure Caregiver–Child Attachment
- Community Violence
- Depressive Symptomology
- Peer Rejection

Risk Factors

Childhood Aggression/ Aggressive Behavior

Mediating Factors

Play Therapy applied here can serve as Intervention to reduce aggressive behavior by bolstering self-concept, relational experiences, and home/school environment.

Potential Long-Term Impact:
- Lower Academic Achievement
- Incarceration
- Adult Impulsivity and Risk Taking
- Unemployment
- Mood and Substance Use Disorders

- Self-Worth/Self-Concept
- Perceived Social Competence
- Positive Relational Experiences
- Family Cohesion
- Parent Training/Caregiver Responsiveness

FIGURE 12.1. Rationale for play therapy to mitigate effects of childhood aggression.

with responding to limits and making choices, a process that eventually externalizes outside of the playroom as greater behavioral regulation and increased self-confidence. Additionally, increased self-worth is also often accompanied by new, less rigid views of self (e.g., "I am capable of being loved" or "I am good at doing some things") and of others (e.g., "Some people can be trusted" or "Not all relationships hurt me"). This releases energy, once preoccupied in a loop of perceived relational threat and subsequent self-protection or self-harm, which can be directed toward more child-appropriate tasks of relationship and play.

Parent Involvement

Children's perceived self-worth and social competence can greatly reduce or heighten the long-term impact of childhood aggression (De Castro,

Brendgen, Van Boxtel, Vitaro, & Schaepers, 2007; McQuade et al., 2016). The degree to which children experience an inner sense of inherent worthiness and perceive relational successes with caregivers and peers helps free those children who demonstrate early aggressive behaviors to develop alternative coping strategies and healthy relationships. Family cohesion and family dynamics are consistently some of the most critical mediating factors between childhood aggressive behavior and longitudinal measures of well-being and aggression (Hamama & Arazi, 2012). Specifically, parenting practices are one of the most impactful factors in the development and advancement of aggressive behaviors during childhood (Hay, Meldrum, Widdowson, & Piquero, 2017).

Baydar and Akcinar (2018) demonstrated that harsh discipline practices versus caregiver responsiveness for children at age 3 were associated with higher or lower levels of aggressive behaviors, respectively, by age 5. A 2018 study by Campaert, Nocentini, and Mesesini further supported this link, reporting that by late childhood into early adolescence, parental harsh discipline and poor monitoring led to moral disengagement. Interestingly, the connection between parental practice and preadolescent behavior was mediated by preadolescents' perceptions of parental approval of aggression. In another study, secure attachment with a primary caregiver buffered the relationship between exposure to community violence and perceived acceptability of aggression (Houston & Grych, 2016).

Parenting/caregiving practices mediate the effects and severity of externalizing behaviors during childhood and adolescence (Gach, Ip, Sameroff, & Olson, 2018), and early intervention is most critical to reduce cumulative risks. Play therapists can provide parent training to help parents gain awareness of their relational impact on their children and learn positive parenting practices, such as new ways to set limits and provide choices. Caregiver training is not limited to parents/caregivers; sometimes play therapists will support residential treatment teams, direct care staff, medical providers, and other mental health providers to develop consistent, positive interpersonal relationships with children at risk for developing or maintaining aggressive behaviors.

Description of the Prescriptive Approach

Children who exhibit more than their fair share of aggressive behavior benefit from a range of therapeutic powers of play (Schaefer, 1995; Schaefer & Drewes, 2013). One such power is *self-expression*. Play therapy not only allows but encourages the free expression of a child, and some children displaying aggressive behavior feel constrained in self-expression. The parents or the teachers may be controlling and/or rigid to a degree that the child is frequently frustrated in self-expression. In family therapy with adolescents, our clinical experience teaches us that these youth complain that no one listens. They do not feel heard, and rage is often the result. Self-expression in play therapy facilitates communication, which helps the child to gain awareness of troubling emotions and distressing memories and thus begin the healing process.

Another therapeutic power of play of benefit to children exhibiting aggressive behaviors is *access to the unconscious*. So much of what drives the aggressive behavior is outside of the child's awareness (Crenshaw & Tillman, 2013). Play reveals and helps to integrate unconscious aggressive wishes and impulses into conscious play and actions. A child, for example, caught in a bitter divorce family triangle may play out his father getting killed in a car accident. He may be aware of the fear of losing his father but unaware of his hostile wishes toward him, due to the father's pressures to align with him against his mother. Only by playing out the car crashes does the child realize that he not only fears the death of his father but has fantasies and unconscious wishes of his father dying to be free of the untenable situation of being caught in the crossfire of a difficult divorce and its attendant loyalty conflicts. This emphasis on motives and conflicts that exist out of the child's awareness is a key component of psychodynamic approaches to play therapy (Crenshaw & Tillman, 2013; Mordock, 2015).

Direct instruction is one of the powers of play identified by Schaefer and Drewes (2013). Teaching self-calming and soothing strategies, positive self-statements, and stress inoculation are often a core component of cognitive-behavioral play therapy (Cavett, 2015), and can be integrated into play therapy focusing on reducing aggressive behaviors. The direct teaching of these skills, which are critical to effective integration of aggressive impulses, is an important component of prescriptive play therapy with children prone to aggressive behaviors.

Indirect teaching, through metaphor and fantasy play, allows ample opportunities to model and teach the skills of self-calming, self-soothing, positive self-talk, and stress inoculation. Indirect teaching also enhances the critical skill of empathy which plays a key role in interrupting the cycle of aggression (Crenshaw & Hardy, 2007; Hardy & Crenshaw, 2008; Hardy & Laszloffy, 2005).

Catharsis and *abreaction* are essential features of psychodynamic play therapy and are often evident when in-depth play therapy is conducted with children whose trauma underlies their acting out of aggressive impulses. Both catharsis and abreaction were dramatically evident in the case of Rashawn, a child who experienced sadistic abuse by his foster father (Crenshaw & Hardy, 2005).

Case Vignette: Luke's Long Road to Reunion with His Mother

Luke at age 12 and his sister Cara at age 10 had been in 10 previous foster homes prior to placement in a group emergency foster care program. The two children differ dramatically in their personalities. Cara is sweet, warm, and friendly, although shy and introverted until she knows you well. Luke is developmentally delayed. In one assessment, the examiner suggested the possibility of autism spectrum disorder, along with attention-deficit/hyperactivity disorder (ADHD), cognitive and learning limitations, and posttraumatic stress disorder (PTSD). Luke was well known for wearing out a young group of male child care workers in the emergency foster care program, even though they dealt with him over three rotating shifts in a 24-hour day. The intensity of his demands, low frustration tolerance, and inability to delay gratification helped the staff appreciate why he was unable to be maintained in any of the 10 prior foster home placements. In one of the foster homes, there was an allegation of sexual abuse in which both children were suspected of being victimized by a foster father. An investigation was inconclusive, but Child Protective Services (CPS) removed the children from the home. In another foster home, the children claimed psychological abuse of Luke that was denied by the foster mother but supported by Cara, and once again the children were removed by CPS and placed in the Group Emergency Foster Care (GEFC) program.

Cara, loyal to her older brother, could have been successful in most of the homes on her own, but she refused to be separated from her brother and tended to be protective of him. This pattern was abruptly broken when, after nearly a year in the GEFC program, the siblings were placed together in yet another foster home. In a matter of 3 months, however, Luke returned to the GEFC program due to disruptive behavior that was overwhelming for the foster mother to handle, but this time Cara elected to remain in the foster home.

The birth parents of these children struggled with problems of substance abuse and domestic violence. The birth father voluntarily surrendered his parental rights after the children were placed in foster care. The mother, however, fought to get her children back and, in the process, participated in a wide range of rehab programs. She received mental health counseling not only for her addiction problems but also her major mood disorder that left her episodically clinically depressed. Many court battles and conflicting opinions among social service caseworkers and officials about the feasibility of family reunification ensued until the mother was approved in the spring of 2018 to resume visits with her children and, at least in the case of Luke, work toward family reunification. Cara was more ambivalent and skeptical about reuniting with her mother and at the point that the mother came back into the picture, was comfortably situated in her foster home, and enjoying a good relationship with her foster mother. The court and social services supervisors decided after much deliberation and discussions with the children to honor the differing loyalties of the two siblings. Luke would work toward family reunification. Cara would continue to live with her foster mother but begin visits with her biological mother on a schedule that was comfortable for her.

It is extremely challenging in this small space to give more than snapshots of the play therapy with Luke which took place weekly over a 4-year period. The snapshots might be considered "Kodak moments" in that they captured an important theme and, in some cases, a turning point in the long-term therapy.

Snapshot 1: During the Early Stages—Intense Struggle with Aggressive Impulses

Luke was one of the most volatile, emotionally dysregulated youth in the therapist's memory when he was placed in the GEFC program at age 10. It has been a point of great emphasis to reduce physical restraints in the residential program, with an aspirational goal of zero restraints. The video clips of every restraint are reviewed by a team of supervisors, including clinicians, to determine if the restraint was done properly and if there was a possibility of avoiding it altogether through some change in approach or intervention. To this day, Luke holds the record of 120 physical restraints in the first 6 months of his placement in the program. It is possible that Luke's record will never be broken because in recent years no one has come close to his astonishing total. To jump ahead to the good news, as of this writing, Luke is at home with his mother on trial discharge and has not had a single physical restraint in the last year of placement.

In the play therapy room, Luke was extremely physical. The struggle with his aggressive impulses was enacted in the safe, contained space of the therapy room and within the safety of the therapeutic relationship. A powerful theme of his therapeutic play was driven by an underlying question: "Are you strong enough to contain my aggression?" Clearly, Luke did not trust his own ability to regulate his impulses. Therefore, to feel safe he needed to know if the therapist would be physically strong enough to keep him and the therapist safe if he were to be triggered and spin out of control. One of his favorite ways of testing the limits of this burning issue was to ask the therapist to play the role of a child care worker and in pretend play restrain him on the floor after he acted out in the cottage in a dangerous way that put other youth at risk. In his scenarios, there was no choice. If the therapist was a responsible child care worker, he could not let him continue in his behavior because someone was going to get hurt, so it met the narrow criteria that not only justified but required physical restraint. Luke would instruct the therapist as to how he was to restrain and hold him on the floor, and he would fight violently against the therapist's attempts. The entire second floor of the Main Building in the residential program knew that the therapist was having his weekly session with Luke because no other play therapy session during the week matched the loudness and intensity of the sessions with Luke.

At times, the therapist did set limits and asked Luke to turn down the dial on his angry, violent struggles. But the authors' reading of what was happening is that he needed the therapist to be strong and competent enough that he could project onto the therapist his seething rage and hold it for him while he was not yet strong enough to contain it himself. There were limits on how physical the therapist was willing to let things go. The therapist was determined that he would not hurt Luke and Luke would not hurt him. When the therapist needed him to dial down the intensity of the rage/violence, Luke was responsive because he shared the same goals. At times, the therapist would leave the sessions perspiring as if he had just left the gym after a vigorous workout. Thankfully, when the issue was settled, in Luke's mind the intensity gradually decreased. Prior to engaging in such physical struggles, the therapist had offered alternatives such as acting out these scenes with puppets, which Luke firmly rejected. Luke was open to acting out some of the scenes for a few sessions using the miniatures children typically use in the play room to create a picture in the sandtray of their world. Luke was not interested in enacting his drama in the sand; he preferred enacting the drama on top of the wooden cover to the sandtray.

Typically, the drama would entail a violent out-of-control person who was a menace to others. Sometimes he would bring the replica of a jail in the playroom into the play. The villain/menace would be in jail but was threatening to break out and sometimes did break out. The theme was consistent with his need for containment of out-of-control scary, aggressive feelings/impulses and the conflict and struggle surrounding this effort.

The scenarios enacted on top of the lid of the sandtray were not satisfying to Luke, and after a few sessions, he preferred to act them out with human actors, typically just Luke and the therapist. However, on a few occasions, with Luke's agreement, we called in interns on short notice to fulfill a role in Luke's script. It was quite fascinating to observe that despite Luke's well-known cognitive limitations and significant learning deficits, he always had a scenario in mind to play out when he arrived in the playroom, often building on the previous session. By way of precaution, the therapist made sure that Luke instructed him on how to restrain him and how much force and pressure he wanted the therapist to use so that it was clear that the therapist was doing this at Luke's direction and under his control. To further reinforce that view, the therapist checked with him frequently and asked, "Am I doing this right?" "Do you want me to let you up?" "Tell me when you want me to loosen my grip on your arms?" If these had been enactments of trauma, he would not have initiated them and would have been triggered by engaging in such physical play.

It could be argued that what was happening during this phase was posttraumatic play. A plausible idea is that Luke was enacting the restraints that were so frequent in his daily life during the first 6 months of placement. When the therapist followed up with him about the restraints, he would never accuse the staff of harshness, although he might blame another youngster for provoking him. At times, Luke would even state that the staff "restrain me to keep me safe." The authors believe that the restraints were not traumatizing but rather that Luke pushed frequently to the limit, requiring restraint so that he could feel safe in the presence of his own internal rage and aggressive impulses. Furthermore, it was decided that he was testing the therapist in the play room to settle the same issue: "Can you keep me safe in light of my murderous rage and impulses?" Interestingly, when the issue was settled and he knew that the therapist could physically contain him if need be, the physical play stopped, and it was not revisited in the 3 years of weekly sessions that followed.

Snapshot 2: The Battles in Court and "To Whom Do I Belong?"

Although Luke and Cara didn't know the details, they were aware that their mother was fighting to get them back and to reunify the family. They knew that there was a lengthy struggle in court because they were interviewed multiple times by the attorney assigned to represent them. On one occasion, the therapist transported Luke and Cara to family court and waited in the waiting room while they were interviewed by the judge in the company of the attorney assigned to them. Luke and Cara told the therapist later that they both had unequivocally told the judge that they wanted to return to their mother. Luke assumed that this would happen right away, but, of course, these issues are only resolved after lengthy court sessions and after testimony from key parties. The decision that Luke would be working toward reconciliation and reunification with his mother was not made until nearly 2 years later. The frustration and rage this provoked in Luke dominated his functioning for more than a year.

Fortunately, Luke had learned to channel his rage into mostly verbal lashing out at staff and sometimes at his therapist and his social worker, who was the primary liaison to his family. During this phase of the play therapy, Luke enacted frequent court scenes, often making the therapist the judge to decide if he could go home to his mother. In one particularly poignant court scene, a couple showed up and made a claim to the judge that they were the actual parents of Luke and that they had papers to prove it.

At first, the papers looked legitimate, but then Luke became impassioned and pleaded for the judge to look more closely because the papers were fake and these people were a fraud. Indeed, that is what the judge determined, and he threw the couple out of the court.

The fraudulent couple and fake documents seemed to symbolize for Luke all the numerous foster home placements that didn't work out and perhaps even his biological parents that in anger he would say chose drugs over him and his sister. During this period, he longed for a home and a family, and he even became open to another foster home. Luke had previously stated that he would never try again after his attempt to be in the same foster home where his sister presently lives had failed. He also asked his therapist and a young man working in his cottage as a child care worker with whom he became attached to adopt him. The young man, who was only 24, patiently explained that he still hadn't finished his education and was not in a secure enough situation to be an adoptive father. The therapist told Luke that, although he was a likeable youngster who had grown in many important ways, the relationship was a special one but a therapeutic one. The therapist could not be his father. The therapist explained that he already had children and grandchildren, but he understood how important it was for Luke to be part of a family and how difficult it was for him to be placed outside of his home. Luke understood, but in the case of both his child care worker and his therapist, it was hard for him to accept.

One area of astonishing growth for Luke during this period was in his academic life. Luke was in a self-contained special education class, and his reading and writing were quite limited. In the stable environment provided by the group care program, he developed greatly improved reading and math abilities and became invested in school for the first time. Luke almost never missed school. In fact, in the most recent school year, the program sent the five youths in the program with the best school attendance records at the end of the year to Disneyworld His academic skill improvement was quite important to Luke because he had been embarrassed, and often humiliated, in the past about his inability to read or to make change.

Snapshot 3: The Need to Be Powerful Driven by a "Flashbulb Memory"

During this phase of his play dramas, Luke wanted to be recognized for his strength and physical skills in a more sublimated form than was evident in *Snapshot #1*. He wanted to act-out a play scenario repeated over many sessions of being the undefeated heavyweight boxing champion of the world. When he pretended to enter the ring, Luke would play his own handpicked music on his phone to accompany his grand entry. At times he would instruct the therapist to be the ring announcer, other times the coach in his corner who would talk to him and encourage him between rounds, and sometimes his body guard. The job of the bodyguard (therapist) was to fend off the autograph seekers and the adoring fans who wanted to get as close as possible to the champ. The fantasy of being king of the boxing world was extremely gratifying to Luke, who faced repeated defeats and humiliations throughout his life. He played it out with great gusto and pride. The feeling in the room was that here was a young boy yearning for acceptance, respect, and admiration when his life had been replete with rejections, loss, and trauma.

Luke's need to view himself as strong and fierce, however, had deeper roots. An indelible memory so vivid in his mind could be considered as a "flashbulb memory" because its emotional impact created a lasting imprint of the quality of a photograph. The memory was one in which his mother was beaten brutally by one of her abusive boyfriends, and all he could do was watch because he was not big enough and strong enough to stop it.

Snapshot 5: Serving a Life Sentence

As court deliberations and the slow, grinding process of looking for alternative placements continued without resolution, Luke now approaching 13 years of age grew more depressed, enraged, and hopeless. This was symbolized in the playroom by a central feature of play therapy, turning the passive into attempts at active mastery, as Luke pretended to be a prison guard and the therapist became the prisoner. The prisoner (therapist) was accused of various crimes but was not given a fair hearing in court to explain his side of the story and was ordered to jail. The cell was the utility closet in the playroom where additional supplies are kept for the playroom. When put in the cell, the prisoner protested and complained loudly that no one was listening to his side of the story and that a great injustice was being done. With each protest and complaint, the prisoner's sentence would get longer. The jailer became the judge and jury, and there was no one to represent the prisoner's interests. (This represented Luke's feelings of betrayal that his attorney did not advocate for his interests in court because she did not support his mother's fight for reunification.) At one point, Luke opened the door and screamed at the prisoner: "You never are going to see your mother again!" At that point, Luke made it crystal clear what this was all about: a boy separated from his mother for what felt like a lifetime, with no reason to hope that there would ever be a reunion.

It became clear to the therapist in his role as the prisoner that he was fighting a losing battle. The therapist experienced in his cell a small degree of the hopelessness that Luke felt but in Luke's case in more intense proportions. The therapist began to voice such feelings: "I've lost hope"; "It doesn't matter what you do to me" (at times the guard was quite harsh). Interestingly, as the therapist reflected with great affect the feelings that he knew intuitively that Luke was feeling, Luke's attitude as the prison guard noticeably softened. He was kinder and offered the prisoner treats rarely offered to the prisoners. Luke's shocking change of attitude culminated in his releasing the prisoner. Luke told the prisoner to never tell, but he (as the guard) had put up his own money to bail the inmate out. The prisoner told the "guard" that he was not surprised because all along, even though the guard could be mean and harsh on the outside, he could always tell that the jailer had a kind and generous heart. The therapist knew well of Luke's kind and generous heart. At the end of the summer work program the previous year that Luke participated in, he earned a check of $450.00; his social worker took him to a bank to cash it. On the way back, Luke spotted a homeless man with a cardboard sign asking for money. Luke wanted to give his entire summer earnings to the man. His social worker was finally able to convince him to give $20 and to save the rest in an account that she supervised for him.

Snapshot 6: A Reprieve from the Powers That Be

The details of how Luke's mother finally won her court battle to reunite with her son is beyond the scope of this chapter and could comprise a whole book itself. The play therapist testified on her behalf and represented the strong, clearly stated wishes of her son, Luke. Finally, through the mother's heroic efforts and her court-appointed public defender, the path was finally cleared for Luke to return to his mother with the requirement that there be ongoing family therapy to enhance the chances of the reunification succeeding. The first time that Luke met with his mother in years was a joy to behold. He was so thrilled to see her. To know that she was alive, that she was clean and had been sober for almost 4 years, and that she was not involved in a relationship of any kind, let alone an abusive one, gave Luke a sense of relief and peace that had eluded him in his 4 years of placement. Likewise, for his mother to lay eyes on him and see that he too was okay and had grown taller than she was, and had developed into this muscular adolescent boy now approaching 14, was moving beyond words to the therapist.

This young man displayed remarkable courage: in family sessions leading up to discharge to his mother, Luke confronted her with his anger that she and his father had let him and his sister down by their drinking, drug abuse, and fighting with each other. Luke also expressed his anger about her choice of abusive boyfriends and his worry that she would make the same mistake again. Luke was greatly relieved that his mother could hear his anger without getting defensive or making excuses. She agreed that their actions had hurt him and his sister in a devastating way. As of this writing, Luke lives at home with his mother, and the weekly family therapy sessions continue to provide support to both Luke and his mother.

Empirical Support for Play Therapy for Aggressive Behaviors

Our search of play therapy outcome research from 1995 to the present resulted in a total of 43 outcome studies. These studies investigated the impact of play therapy on reducing externalizing problems across varying populations of children, presenting concerns, and play therapy modalities, via the online play therapy research database, play therapy publications, and personal communication with play therapy researchers (Bratton et al., 2015; Bratton & Swan, 2017). Forty-two of the studies that measured change in externalizing problems reported observable reduction in externalizing problems, including rule-breaking and aggressive behaviors, after receiving play therapy intervention. Five outcome studies in the past decade specified recruitment to children demonstrating "aggressive behaviors," all of which reported decreases in these behaviors (Momeni & Kahrizi, 2015; Ray, Blanco, Sullivan, & Holliman, 2009; Ritzi, Ray, & Schumann, 2017; Schumann, 2010; Wilson & Ray, 2018).

Wilson and Ray (2018) conducted a large randomized controlled study using descriptive discriminant analysis to investigate the impact of receiving child-centered play therapy (CCPT) for children referred for aggressive behaviors. Parents perceived their children as less aggressive, more self-regulated, and more empathic through participating in CCPT compared to the waitlist control group. Results confirmed that participation in play therapy was predictive of a decline in aggressive behaviors (Wilson & Ray, 2018). In conjunction with reducing aggressive behaviors, play therapy also bolsters children's self-concepts and enriches children's interpersonal relational connections, establishing a reservoir of inner resources that children can access during future experiences of pain or loss.

Play therapy is a well-established school intervention for improving children's behavior, with over 56 outcome studies documenting its effect on child behavior in school settings (Bratton et al., 2015). Alternative school-based play therapy interventions demonstrate positive influence for children who exhibit externalizing behaviors, such as play-based school mentor, parent, and teacher support programs (Ceballos & Bratton, 2010; Jones, Rhine, & Bratton, 2002; Morrison & Bratton, 2011; Sheely & Bratton, 2010).

Conclusion

Aggressive behavior is an external communication of children's internal anger and rage. Play therapists listen to children's behavior as witnesses to their frustrations and provide containment and safety for children to express unspoken pain through play. Like Luke in the case vignette, children who experience adverse life events may begin to anticipate relationships to be unsafe, distrustful, unstable, and threatening. Relational trauma can underlie children's intense and valid anger/rage, externalized as observable aggressive behaviors. Play therapists provide a safe therapeutic environment in which children can begin to integrate their aggressive impulses and unconscious desires into conscious play and action. In play therapy, Luke was allowed the freedom to express his aggression and rage within the physical safety and emotional containment of the therapeutic relationship. Luke's story was a journey of working through and processing his aggression and deep relational hurts through self-directed play and corrective relational experiences.

Play therapy research demonstrates positive therapeutic outcomes for children who exhibit aggressive behaviors. Play therapy may last as short as 16 sessions, as in aggression research studies, and as long as 4 years, as in the case example of Luke. Play therapy can be delivered as prevention to children identified as at risk for developing aggressive behaviors and as intervention to mitigate the long-term effects of pervasive aggressive behaviors resulting from relational trauma.

REFERENCES

Achenbach, T. M. (1994). Child Behavior Checklist and related instruments. In M. E. Maruish (Ed.), *The use of psychological testing for treatment planning and outcome assessment* (pp. 517–549). Hillsdale, NJ: Erlbaum.

Augsburger, M., Dohrmann, K., Schauer, M., & Elbert, T. (2016). Relations between traumatic stress, dimensions of impulsivity, and reactive and appetitive aggression in individuals with refugee status. *Psychological Trauma, 9*(1), 137–144.

Barnes, S., Howell, K., Thurston, I., & Cohen, R. (2017). Children's attitudes toward aggression: Associations with depression, aggression, and perceived maternal/peer responses to anger. *Journal of Child and Family Studies, 26*(3), 748–758.

Baydar, N., & Akcinar, B. (2018). Reciprocal relations between the trajectories of mothers' harsh discipline, responsiveness and aggression in early childhood. *Journal of Abnormal Child Psychology, 46*(1), 83–97.

Boxer, P. (2007). Aggression in very high-risk youth: Examining developmental risk in an inpatient psychiatric population. *American Journal of Orthopsychiatry, 77*(4), 636–646.

Bratton, S. C., Dafoe, E., Swan, A., Opiola, K., McClintock, D., & Barcenas, G. (2015). Evidence-based child therapy: Play therapy outcome research database. Retrieved from *http://evidencebasedchildtherapy.com/research*.

Bratton, S. C., & Swan, A. (2017). Status of play therapy research. In R. L. Steen (Ed.), *Emerging research in play therapy and consultation* (pp. 1–18). Hershey, PA: IGI Global.

Campaert, K., Nocentini, A., & Menesini, E. (2018). The role of poor parenting and parental approval for children's moral disengagement. *Journal of Child and Family Studies, 27*(8), 2656–2667.

Card, N. A., Stucky, B. D., Sawalani, G. M., & Little, T. D. (2008). Direct and indirect aggression during childhood and adolescence: A meta-analytic review of gender differences, intercorrelations, and relations to maladjustment. *Child Development, 79*(5), 1185–1229.

Cavett, A. (2015). Cognitive-behavioral play therapy. In D. A. Crenshaw & A. L. Stewart (Eds.), *Play therapy: A comprehensive guide to theory and practice* (pp. 83–88). New York: Guilford Press.

Ceballos, P. L., & Bratton, S. C. (2010). Empowering Latino families: Effects of a culturally responsive intervention for low-income immigrant Latino parents on children's behaviors and parental stress. *Psychology in the Schools, 47*(8), 761–775.

Chng, B., & Tan, C. (2017). The effect of perceived racial discrimination on aggression. *Journal of Social Science and Humanities, 25*(1), 461–472.

Crenshaw, D., & Hardy, K. V. (2005). Fawns in gorilla suits: Understanding and treating the aggression of children in the foster care system. In N. B. Webb (Ed.), *Working with traumatized youth in child welfare* (pp. 171–195). New York: Guilford Press.

Crenshaw, D., & Hardy, K. V. (2007). The crucial role of empathy in breaking the silence of traumatized children in play therapy. *International Journal of Play Therapy, 16*(2), 160–175.

Crenshaw, D. A., & Tillman, K. S. (2013). Access to the unconscious. In C. E. Schaefer & A. A. Drewes (Eds.), *The therapeutic powers of play: 20 core agents of change* (pp. 25–38). Hoboken, NJ: Wiley.

Cui, L., Colasante, T., Malti, T., Ribeaud, D., Eisner, M., & Eisner, M. P. (2016). Dual trajectories of reactive and proactive aggression from mid-childhood to early adolescence: Relations to sensation seeking, risk taking, and moral reasoning. *Journal of Abnormal Child Psychology, 44*(4), 663–675.

Cullerton-Sen, C., Cassidy, A. R., Murray-Close, D., Cicchetti, D., Crick, N. R., & Rogosch, F. A. (2008). Childhood maltreatment and the development of relational and physical aggression: The importance of a gender-informed approach. *Child Development, 79*(6), 1736–1751.

De Castro, B. O., Brendgen, M., Van Boxtel, H., Vitaro, F., & Schaepers, L. (2007). "Accept Me, or Else . . .": Disputed overestimation of social competence predicts increases in proactive aggression. *Journal of Abnormal Child Psychology, 35*(2), 165–178.

Finzi, R., Ram, A., Har-Even, R., Shnit, D., & Weizman, A. (2001). Attachment styles and aggression in physically abused and neglected children. *Journal of Youth and Adolescence, 30*(6), 769–786.

Gabriel, L., James, H., Cronin, D. J., Tizro, Z., Beetham, T., Hullock, A., & Raynar, A. (2017). Reflexive research with mothers and children victims of domestic violence. *Counselling and Psychotherapy Research, 17*(2), 157–165.

Gach, E. J., Ip, K. I., Sameroff, A. J., & Olson, S. L. (2018). Early cumulative risk predicts externalizing behavior at age 10: The mediating role of adverse parenting. *Journal of Family Psychology, 32*(1), 92–102.

Halperin, J. M., & McKay, K. E. (2012). *CAS Children's Aggression Scale: Professional manual.* Lutz, FL: Psychological Assessment Resources.

Hamama, L., & Arazi, Y. (2012). Aggressive behaviour in at-risk children: Contribution of subjective well-being and family cohesion. *Child and Family Social Work, 17*(3), 284–295.

Hardy, K. V., & Crenshaw, D. A. (2008). Healing the wounds to the soul camouflaged by rage. In D. A. Crenshaw (Ed.), *Child and adolescent psychotherapy* (pp. 15–20). Lanham, MD: Jason Aronson/Rowman & Littlefield.

Hardy, K. V., & Laszloffy, T. A. (2005). *Teens who hurt: Clinical interventions to break the cycle of adolescent violence.* New York: Guilford Press.

Harrison, A., Genders, R., Davies, H., Treasure, J., & Tchanturia, K. (2011). Experimental measurement of the regulation of anger and aggression in women with anorexia nervosa. *Clinical Psychology and Psychotherapy, 18*(6), 445–452.

Hay, C., Meldrom, R., Widdowson, A., & Piquero, A. (2016). Early aggression and later delinquency: Considering the redirecting role of good parenting. *Youth Violence and Juvenile Justice, 15*(4), 374–395.

Houston, J., & Grych, J. (2016). Maternal attachment buffers the association between exposure to violence and youth attitudes about aggression. *Journal of Clinical Child and Adolescent Psychology, 45*(5), 605–613.

Jansen, E., Miller, A. L., Lumeng, J. C., Kaciroti, N., Herb, H. E. B., Horodynski, M. A., et al. (2017). Externalizing behavior is prospectively associated with intake of added sugar and sodium among low socioeconomic status preschoolers in a sex-specific manner. *International Journal of Behavioral Nutrition and Physical Activity, 14*, 135.

Jones, L., Rhine, T., & Bratton, S. (2002). High school students as therapeutic agents with young children experiencing school adjustment difficulties: The effectiveness of a filial therapy training model. *International Journal of Play Therapy, 11*(2), 43–62.

Kokko, K., & Pulkkinen, L. (2000). Aggression in childhood and long-term unemployment in adulthood: A cycle of maladaptation and some protective factors. *Developmental Psychology, 36*(4), 463–472.

Mazurek, M., & Sohl, K. (2016). Sleep and behavioral problems in children with autism spectrum disorder. *Journal of Autism and Developmental Disorders, 46*(6), 1906–1915.

McQuade, J. D., Breaux, R. P., Gómez, A. F., Zakarian, R. J., Weatherly, J., & Gómez, A. F. (2016). Biased self-perceived social competence and engagement in subtypes of aggression: Examination of peer rejection, social dominance goals, and sex of the child as moderators. *Aggressive Behavior, 42*(5), 498–509.

Merrell, K. W. (2011). *Social Emotional Assets and Resilience Scale: Professional manual.* Lutz, FL: Psychological Assessment Resources.

Momeni, K., & Kahrizi, S. (2015). The effectiveness of sand play therapy on the reduction of the aggression in preschool children. *Journal of Iranian Psychologists, 11*(42), 147–158.

Mordock, J. B. (2015). Psychodynamic play therapy. In D. A. Crenshaw & A. L. Stewart (Eds.), *Play therapy: A comprehensive guide to theory and practice* (pp. 66–82). New York: Guilford Press.

Morrison, M., & Bratton, S. C. (2011). The effects of child teacher relationship training on the children of focus: A pilot study. *International Journal of Play Therapy, 20*(4), 193–207.

Neller, D. J., Denney, R. L., Pietz, C. A., & Thomlinson, R. P. (2006). The relationship between trauma and violence in a jail inmate sample. *Journal of Interpersonal Violence, 21*(9), 1234–1241.

Ostrov, J. M., & Crick, N. R. (2007). Forms and functions of aggression during early childhood: A short-term longitudinal study. *School Psychology Review, 36*(1), 22–43.

Piché, G., Huỳnh, C., Clément, M., & Durrant, J. E. (2017). Predicting externalizing and prosocial behaviors in children from parental use of corporal punishment. *Infant and Child Development, 26*(4), 1–18.

Prinstein, M., & La Greca, A. (2004). Childhood peer rejection and aggression as predictors of adolescent girls' externalizing and health risk behaviors: A 6-year longitudinal study. *Journal of Consulting and Clinical Psychology, 72*(1), 103–112.

Ray, D. C., Blanco, P. J., Sullivan, J. M., & Holliman, R. (2009). An exploratory study of child-centered play therapy with aggressive children. *International Journal of Play Therapy, 18*(3), 162–175.

Reef, J., Diamantopoulou, D., van Meurs I., Verhulst, F., & van der Ende, J. (2011). Developmental trajectories of child to adolescent externalizing behavior and adult DSM-IV disorder: Results of a 24-year longitudinal study. *Social Psychiatry and Psychiatric Epidemiology, 46*(12), 1233–1241.

Ritzi, R. M., Ray, D. C., & Schumann, B. R. (2017). Intensive short-term child-centered play therapy and externalizing behaviors in children. *International Journal of Play Therapy, 26*(1), 33–46.

Rubens, S., Evans, S., Becker, S., Fite, P., Tountas, A., Rubens, S. L., et al. (2017). Self-reported time in bed and sleep quality in association with internalizing and externalizing symptoms in school-age youth. *Child Psychiatry and Human Development, 48*(3), 455–467.

Sacco, P., Bright, C., Jun, H.-J., & Stapleton, L. (2015). Developmental relations between alcohol and aggressive behavior among adolescents: Neighborhood and sociodemographic correlates. *International Journal of Mental Health and Addiction, 13*(5), 603–617.

Schaefer, C. E. (1995). *The therapeutic powers of play.* New York: Jason Aronson.

Schaefer, C. E., & Drewes, A. A. (Eds.). (2013). *The therapeutic powers of play: 20 core agents of change.* Hoboken, NJ: Wiley.

Schumann, B. (2010). Effectiveness of child centered play therapy for children referred for aggression in elementary school. In J. Baggerly, D. Ray, & S. Bratton (Eds.), *Child-centered play therapy research: The evidence base for effective practice* (pp. 193–208). Hoboken, NJ: Wiley.

Scott, B. G., Lapré, G. E., Marsee, M. A., & Weems, C. F. (2014). Aggressive behavior and its associations with posttraumatic stress and academic achievement following a natural disaster. *Journal of Clinical Child and Adolescent Psychology, 43*(1), 43–50.

Sheely, A. I., & Bratton, S. C. (2010). A strengths-based parenting intervention with low-income African American families. *Professional School Counseling, 13*(3), 175–183.

White, B. A., & Kistner, J. A. (2011). Biased self-perceptions, peer rejection, and aggression in children. *Journal of Abnormal Child Psychology, 39*(5), 645–656.

Wilson, B. J., & Ray, D. (2018). Child-centered play therapy: Aggression, empathy, and self-regulation. *Journal of Counseling and Development, 96*(4), 399–409.

PART V

Clinical Applications of Prescriptive Play Therapy for Other Disorders

CHAPTER 13

Play Therapy for Children with Autism Spectrum Disorder

Robert Jason Grant

Description of the Disorder

Autism spectrum disorder (ASD) is a neurodevelopmental disorder characterized by communication and social deficits. Children with ASD tend to have communication deficits, such as responding inappropriately in conversation, or difficulty building friendships. They may be overly dependent on routines, sensitive to changes in their environment, or intensely focused on certain items (Hillman, 2018). Children with ASD struggle to develop and grow socially and emotionally in a pattern similar to their typically developing peers. They frequently have difficulties initiating and joining in play, understanding turn taking, building friendships, and participating in reciprocal social interactions (Salter, Beamish, & Davies, 2016).

The Centers for Disease Control and Prevention (2018) stated that 1 in 59 children is estimated to have ASD. It is three to four times more common in boys than in girls. ASD is a lifelong condition, but many children diagnosed with ASD go on to live independent, productive, and fulfilling lives, especially with the benefit of early and continuous intervention and therapies. The American Psychiatric Association (2013) has defined ASD as a complex developmental condition that involves persistent challenges in social interaction, speech and nonverbal communication, and restricted/repetitive behaviors. The effects of ASD and the severity of symptoms are different in each person. The characteristics of ASD fall into two categories:

1. Social interaction and communication problems, including difficulties in normal back-and-forth conversation, reduced sharing of
   interests or emotions, challenges in understanding or responding to
   social cues such as eye contact and facial expressions, and deficits
   in developing/maintaining/understanding relationships.
2. Restricted and repetitive patterns of behaviors, interests, or activities, including hand-flapping and toe-walking, playing with toys
   in an uncommon way (such as lining up cars or flipping objects),
   speaking in a unique way (such as using odd patterns or pitches
   in speaking or "scripting" from favorite shows), having significant
   need for a predictable routine or structure, and exhibiting intense
   interests in activities that are uncommon for a similarly aged child.

According to Howard, Copeland, Lindaman, and Cross (2018), children with ASD typically show deficits in early infancy, namely, in the areas
of play, stereotypical behaviors, and shared attention. They tend to struggle
with symbolic play and prefer to play alone, and they show a preference for
toys based on sensory stimulation. Children with ASD also display a repetitive and stereotypical quality to their play and it can be challenging for
peers to navigate when they are trying to engage with the child with ASD.
Further, deficits in joint attention and theory of mind skills contribute to
social struggles that impede successful peer interactions.

Developmental delays and differences in underlying capacities for joint
attention, imitation, and social reciprocity are all closely intertwined with
an emerging capacity for play. Research suggests that children with ASD
have specific impairments in regard to symbolic, pretend, and peer (group)
play (Kossyvaki & Papoudi, 2016; Stagnitti & Pfeifer, 2017; Banerjee &
Ray, 2013). Children with autism present unique profiles that manifest in
spontaneous engagement with toys, activities, and themes. Their play often
becomes fixated (Wolfberg, Bottema-Beutel, & DeWitt, 2012). Pretend and
spontaneous play is often limited, with the child usually relying heavily
on adult prompts. Through pretend play and peer interactions, typically
developing children explore social roles and rules to build mutual meaning.
They develop understanding of the relationships between peers and adults
and the ability to infer others' needs, beliefs, and intentions (Hess, 2006).

Wolfberg (1999) proposed that children must be able to enter a social
group and coordinate the mutual activity to engage in play with peers or
other partners. Play supports the exploration of social roles when children
learn to compromise and become aware of and understand the mental states
of others. Children with ASD who lack play skills, specifically in the areas
of pretend, symbolic, and peer play, are highly susceptible to being left out
and rejected by neurotypical peers. They are likely to be socially isolated
and bullied, and to develop a negative self-worth. Further, they miss out not

only on peer social benefits of play but a whole host of other learning and problem-solving mechanisms that are typically developed through play.

An ASD diagnosis typically accompanies play challenges as well as difficulties in relating and forming relationships, verbal and nonverbal communication, and executive functioning skills. ASD is a complex developmental disorder. Problems can express themselves differently and can appear in various combinations. Not every child with the same generic diagnostic label has all these problems to the same degree (Greenspan & Wieder, 2006). ASD ranges from severe to mild in terms of an individual's impairment. A child on the severe end of the spectrum may be unable to speak and may also have more serious developmental delays. A child on the mild end of the spectrum may be able to function in a regular classroom at school and may eventually reach a point where he or she no longer meets the criteria for ASD. Even if two children have the same diagnosis, no two children with an ASD are alike (Grant, 2017a).

Considering that children with ASD present on a spectrum that produces several "looks" of autism, it is necessary that interventions and therapies be adaptable and flexible to meet the various manifestations of ASD. The individual child and how his or her ASD affects his or her functioning must be assessed and considered when choosing the best, most appropriate course of treatment. Skill strengths and deficits will widely differ from child to child, as well as according to family resources and access to therapies. The ASD play therapist must be prepared for such variance and be willing and able to take a prescriptive play therapy approach to addressing ASD issues.

Rationale for Prescriptive Play Therapy

Play is the natural language of children, including children with ASD. It is often the easiest way for children to express troubling thoughts and feelings that are both conscious and unconscious. By making learning an enjoyable and engaging experience, therapists are best able to impart the information children need to overcome knowledge and skill deficits (Schaefer & Drewes, 2014). The therapeutic powers of play refer to the specific change agents in which play initiates, facilitates, or strengthens the therapeutic effect. These play powers act as mediators that positively influence the desired change in the client (Barron & Kenny, 1986) and provide the foundational framework for the clinical understanding and use of play therapy (VanFleet & Faa-Thompson, 2017).

Prescriptive play therapy is a therapist-informed method of selecting and implementing a particular play therapy approach that research has indicated is likely to be the most effective for a specific problem or symptom.

The basic premise underlying prescriptive play therapy, a therapy created by Charles Schaefer (2001), is the notion that all play therapy approaches have the potential to be the one most useful for some children, and that no single approach is the best fit for all children. The goal of treatment in prescriptive play therapy is to identify the best possible evidence-based intervention or strategy to maximize symptom reduction and promote overall therapeutic gain (O'Connor & Braverman, 2009). A prescriptive play therapy approach is particularly concerned with identifying the unique aspects of clinical theory and application having the greatest potential for a positive impact on the target problem or issue. A prescriptive approach does not require therapists to adhere strictly to the initial treatment chosen. Because the overarching goal is symptom relief, therapists explore alternative treatments if the initial choice proves unsuccessful (Schaefer, 2001).

Several play therapy approaches have shown success in treating children with ASD, most notably filial therapy (VanFleet, 2012), Theraplay® (Booth & Jernbeg, 2010), child-centered play therapy (Hillman, 2018), and AutPlay® Therapy (Grant, 2017a). Multiple research has promoted the importance of play for children with ASD (Kuhaneck & Britner, 2013; Barry et al., 2003; Wolfberg et al., 2012; Hess, 2006; Overley, Degges-White, Snow, Mossing, & Holmes, 2018). Play therapy is continuing to grow in importance as a valid and needed treatment approach for children with ASD. Play therapy has been shown to help children with ASD increase their social play skills, improve emotional expression, decrease unwanted behaviors (Salter et al., 2016), improve reactive and symbolic play, communication, specific social interactions with peers, and provide improvement in the parent–child relationship (Howard et al., 2018).

Banerjee and Ray (2013) proposed that some core ASD deficits can be addressed through play therapy such as communication improvements, relationship development, and recognition and expression of emotion. Further, they reported that play therapy can be effective for gains in sensorimotor play, constructive play skills, pretend play skills, functional play, and socialization skills, and for reducing problem behaviors. Kasari, Chang, and Patterson (2013) reported that play interventions for children with ASD are critical to later developmental outcomes, including language, cognitive, and social abilities. Children with ASD need the opportunity for and interventions for increasing play skills that have the potential for a whole host of benefits. Grant (2018) reported that play therapy approaches such as AutPlay Therapy are showing increasing evidence that play-based interventions are effective in treating children and their families affected by ASD. Play provides a natural and engaging element for all children, and play therapy interventions provide the skill component that children need to increase their functioning ability. The combination of play and skill-based interventions is not only gaining research support, but also presents a logical approach to treating children and families dealing with ASD issues.

Although research has demonstrated the success of play therapy approaches for working with children with ASD, the research covers a wide range of play therapy theories and models. Several of the studies cited in this chapter cover a range of models, including child-centered play therapy, filial therapy, Theraplay, developmental play therapy, sensorimotor play therapy, family play therapy, and behavioral-based play therapy. These studies show positive results for the greater field of play therapy but also emphasize the need for a prescriptive play therapy approach when working with children with ASD. As several play therapy models have been shown to be effective, it is important for the ASD play therapist to ask, "What approach is the best approach for the individual child I am working with?" and for the ASD play therapist to understand that the approach will likely change from child to child, even within the same diagnosis category of ASD.

Schaefer and Drewes (2014) presented 20 core change agents of the therapeutic powers of play. These change agents include self-expression, access to the unconscious, direct teaching, indirect teaching, catharsis, abreaction, positive emotions, counterconditioning fears, stress inoculation, stress management, therapeutic relationship, attachment, social competence, empathy, creative problem solving, resiliency, moral development, accelerated psychological development, self-regulation, and self-esteem. The change agents highlight the prescriptive play therapy approach. Being able to identify the specific needs of the child and finding the right approach with the most effective change agents will produce the best outcome. Through specific consideration and selection of the cores change agents, children with ASD can learn social skills, develop relationships, learn how to communicate and express themselves through verbal and nonverbal means, improve emotional regulation ability, and develop problem-solving abilities.

AutPlay® Therapy

AutPlay Therapy is an integrative approach that follows a prescriptive play therapy formula. Each child is individually assessed to identify skill strengths, deficits, developmental level, and family resources to guide further implementation of treatment. Each child will have his or her own prescribed treatment plan implementing evidence-based practices and a methodology that appears to be the best, most effective approach for that child. AutPlay Therapy (Grant, 2017a) is a play therapy and behavioral therapy approach for working with children and adolescents with ASD and other neurodevelopmental disorders. AutPlay Therapy involves both the child and the parent in the therapeutic process. Using a play therapy base that is a natural language for the child enables parents to be involved with their child in a way that teaches skills and increases abilities within a enjoyable and connecting process. The child and parents work through three phases of treatment: intake and assessment phase, structured intervention phase, and termination phase. Treatment approaches and goals typically focus on six struggle areas common to ASD: emotional regulation, social functioning, connection (relationship development), anxiety reduction, sensory processing, and behavior change.

The AutPlay Therapy protocol can potentially incorporate and address any of the 20 core agents of change of the therapeutic powers of play. AutPlay utilizes structured play therapy interventions that are specifically chosen or created for the individual child. Each intervention embodies one or more of the 20 core agents of change, depending on the child's assessed needs. Although any of the core change agents could be identified and addressed with a child with ASD, typically children with an ASD diagnosis benefit from a focus on direct teaching, positive emotions, stress management, stress inoculation, empathy, therapeutic relationship, positive peer relationship, counterconditioning fears, social competence, and self-regulation.

AutPlay Therapy Intervention and the Therapeutic Powers of Play

Action Identification (Grant, 2017a) is an AutPlay intervention designed for both children and adolescents to address social skill improvement and behavior change. The intervention can be implemented using index cards and something to write with, or it may be implemented with no materials. Children with ASD often struggle with expected and unexpected behaviors in various situations. Action Identification is an engaging and interactive intervention that helps children recognize expected versus unexpected behavior in certain situations (context) and provides the opportunity to practice expected responses.

The therapist explains to the child that they will begin by writing behaviors on index cards. The therapist takes two index cards and in turn gives the child two index cards. Both the therapist and the child then write two common child behaviors on the index cards. The behaviors the therapist writes down should be those that the child is currently struggling with in some setting. The child can write whatever behaviors come to mind. Some examples of behaviors might include shoving people while waiting in line, running out of the school building, yelling at one's sister, taking one's clothes off in public, and interrupting the teacher when she is talking.

Once the behaviors have been written down, the therapist explains that they will each act out the behaviors they have written on the cards and the other person has to guess what the behavior is. The person who guessed the behavior has to explain when and where the behavior would be expected and when and where the behavior would not be expected. For example, the therapist might write down running out of the classroom at school. The therapist would then act out running out of the room. Once the child guessed the behavior correctly, the child would have to share with the therapist when or where this behavior would be expected (playing a game of hide and go seek) and when and where the behavior would not be expected (while sitting in a classroom at school). The child would then act out one of his or her behaviors and the therapist would have to guess, etc. The therapist and child can go through several different behaviors and continue playing the intervention until the child is no longer interested.

There is no specific number of behaviors to begin with; for example, the therapist could use three index cards and do three behaviors. The therapist could even make no use of cards and could simply tell the child to think of a common behavior children do and then act out the behavior; the therapist would then try to guess the behavior. This is a more appropriate version for children who do not write because of age or developmental issues. The therapist will want to apply the behaviors to the child's real life if applicable in order to help the child decrease unexpected behaviors. If the child is struggling to identify the expected versus unexpected situations (context), the practitioner should assist the child.

Children enjoy acting out the behaviors, by both the therapist and themselves. The therapist should incorporate their playful instinct when acting out the behaviors. It is acceptable to be silly and somewhat over the top with the acting-out portion of this intervention. Children will respond better to the discussion of expected and unexpected behaviors if they are enjoying the intervention. Action Identification helps develop social skills, specifically helping children identify when certain behaviors are expected or not expected and in what context or situations behaviors would be expected or unexpected. If the therapist is unsure of behaviors to work on with the child, then asking the parents for suggestions would be appropriate. Parents are taught this intervention and are instructed to play the intervention at home each day focusing on a few specific behaviors the child is having difficulty with.

Action Identification represents one of many play therapy interventions that might be chosen to address the specific needs of the child with ASD. This intervention highlights several of the core change agents of the therapeutic powers of play (Schaefer & Drewes, 2014).

- *Direct teaching*—involves receiving instruction, observing another individual modeling a skill, and participating in guided practice while experiencing positive reinforcement (Fraser, 2014). Action Identification is most present with this change agent. This intervention is heavily laden with observation, modeling, and practice, all of which are evidence-based practices for working with children with ASD.

- *Positive emotions*—involves the child experiencing, recognizing, and expressing positive emotions such as calm, satisfied, loved, and accepted (Kottman, 2014). Action Identification purposefully removes judgment about unexpected behaviors. Behaviors just are, and the focus is on when and where they are expected or not expected. Using the terminology expected/unexpected mitigates the feeling that the child exhibited "bad" behavior. Children can look at their behaviors more positively and feel empowered for change.

• *Stress inoculation*—involves children learning about and managing anxious feelings related to future events that are likely to be stressful (Cavett, 2014). Many children with ASD express unexpected behaviors due to unregulated stress and anxiety, much of which can come from not knowing what to do or think in a given situation. Action Identification gives children a tool to practice and understand what to do, which can decrease future stress and anxiety.

• *Therapeutic relationship*—involves a therapeutic alliance between the therapist and child which communicates value, nonjudgment, acceptance, and importance to the child (Steward & Echterling, 2014). Action Identification, as with any AutPlay intervention, accepts the child where he or she is at and always views skill deficits in a nonjudgmental capacity, but it is the greater protocol in AutPlay that highlights this change agent throughout each intervention. Structured interventions do not begin in AutPlay® until Session 5 or 6. Sessions prior to this are heavily focused on relationship development. In AutPlay, it is the relationship between the therapist and child that fosters the success of structured interventions.

• *Social competence*—involves the acquisition and successful utilization of social skills (Nash, 2014). Action Identification at its core is a social skill role play and practice intervention. The majority of evidence-based procedures for increasing social skills in children with ASD includes role play and repetitive practice.

• *Moral development*—involves the child's ability to be aware of and place value on rules or expectations and to weigh values relative to his or her developmental levels (Packman, 2014). Moral development is challenging for children with ASD. Socially decided-upon rules of right and wrong are often confusing for children with ASD. Action Identification helps children with ASD begin to understand social expectations and expected behaviors as the 'right" thing to do not only for themselves but also for others around them.

• *Self-regulation*—involves the ability of children to subordinate or regulate their actions, feelings, and thoughts, especially in response to their surroundings (Yeager & Yeager, 2014). Self-regulation is a valuable and challenging process for children with ASD. Action Identification begins the process of helping children understand that their actions/thoughts/feelings sometimes need to be managed or controlled, especially in certain contexts.

Parent and Family Involvement

The National Autism Center (2018) national standards project identified 27 evidence-based practices for working with children with ASD. One of the evidence-based practices is parent training and parent-implemented intervention. Multiple research has supported the importance of parent involvement in working with children with ASD (Solomon, Ono, Timmer, & Goodlin-Jones, 2008; Rogers et al., 2012). Parent involvement in the treatment of children with ASD is not a new concept. For decades, autism-focused treatments have included parents in the treatment process. Parental involvement may vary from treatment to treatment, but often parents are gaining education and awareness, being taught to advocate for their child, participating in therapy sessions with their child, and learning approaches and activities to implement with their child at home.

Research supports the need for therapists to work with parents who have a child with ASD and shows several benefits of working with parents, including providing familiarity and consistency, strengthening the parent–child relationship, and reducing parental stress. Many play-based ASD treatments involve parents and other family members in the treatment process (Greenspan & Wieder, 2006; MacDonald & Stoika, 2007; Solomon, 2012). Including parents in treatment for children with ASD offers many benefits: parents become the representative of what is outside the child and the foundation for reality; and the parent's ability to enter the child's symbolic world becomes the critical vehicle for fostering emotional differentiation and higher levels of abstract and logical thinking. The benefits of including parents and other family members in a family treatment process reach across the system, helping the child, parents, and other family members to achieve individual and family goals in a true systemic process (Grant, 2015; Greenberg & Wieder, 2006).

Family play therapy approaches such as Theraplay have produced some of the most substantial play therapy research for working with children with ASD (Howard et al., 2018). Family play therapy approaches and play approaches implementing parent training have been found to be effective in treating a wide range of presenting child problems. They embody directive and nondirective elements and focus on improving the parent–child relationship (Gil, 2015). Parent–child interaction therapy (PCIT) and parent–child psychotherapy (PCP) incorporate parent training and involvement, and both are considered evidence-based practices. Filial therapy, child–parent relationship therapy (CPRT), Theraplay, and AutPlay Therapy are all play therapy approaches, and all have substantial research to support positive treatment outcomes for children and families affected by ASD.

AutPlay Therapy is an integrative family play therapy approach that makes use of the methodology from other family play therapy approaches such as Theraplay, filial therapy, family play therapy, and cognitive-behavioral play therapy. Although play therapy as a whole is the base for AutPlay Therapy, the above-mentioned approaches have specific elements and constructs that have more directly impacted the work of AutPlay Therapy. The play therapy approaches of Theraplay, filial therapy, and family play therapy all provide a comprehensive treatment approach to working with child and parents in a family play therapy approach designed to create healthy relationship connection, problem solving, behavior modification, and, to some degree, skill development. These play therapy approaches focus on the child's ability to develop healthy and lasting relationships, with the primary focus of relationship development being the relationship between child and parent. Through this process, other issues such as reducing unwanted behaviors and improving skill development can also be mastered.

The AutPlay Therapy approach views parents as co-change agents with the play therapist. Parents are be encouraged, supported, and empowered to work with their child in ways that will be productive to established treatment goals. The therapist trains parents to implement structured play therapy interventions at home with their child. These interventions are typically chosen by the therapist (although parents often participate in choosing interventions) as interventions directly related to developing the child's identified skill deficits. Parent involvement fluctuates, depending on the child's specific needs and presenting issues. Parental involvement is a standard piece of the AutPlay protocol but may look different depending on the child's functioning level and skill deficits. The AutPlay therapist continues to work with both the child and the parents until treatment goals have been met.

Case Vignette: Calvin

Calvin entered play therapy when he was 6 years old. Three years earlier, he had been evaluated by a neuropsychologist and was diagnosed with autism spectrum disorder. He had participated in an early intervention program, and his parents stated that Calvin had been making steady improvements in communication and social development during the past few years. At the time Calvin began play therapy, he was halfway through his kindergarten school year. Calvin was attending a public school and was participating in an individualized education program that was providing him some accommodations at school. He was not participating in any other interventions when he began play therapy.

Calvin's parents brought him to therapy because they felt that AutPlay Therapy would help him improve his social skill deficits, especially social deficits related to interacting with his peer group. His parents expressed that Calvin had difficulty engaging in play with his peers and in talking with and interacting in meaningful ways with them. He also presented minor behavior problems when situations did not go the way he wanted. His parents described Calvin as mostly being socially isolated. He did not engage with other children, and when other children would try to interact with him, he would often ignore them or he would begin to participate and then abruptly leave the peer situation. Calvin appeared to be in his own thoughts and preferred to play independently. He also preferred to be in control of situations and became unhappy when others would implement any level of change or control in the way he wanted things to happen. Calvin's behaviors might escalate to yelling at or hitting another child or possibly even running away. His parents wanted AutPlay Therapy to help Calvin improve his play skills with others, especially his peers. They also wanted to see Calvin work and play cooperatively with other children, produce successful reciprocal play, and manage others being in control without displaying behavior problems.

Calvin lived with his biological father and mother and two older brothers (ages 10 and 11). His older brothers were both neurotypical. Calvin appeared to have a strong family support system. His parents were heavily invested in participating in therapy. Calvin and his family had an active social life and Calvin would, at times, participate in "play dates" with a family friend. Calvin's two older brothers were involved in soccer, and the family spent a great deal of time attending soccer practices and games.

Play Therapy sessions began with a phone intake that obtained information about Calvin's diagnosis and functioning level. An in-person intake session was scheduled, and the therapist emailed the family a social story about going to see a play therapist. The family was instructed to read the social story to Calvin daily until his appointment day (see Figure 13.1). The social story was designed to help Calvin become familiar with the therapy clinic, playroom, and therapist before arriving for his first appointment.

The first three play therapy sessions followed the AutPlay Therapy protocol for the intake and assessment phase. In this first phase of treatment, assessment procedures were implemented to gain more specific information about Calvin and were designed to help him and his parents build rapport with the play therapist. Calvin participated in a child observation session during which the play therapist observed him and his mother together in a child–parent interaction. Both observations were conducted in a play therapy room. Calvin's parents also completed four AutPlay Therapy

A play therapist is someone who plays with kids and tries to help them with their problems.

My mom or dad or both may take me to see the play therapist.

The play therapist usually has an office.

Sometimes my parents may see the play therapist with me.

Sometimes I may see the play therapist by myself.

There are toys to play with and other things to do at the play therapist's office.

I can play with the toys, games, and art materials.

The play therapist may talk to me.

I can talk to the play therapist, and that's okay.

I don't have to talk to the play therapist, and that's okay.

I can go to the play therapist's office and not feel nervous.

I can go to the play therapist's office and have fun.

I will try to go to the play therapist's office and feel better.

FIGURE 13.1. Calvin's social story: Going to see a play therapist.

inventories: the AutPlay Social Skills Inventory (child version), the AutPlay Emotional Regulation Inventory (child version), the AutPlay Connection Inventory (child version), and the AutPlay Assessment of Play Inventory. All inventories were administered to identify Calvin's skill strengths and deficits in the areas of social skills, emotional regulation ability, connection with others, and play functioning. Calvin's assessment sessions demonstrated that he was able to participate, on a limited level, in directive instruction. Advanced instruction or activities beyond his limited skill level triggered discomfort, resulting in Calvin withdrawing and ignoring others around him. It was further observed that Calvin lacked interactive social engagement and the ability to participate in reciprocal play. He appeared to understand some pretend play and functional play, but he significantly lacked social play skills.

After the intake and assessment phase was completed, treatment goals were established, and it was determined that Calvin and his mother would participate in the AutPlay Follow Me Approach, which is designed for children who struggle with attunement and engagement ability. Treatment goals included increasing reciprocal interaction and engagement with others, tolerating and participating in other people's ideas and activities, and improving social interaction and play with peers. At Session 4, Calvin and his mother began participating in the Follow Me Approach. The play therapist facilitated the approach with Calvin, while his mother observed to learn the approach.

Grant (2017a) defines the AutPlay Follow Me Approach as a relational and skill development approach that moves the child from an inability to focus and complete structured instruction to fully participating in therapist- and parent-led structured play interventions. The therapist teaches the parents how to stage Follow Me play times at home with their child. The Follow Me Approach is typically conducted in a play room or play space that has been established for the child. A Follow Me play session typically takes approximately 20–30 minutes. The primary components of this approach include the child leading the play time, the adult periodically making tracking and reflective statements, the adult periodically asking the child questions, the adult trying to engage with the child in whatever he or she is playing, and the adult being mindful of the child's tolerance level.

Calvin's mother observed the play therapist conducting the Follow Me Approach for three sessions, and at Session 7, she conducted the approach herself while the therapist observed. At this point, Calvin and his mother were ready to begin having Follow Me play times at home. The therapist established with Calvin's mother that they would implement a Follow Me play time every other day for 30 minutes and that the play time would be facilitated in the family-designated play room. Calvin and his mother were participating in at-home Follow Me play times conducted by his mom, and in addition, they were both seeing the play therapist every week, at which time the therapist conducted the approach with Calvin.

Calvin was progressively improving in his engaging skills with his mother and the therapist. He was also increasing his ability to let others make decisions in the play and to follow the lead of others. At Session 18, the therapist introduced the next step in treatment: connection games. These games are designed to help the child respond to and participate with another person who has initiated an activity or game. Connection games are simple, usually one-step instruction games that the therapist or parent initiates with the child. Calvin had progressed enough in his engagement ability to introduce connection games and to see how Calvin would respond. The therapist and Calvin's mother decided to begin with an AutPlay bubble-blowing intervention called Body Bubbles (Grant, 2017a). Calvin's mother would elicit his attention and let him know they were going to play a bubble-blowing game. His mom would blow the bubbles and instruct Calvin to pop the bubbles with different body parts. His mother would work on taking turns blowing and popping the bubbles with Calvin. She introduced the intervention at Session 19. Calvin responded to her initiation and participated in the intervention for approximately 1 minute and then left the interaction and began playing on his own. The therapist instructed Calvin's mother to keep playing the intervention during their home play times and see if Calvin's participation increased.

At Session 21, Calvin was participating in the Body Bubbles intervention for approximately 10–12 minutes at a time. He was successfully taking turns with both his mother and the therapist. His mother had also gotten his two older brothers involved, and they would all play the Body Bubbles intervention with Calvin. The therapist introduced additional connection games, and the therapist and Calvin's mother implemented other connection games in the Follow Me play times. Calvin responded positively, showing increased ability to attune and engage in the interventions initiated by another person. At Session 28, the therapist discussed with Calvin's mother the next step in the treatment process (phase two of AutPlay® Therapy), introducing specific structured interventions to target skill gains.

At Session 29, focus shifted from the Follow Me Approach to introducing structured play interventions designed to further address Calvin's treatment goals. His older brothers were further incorporated into this phase of treatment. The therapist began by facilitating an AutPlay intervention called What Am I (Grant, 2017b). The therapist explained to Calvin that they would be playing a game together. The therapist had Calvin's mom write down some simple objects on two index cards, one for the therapist and one for Calvin. Mom taped one card on the therapist's shirt and one card on Calvin's shirt. The therapist and Calvin had to take turns asking each other questions to try and guess what object was written on the index card taped to their shirt. Once the objects were guessed, new ones were created, and the game continued. The objects were simple and age appropriate such as apple, ball, and bike. Calvin's mother observed and learned the intervention and began implementing the intervention at home during their play times. She also taught the intervention to her other sons, and they all played with Calvin.

The therapist periodically introduced new play interventions to address Calvin's treatment goals. The therapist would facilitate the interventions to Calvin and his mother, and in turn she would teach the interventions to his brothers. They all would play the interventions with Calvin at home between therapy sessions. This process continued until Session 40, after which treatment progress was assessed. Calvin had progressed and was successfully displaying all of the skills that were part of his original treatment goals. His mother reported that Calvin was engaging with and playing with other children at school, especially at recess. Prior to beginning therapy, Calvin would be wandering by himself during recess, not engaging with or playing with any other children. His mother also reported that Calvin was more fully participating with other children during their play dates. He was now able to follow the lead of other children, participate in play initiated by other children, take turns, and stay engaged in play with other children. The therapist and mother established a termination date for therapy as Calvin had progressed and had met his initial treatment goals. No new goals were established.

The termination phase of AutPlay Therapy was initiated at Session 41. In this session, the therapist discussed with Calvin that his counseling time would be ending at Session 48, when they would be having a party to celebrate his accomplishments. The sessions leading up to his termination were used to continue to strengthen his skill gains with therapy and at-home play times. At Session 47, the therapist and Calvin's mother discussed how she would continue to have specific play times at home to help Calvin maintain his skill gains and continue to gain age-appropriate skills. His mother was told that she could contact the therapist if she had any issues or questions and that treatment could resume if needed. And so Session 48, Calvin's final session, arrived, and a celebration party was held, which also included his parents and brothers.

Empirical Support for Play Therapy Interventions

Parker and O'Brien (2011) stated that the literature abounds with case studies noting changes in behavior resulting from interventions using play therapy. The issues treated with play therapy approaches include learning disabilities, speech difficulties, anxiety, child abuse, trauma, family, and autism.

Multiple case studies and clinical outcomes have shown that children who participate in AutPlay Therapy once a week for 6 months show skill gains in preassessed target areas of treatment. Parent rating scales also support skill gains for children who have participated in AutPlay Therapy once a week for 6 months. Following these treatments, parents also report feeling more knowledgeable and empowered in their parenting abilities and experiencing less stress regarding their child's ASD issues.

The National Autism Center and the National Standards Project (2018) have reviewed literature to establish evidence-based practices for individuals with ASD between birth and 22 years of age. Both reviews included literature up to and including 2007, and both applied rigorous criteria when determining which studies would be included as evidence of efficacy for a given practice. In 2014, the National Autism Center conducted an expanded and updated review, which yielded a total of 27 evidence-based practices. AutPlay Therapy incorporates several of the approaches identified as evidence-based practices for treating children and adolescents with ASD. Practices incorporated into the AutPlay Therapy protocol include cognitive-behavioral intervention, modeling, naturalistic intervention, parent-implemented intervention, prompting, reinforcement, scripting, self-management, social narratives, social skills training, and visual supports.

Conclusion

Literature support for using play therapy with children with ASD has been growing substantially with each passing year. As we learn more about various play therapy approaches and the power of the therapeutic core change agents in play, we can recognize the protocol, effectiveness, and purpose of play therapy with ASD. Although research continues to show gains for implementing play therapy approaches such as AutPlay Therapy for children with ASD, more randomized controlled studies specifying a prescriptive play therapy approach are needed. Further, research defining the core agents of change and how they manifest themselves within a play therapy approach or intervention are also needed. As play is the natural language of children, harnessing that language into understanding the therapeutic powers of play holds unlimited possibilities in transforming the lives of children and families affected by ASD.

REFERENCES

American Psychiatric Association. (2013). *Diagnostic and statistical manual of mental disorders* (5th ed.). Arlington, VA: Author.

Banerjee, M., & Ray, S. G. (2013). Development of play therapy module for children with autism. *Journal of the Indian Academy of Applied Psychology, 39,* 245–253.

Barron, R., & Kenny, D. (1986). The moderator-mediator variable distinction in social psychological research: Conceptual, strategic, and statistical considerations. *Journal of Personality and Social Psychology, 5,* 1173–1182.

Barry, T. D., Klinger, L. G., Lee, J. M., Palardy, N., Gilmore, T., & Bodin, S. D. (2003). Examining the effectiveness of an outpatient clinic-based social skills group for high functioning children with autism. *Journal of Autism and Developmental Disorders, 33,* 685–701.

Booth, P. B., & Jernberg, A. M. (2010). *Theraplay.* San Francisco: Jossey-Bass.

Cavett, A. M. (2014). Stress inoculation. In C. E. Schaefer & A. A. Drewes (Eds.), *The therapeutic powers of play: 20 core agents of change* (pp. 131–141). Hoboken, NJ: Wiley.

Centers for Disease Control and Prevention. (2018). Autism spectrum disorder (ASD) data and statistics. Retrieved from *www.cdc.gov/ncbddd/autism/data. html.*

Fraser, T. (2014). Direct teaching. In C. E. Schaefer & A. A. Drewes (Eds.), *The therapeutic powers of play: 20 core agents of change* (pp. 39–50). Hoboken, NJ: Wiley.

Gil, E. (2015). *Play in family therapy.* New York: Guilford Press.

Grant, R. J. (2015). Family play counseling with children affected by autism. In E. J. Green, J. N. Baggerly, & A. C. Myrick (Eds.), *Counseling families: Play-based treatment* (pp. 109–125). Lanham, MD: Rowman & Littlefield.

Grant, R. J. (2017a). *AutPlay therapy for children and adolescents on the autism spectrum: A behavioral play-based approach.* New York: Routledge.

Grant, R. J. (2017b). *Play-based interventions for autism spectrum disorders and other developmental disabilities.* New York: Routledge.

Grant, R. J. (2018). AutPlay therapy with preadolescents affected by autism. In E. Green, J. Baggerly, & A. Myrick (Eds.), *Play therapy with preteens* (pp. 123–139). Lanham, MD: Rowman & Littlefield.

Greenspan, S., & Wieder, S. (2006). *Engaging autism.* Cambridge, MA: Da Capo Press.

Hess, L. (2006). I would like to play but I don't know how: A case study of pretend play in autism. *Child Language Teaching and Therapy, 22,* 97–116.

Hillman, H. (2018). Child-centered play therapy as an intervention for children with autism: A literature review. *International Journal of Play Therapy, 27,* 198–204.

Howard, A. R., Copeland, R., Lindaman, S., & Cross, R. (2018). Theraplay impact on parents and children with autism spectrum disorder: Improvements in affect, joint attention, and social cooperation. *International Journal of Play Therapy, 27,* 56–68.

Hull, K. (2011). *Play therapy and Aspergers syndrome.* Lanham, MD: Jason Aronson.

Kasari, C., Chang, Y. C., & Patterson, S. (2013). Pretending to play or playing to pretend: The case of autism. *American Journal of Play, 6,* 124–135.

Kossyvaki, L., & Papoudi, D. (2016). A review of play interventions for children with autism at school. *International Journal of Disability, Development, and Education, 63,* 45–63.

Kottman, T. (2014). Positive emotions. In C. E. Schaefer & A. A. Drewes (Eds.), *The therapeutic powers of play: 20 core agents of change* (pp. 103–120). Hoboken, NJ: Wiley.

Kuhaneck, H. M., & Britner, P. A. (2013). A preliminary investigation of the relationship between sensory processing and social play in autism spectrum disorder. *Occupational Therapy Journal of Research, 33,* 159–167.

MacDonald, J., & Stoika, P. (2007*). Play to talk: A practical guide to help your late-talking child join the conversation.* Madison, WI: Kiddo.

Nash, J. B. (2014). Social competence. In C. E. Schaefer & A. A. Drewes (Eds.), *The therapeutic powers of play: 20 core agents of change* (pp. 185–193). Hoboken, NJ: Wiley.

National Autism Center. (2018). National standards project. Retrieved form *www. nationalautismcenter.org/national-standards-project.*

O'Connor, K, J., & Braverman, L. D. (2009). *Play therapy theory and practice: Comparing theories and techniques.* Hoboken, NJ: Wiley.

Overley, L. C., Degges-White, S., Snow, M. S., Mossing, S. L., & Holmes, K. P. (2018). Exploring the experiences of play therapists working with children diagnosed with autism. *International Journal of Play Therapy, 27,* 14–24.

Packman, J. (2014). Moral development. In C. E. Schaefer & A. A. Drewes (Eds.), *The therapeutic powers of play: 20 core agents of change* (pp. 243–254). Hoboken, NJ: Wiley.

Parker, N., & O'Brien, P. (2011). Play therapy reaching the child with autism. *International Journal of Special Education, 26,* 80–87.

Rogers, S. J., Estes, A., Lord, C., Vismata, L., Winter, J., Fitzpatrick, A., Guo, M., et al. (2012). Effects of a brief early start Denver model (ESDM) based parent intervention on toddlers at risk for autism spectrum disorders: A randomized control trial. *Journal of the American Academy of Child and Adolescent Psychiatry, 51,* 1052–1065.

Salter, K., Beamish, W., & Davies, M. (2016). The effects of child centered play therapy (CCPT) on the social and emotional growth of young children with autism. *International Journal of Play Therapy, 25,* 78–90.

Schaefer, C. E. (2001). Prescriptive play therapy. *International Journal of Play Therapy, 10*(2), 57–73.

Schaefer, C. E., & Drewes, A. A. (2014). *The therapeutic powers of play: 20 core agents of change.* Hoboken, NJ: Wiley.

Solomon, M., Ono, M., Timmer, S., & Goodlin-Jones, B. (2008). The effectiveness of parent child interaction therapy for families of children on the autism spectrum. *Journal of Autism and Developmental Disorders, 38*(9), 1767–1776.

Solomon, R. (2012). The play project: A train-the-trainer model of early intervention for children with autism spectrum disorder. In L. Gallo-Lopez & L. C. Rubin (Eds.), *Play-based interventions for children and adolescents with autism spectrum disorders* (pp. 249–269). New York: Routledge.

Stagnitti, K., & Pfeifer, L. I. (2017). Methodological considerations for a directive play therapy approach for children with autism and related disorders. *International Journal of Play Therapy, 26,* 160–171.

Steward, A. L., & Echterling, L. G. (2014). In C. E. Schaefer & A. A. Drewes (Eds.), *The therapeutic powers of play: 20 core agents of change* (pp. 157–169). Hoboken, NJ: Wiley.

VanFleet, R. (2012). Communication and connection: Filial therapy with families of children with ASD. In L. Gallo-Lopez & L. C. Rubin (Eds.), *Play-based interventions for children and adolescents with autism spectrum disorders* (pp. 193–208). New York: Routledge.

VanFleet, R., & Faa-Thompson, T. (2017). *Animal assisted play therapy.* Sarasota, FL: Professional Resource Press.

Wolfberg, P. (1999). *Play and imagination in children with autism.* New York: Teachers College Press.

Wolfberg, P., Bottema-Beutel, K., & DeWitt, M. (2012). Including children with autism in social and imaginary play with typical peers. *American Journal of Play, 5,* 55–80.

Yeager, M., & Yeager, D. (2014). Self-regulation. In C. E. Schaefer & A. A. Drewes (Eds.), *The therapeutic powers of play: 20 core agents of change* (pp. 269–293). Hoboken, NJ: Wiley.

CHAPTER 14

Play Therapy for Children with Attachment Disruptions

Paris Goodyear-Brown

Description of Attachment Disorders and the Need for a Diagnostic Continuum

Diagnostic criteria for attachment problems in children is notably limited. While clinicians work daily with children and families with a variety of attachment disturbances, we don't have a nuanced classification system that is recognized by third-party payment sources. The only DSM-5 diagnosis specifically focused on a child's clinical disorder of attachment is reactive attachment disorder (RAD; American Psychiatric Association, 2013). It is currently classified as a stressor-related disorder. This disorder was originally introduced in DSM-III, and while it has had several iterations of evolution, it continues to have significant diagnostic limitations, including its dependence on documented parental neglect and narrow categories of how an attachment disturbance presents. The two subtypes of RAD characterize the child as either inhibited (hypervigilant, withdrawn, seeking close and sometimes bizarre proximity to caregivers) or indiscriminate (seeking care from any available caregiver). ICD-11, the diagnostic system of the World Health Organization, describes RAD as grossly abnormal attachment behaviors, marked by an inability to receive care when it is offered (ICD-11 for Mortality and Morbidity Statistics, 2019). They offer a second set of criteria for children who present with disinhibited social engagement disorder, which is characterized by grossly abnormal social behavior, including indiscriminate approach to adults and overfamiliarity. Both of these diagnoses are only applicable to children and must have features that develop after a developmental age of 9 months and before a child has turned 5.

These categories of disordered attachment are limited and in all cases are diagnostically dependent on grossly inadequate care. For real-world practitioners, these categories do not begin to describe the nuance of attachment disturbances we see within family systems. Even when dealing with a child who has experienced severe neglect, maltreatment, or institutional care, many practitioners are hesitant to use the RAD diagnosis because of the way in which it pathologizes the child, its wide if perhaps misguided association with a poor prognosis among caregivers, and the potential negative impact on parents' perceptions of the child in their care.

The paucity of diagnostic language and evidence-based methods for treating attachment disturbances led to a proliferation of attachment therapies, some of which were fraught with peril. In 2006, the American Professional Society on the Abuse of Children published a report by a task force created to offer reflections, cautions, and practice guidelines regarding attachment therapies, RAD, and attachment problems. The dearth of consensus on what constitutes an attachment disorder presents grave challenges for creating and testing evidence-based treatments for attachment disturbances.

If we approach the consequences of attachment disruptions through the lens of the Adverse Childhood Experiences (ACE) study, we find a wealth of data trumpeting the long-lasting traumagenic impact of early attachment disruptions (Anda et al., 2006; Dube et al., 2003; Felitti et al., 1998). Each of the ACEs—physical, emotional, or sexual abuse; physical or emotional neglect; incarceration of a parent, mental illness of a parent, or violence against a parent; substance abuse; and divorce—represents a rupture in the consistent, nurturing, attuned caregiving relationship that leads to a secure attachment between child and caregiver. As the number of ACEs (number of attachment-disrupting experiences) increases, so do risk factors for lifelong mental and physical health problems. Each of the ACEs creates toxic stress for the caregiver, the child, or both, and can create cascading posttraumatic stress effects, hindering the potential for the parent to open and close circles of communication with the child. Healthy attachment interactions, those that result in a trust foundation for children, derive from needs being met over and over again thousands of times. Contingent reciprocity, or serve and return interactions, allow for the child's needs to be met and trust to be built. Attachment disruptions of an ongoing or compounded nature make children sick.

Play therapists who have worked with a variety of families experience the lack of goodness of fit that can exist between a parent and child, perhaps due to personality, perhaps due to temperament, sometimes due to the parents' attachment style, and sometimes resulting from parental psychopathology, stressors, or addictions. All children work hard to figure out a strategy for remaining close to their caregiver. The work of John Bowlby and Mary Ainsworth continues to provide the scaffolding for modern attachment theory (Ainsworth & Bowlby, 1991). Mary Ainsworth's work informed our initial understanding of secure and insecure attachments. These classifications were expanded by Mary Main (Main & Hesse, 1990) to create an initial lexicon for how we talk about the attachment behaviors of children. Her early classifications of secure, avoidant, ambivalent, and disorganized attachment patterns as a way to begin describing what is happening in a dyad are often seen as being more clinically useful than our standardized diagnostic systems.

In our current managed care environment, it would be helpful to translate these clinical insights to diagnostic categories that are more nuanced than the single disorder of attachment now referenced in the DSM. Children do not need to have received grossly inadequate care to have disturbances in their attachment relationships or to need clinical help. As our Nurture House staff supervises other clinicians and consults with other mental health agencies that specialize in treating attachment problems, we often discuss the potential value of creating a spectrum of attachment disturbance within the DSM, much like the autism spectrum. Categorizing attachment problems along a continuum of severity or quality of disturbance would be useful to the many practitioners working to support families experiencing attachment disruption.

As we continue to advocate for new levels of refinement to our current diagnostic criteria for attachment disorders, we can turn our attention to better understanding other existing diagnoses through the lens of attachment. Attachment insecurity and disorganization increase risks from infancy through adolescence for both internalizing and externalizing clinical problems and contribute to multiple forms of psychopathology (Bizzi, Cavanna, Castellano, & Pace, 2015; Dubois-Comtois, Moss, Cyr, & Pascuzzo, 2013; Fearon, Bakermans-Kranenburg, van IJzendoorn, Lapsley, & Roisman, 2010; Groh, Roisman, van IJzendoorn, Bakermans-Kranenburg, & Fearon, 2012; Lecompte & Moss, 2014; Madigan, Atkinson, Laurin, & Benoit, 2013). The overarching goal in a healing process then becomes the enhancement of attachment security within families. Given the complexity of family systems and in order to maximize therapeutic benefits of reparative attachment work (work aimed at enhancing the quality, frequency, and duration of connected, supportive moments between a parent and child), we must support several forms of therapeutic work at once. A prescriptive approach in which individual families are assessed and treatment components are chosen specifically for their needs is the most clinically sound, yet flexible, way to provide nuanced care for families who present with attachment disruptions.

Rationale for Nurturing Engagement for Attachment Repair

Nurturing Engagement for Attachment Repair (NEAR) is a prescriptive play therapy model designed to target the attachment distress within a family system, provide attachment repair or enhancement as needed, and help parents become partners in the child's healing process. NEAR can be used as a stand-alone approach if attachment enhancement and low-level attachment repair is all that is needed. However, when clinicians are treating family systems with complex trauma, neglect, or maltreatment, NEAR is usually embedded within the larger TraumaPlay model. TraumaPlay, my flexibly sequential play therapy model for treating traumatized children, encourages the integration of caregivers in a supportive way at any point along the continuum of treatment. While caregiver involvement is always valued, assisting the parent in becoming a soothing partner is a specific treatment goal embedded within the larger treatment focus of soothing the physiology. The components of TraumaPlay are summarized in Figure 14.1.

Many of the children we see at Nurture House have attachment trauma as an integral part of their trauma story. Helping these children grow in trust and connection with their caregivers, helping them receive and respond to the coregulation of their parents, and helping parents better understand the needs underlying the behaviors are foundational pieces of their overarching trauma recovery journey, and one that we often prioritize as needing attention before we dive into trauma content. When we are supervising clinicians in TraumaPlay, we are often asked, "Do we work on the trauma content first or on building up the family system (strengthening the attachment relationships) first?" We have wrestled clinically with this question and in most cases believe that enhancing the role of parents as soothing partners prior to any play-based gradual exposure work is safest and most effective. *Why?* It is easier for children to approach trauma content when we have already enhanced safety and security and augmented adaptive coping. The caregiver may be our best bet for enhancing security and for providing coping comfort. The connected caregiver often becomes the most effective history keeper, or put another way, the keeper of the child's story. Enhancing the parent's ability to hold the hard story both prepares them for trauma narrative work and supports the likelihood that the story of what happened can continue to be held long after therapy has ended.

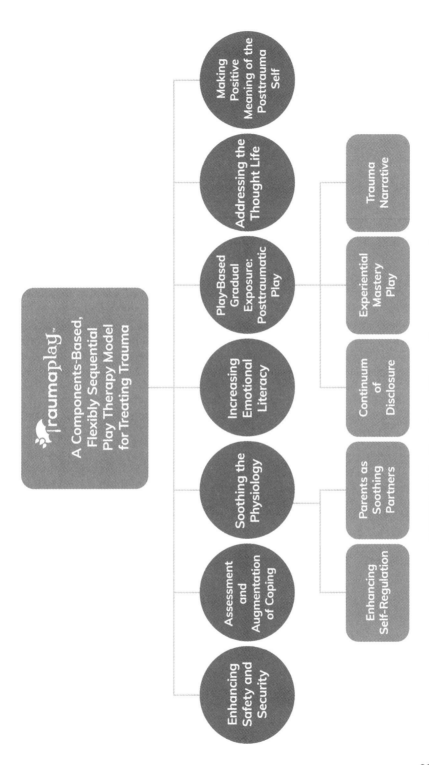

FIGURE 14.1. Flowchart of TraumaPlay treatment goals.

Parents as Soothing Partners serves as an umbrella under which we make room for the parent work codified in NEAR. NEAR is prescriptive in that it invites the selective use of the following:

1. Psychoeducation for both parents and children.
2. Coregulation strategies.
3. Therapist modeling of delight as a parallel process.
4. Therapist facilitation of nurturing dyadic activities within the session.
5. Work around enhancing reflective capacity for parent and/or child.
6. Coherent narrative building within the dyad or family.
7. Parent coaching in all of the above.

In some cases, all of these methods will be used. Clinicians may also choose the components of NEAR that are most likely to provide the corrective emotional experiences needed by the system or the most powerful paradigm shifts needed for parent, child, or both.

While we see many complex attachment/trauma cases at Nurture House, we also see biologically intact families at Nurture House, who, for a variety of reasons, are seeking attachment repair or attachment enhancement. Simply put, when a child has an unmet need, or when a parent responds to a child in an over- or underresponsive way, there is the potential for an attachment rupture to occur. The underpinnings of attachment rupture are endless. An anxious child needs more structure than his mom (who tends to "go with the flow" and is wired for spontaneity) can provide him. The reverse situation, in which the highly exploratory child has a highly anxious mother who only feels good when he is close to the child, is another kind of mismatch. In each of these presentations, this lack of goodness-of-fit between Mom's way and the child's way of meeting the world often results in a pattern of misattunement that creates emotional distress in both, followed by distance or demand, judgment, and loneliness. Eventually, this continued misattunement leads to the creation of maladaptive coping strategies in both mom and child to get their needs met. NEAR embraces the complexity of family systems and the potential nuances needed in treating parts of the system, while keeping as the central question for both parent and child, "What is the underlying need that is not being met here?"

Step-by-Step Details of the Intervention

The Nurture House Dyadic Assessment

In order to be prescriptive in our treatment choices, we must have a robust assessment process that helps us to capture the clinical data needed to engage in case conceptualization. We have developed an in-house clinical tool, the

Nurture House Dyadic Assessment (NHDA), that helps us to refine our understanding of each family's needs, so that we can more selectively choose the components of NEAR that are likely to create the most efficient and effective changes within a family system. The NHDA captures parent–child interactions in a variety of ways. It begins with a quick observation of the parent and child in the waiting room (are parent and child physically close or distant, engaged in play together or entertaining themselves independently? how have they negotiated snacks, drinks, and the free gumball machine?). The clinician escorts the parent and child into a playroom and invites them to have 5 minutes of playtime during which the child is in charge and then 5 minutes of playtime during which the parent is in charge, followed by a prompt to have the parent and child clean up. While we code for different dynamics, the structure of that part of the assessment is very similar to that of the Dyadic Parent–Child Interaction Coding System (DPICS; the parent–child interaction therapy [PCIT] assessment tool). When clean-up appears to be finished (this can range from 30 seconds to 3 minutes), the therapist gestures to the bin of envelopes that include prompts from the Marschak interaction method (Marschak, 1960; Lindaman, Booth, & Chambers, 2000), the primary assessment tool of Theraplay (Booth & Jernberg, 2009), and prompts that begin to assess the dyad's strategies for dealing with harder content. For example, one of our additional prompts states, "Adult tells the child about a time when the adult made a mistake and then asks the child to tell about a time the child made a mistake." A second prompt encourages parent and child to talk about "a hard thing that happened." While we are not wanting to open up significant trauma content in this initial assessment, we are interested to see if parent and/or child are able to reflect on difficult moments in their own lives or in the family and how they navigate the approach to more challenging content.

Unlike other dyadic assessments in which the best-practice scenario has the parent and child in a room with a one-way mirror and the therapist is observing from another room, the NHDA is intentionally administered with the therapist in the room. This is in part because we are working to establish the counselor as an anchor point, a grounding presence, from the start of the therapeutic process. The therapist's physical presence in the midst of this new environment and potentially anxiety-provoking tasks has the added benefit of yielding rich information about how each party relates to this third party. In some cases, parent and child barely acknowledge the therapist as they play together. In other cases, either the parent or child may be looking for clarity, permission, validation, or any number of other things from the therapist. Paying attention to these interactions during assessment can help prepare the therapist to help hold or challenge the system more prescriptively. The therapist will continue to form a third point of the triangle throughout treatment, using this therapeutic triangulation to create shift in the system.

The Power of Parallel Process

Parents need multiple forms of equipping; therefore, NEAR therapists are always functioning on multiple levels of interaction with parents and children simultaneously. Throughout our interactions with parents and children, we are aware of the parallel process that is occurring. At some points in session, we are acting as embodied conveyors of delight in the child, communicating the child's preciousness in ways that can be osmosed by the caregiver. Parents of children with difficult behaviors often have their hearts and minds soothed as they watch a NEAR clinician bringing genuine delight to the child who is often the recipient of correction and censure at school or in other organized settings. We are mindful of the two basic roles we play in need meeting with children, and before we even offer psychoeducational materials from the Circle of Security project (Powell, Cooper, Hoffman, & Marvin, 2009), we become a secure base and a safe haven for both parents and child.

Targeted expansion of any essential quality of a parent's attachment behavior begins by the therapist modeling that quality with the parent. One of my life mantras is that you can only give what you have received. Some of the parents we see at Nurture House have not been delighted in, and so we delight in them. We celebrate their successes, we point out and affirm the strengths that are present in their parenting, we laugh with them, and we hold their big feelings, giving them doses of experience that can be passed on to their children. Sometimes the family therapist is the first safe attachment figure for a parent, and in that way we provide the corrective emotional experiences to a parent that allow her to open herself to interacting differently with her child.

Shifting Parents' Paradigms: Playful Psychoeducation

The goal of psychoeducation at Nurture House is not expanded head knowledge but expanded heart knowledge. Our clinicians find that when parents receive the shift in understanding that a nugget of psychoeducation can bring, their internal compassion wells are refilled. By the time parents enter treatment, they are often disappointed, exhausted, and sometimes even disgusted with themselves or their child. They inevitably need nurture themselves while on the journey to making shifts in their parenting paradigms.

One of the paradigm shifts we are hoping to help parents make is from seeing themselves as enforcers to seeing themselves as coregulators. Many parents have as their highest priority a desire for their child to stay calm. Sometimes parents see their job as protector from all pain, other times as enforcer of all rules. Our job is to help discern where each parent may be over- or underresponsive, help them become curious and compassionate with themselves and their children, and give them room to fail without shame while revamping their parenting responses. A NEAR therapist may unpack concepts of healthy development and the basic needs of children/ roles of parents (Circle of Security); concepts specific to neurobiology and trauma; the coregulation strategies codified in the acronym SOOTHE (Goodyear-Brown, 2010, 2019); the empowering, connecting, and correcting principles of trust-based relational intervention (Purvis, Cross, & Sunshine, 2007); and how to see their children's behaviors through the lens of their window of tolerance for stress (Siegel, 1999). All of these psychoeducational pieces serve the dual purpose of helping parents see under the behaviors to the real child while refilling their compassion wells.

Skill Building and Parent Coaching

The NHDA highlights areas in which a parent needs coaching in specific skill sets. When a parent needs to have a particular skill set expanded, we provide live coaching, prescriptively using one of several evidence-based approaches. Families who have had their joy stolen by trauma or parents who need support in delighting in their children in session respond well to an integration of Theraplay® into their treatment plan. When the assessment yields data that the parent needs support in attuning to the child and being fully present with the child, we find an integration of filial therapy or child–parent relationship therapy to be very helpful. These models are also especially helpful when a parent needs help in releasing control in the relationship and learning to follow the child's lead. Skills such as tracking, reflecting, and describing receive lots of attention and are practiced by the parent. In other families, the dyadic assessment reveals a parent who is highly critical or lacking in praise. In these families, we have found the codification of the PRIDE (praise, reflection, imitation, description, and engagement) skills offered in PCIT, the trio of communications to avoid, supported by live coaching, as well as the paremeters for 5-minute special playtimes at home to be invaluable aids in growing a parent's ability to pay attention to the positive instead of the negative.

Attachment Enhancement Games

NEAR therapists are encouraged to receive training in Theraplay, which is now on the Evidence-Based Treatments list of the Substance Abuse and Mental Health Administration. This attachment-based structured play therapy intervention offers a rich set of dyadic games that can be selectively used to enhance structure, nurture, engagement, or challenge and sometimes all of those at once! If the NHDA reveals that the parent's ability to provide structure and the child's ability to receive it need enhancement, the structure-enhancing games offered in Theraplay are immensely helpful to children with early attachment ruptures. These games encourage children to wait on their caregiver's cue in order to get what the NEAR therapist refers to as the "joyful payoff" for sharing control. For example, when a Theraplay therapist places a Beanie Baby on her head and tells the child she's going to drop it when she says a silly word like wiggle—and the child can catch it—the "payoff," the neurochemical surge of competence that comes when the child completes the action of catching the Beanie Baby, reinforces the rightness of the risk to share control with the parent. These games can be particularly powerful with children who have developed a control foundation, based on early neglect or trauma. For these children, their deep and abiding belief, perhaps unarticulated, is "I must control everything at all costs or I'll die." As these children grow in their ability to trust and share power, the therapist will move from the verbal prompts of Theraplay to nonverbal cues that require more intensity of eye gaze in order for the child to play the game successfully. The high-nurture games of Theraplay—taking care of hurts, rocking in a blanket, hide-and-seek feeding games—are also powerful tools for use in NEAR sessions when the NHDA has revealed a need to enhance the nurture dimension between parent and child.

I have also developed prop-based attachment enhancement games—Delighting-In games—that can be incorporated into NEAR sessions. Part of our psychoeducation with parents involves helping them expand their concept of how they love their children. While most parents would agree that communicating unconditional love is important, they may not understand that the ways in which we receive love are prescriptive. That is, one size does not fit all when it comes to how each of us likes to be loved. So part of the NEAR model is helping families explore various ways to love each other more effectively. The Delight-in-Me Dice game is one of these ways. We start with one large, blank foam cube and slowly unpack the five love languages for children (Chapman & Campbell, 2008): Words of Affirmation, Quality Time, Acts of Service, Physical Touch, and Gifts. We write one of the love languages on each side as we go, and on the sixth side is written the words "Choose one." If a family needs more structure around expressing love to each other, we will create a series of five foam die, one for each love language. If the mother's love language is Acts of Service, we have a discussion about which Acts of Service mean the most to her, pick the top six, and write each one on a different side of the cube. An Acts of Service die might end up saying, *Unload the dishwasher, Take out the trash,* and so on. If the child's love language is Quality Time, the NEAR therapist helps identify six favorite activities, such as *Read a book together, Play a game of Uno together, or Bake cupcakes together.*

The importance of physical touch in enhancing the attachment bond between parent and child has been well researched (Courtney & Nolan,

2017). Hugs can provide contact comfort and enhance a sense of safety and well-being for some children or parents—but not for others. Therefore, we explore with the dyad or the family the ways that each member gives and receives nurturing touch. A personalized foam die is used as an anchor for the activity, and one agreed upon form of physical affection is written on each side. The physical touch die might say *Give a hug, High-five, Fist bump, Eskimo kiss,* and so on. The parent is asked to carve out 2 to 3 moments a day when the child can roll the die and a nurturing touch can be intentionally shared.

The Rhythm of a Parent–Child NEAR Session

The goals of a dyadic NEAR session can be narrowed down to three primary categories:

1. Providing *in vivo* experiences of shared delight, of nurturing and being nurtured, for both the parents and children.
2. Coaching parents to enhance skill sets, both attachment-focused coregulation skill sets: matching, attunement, the sharing of power, and the SOOTHE strategies, and more behavioral strategies: limit setting, offering choices and consequences, and offering clear directions.
3. Enhancing the family's narrative nuance related to traumatic events, promoting the parent to the position of his-story or her-story keeper.

Since the goals are threefold, a dyadic NEAR session is often broken down into several parts.

The first 5 minutes are spent greeting the parent and child in a fun, connecting way and in reviewing any therapeutic homework that may have been given. The next 15–20 minutes are then spent coaching parent–child interaction with the therapist in a supportive role. In this part of the session, clinicians will have previously chosen a dyadic, coachable skill set, such as the PRIDE skills, filial therapy skills, or trust-based relational intervention skills (TBRI) and will be providing support and coaching of parental attunement skills throughout this time. The next 15–20 minutes are spent engaging in therapist-facilitated nurturing dyadic game play between parent and child. These games may be pulled from Theraplay or from the menu of Delighting-In games that the staff of Nurture House is continually creating. There are an endless number of ways to show care, to communicate love, and to help relationships thrive. All pathways to attachment enhancement are welcome and prescriptively applied in the NEAR model. The last 5 minutes of the NEAR session is reserved for an "I Remember

When" story, in which the parent and child share a snack while the parent tells a story about the child out loud.

The sessions described above are typical for early sessions, but the kinds of stories being told by a caregiver or therapist evolve over the course of treatment. The first stories help set up the caregiver as a history keeper for the child, and cover content related to the child's firsts, like the first time the child walked or said Mommy or rode a bike. The stories may also include adorable or silly moments of shared delight. This kind of storytelling helps both parent and child get used to shared storytelling in a safe way. As the parent shifts her paradigm and the child begins responding differently to stressful situations, the stories shift to celebrations of these new competencies. Once the storytelling scaffolding has been built and the family's window of tolerance for holding hard things has expanded, the therapist begins to weave storytelling around the traumagenic material into the sessions. Sometimes a behavior observed even earlier in the same session (like a child having difficulty receiving a band-aid for a boo-boo from a parent) can be named and connected to the child's early experience. Trauma content is revisited in carefully titrated doses, as both parents and children can tolerate them. Parents are sometimes skeptical about how much a hurt child in their care can tolerate hearing about their own story, and they are often surprised by the intensity with which the child listens and absorbs.

Parent Involvement

In the NEAR model, parents are involved every step of the way. From the NHDA all the way through to the Family Graduation Celebration, parents are delighted in, supported, educated, and coregulated themselves. In addition to the parent–child NEAR sessions described above, goals related to expanding reflective capacity and some aspects of psychoeducation and narrative work require the scheduling of collateral sessions with parents only. The best psychoeducational material will end up falling on deaf ears if all we do is talk *at* parents. Many of the parents whom we see were parentified themselves and did not get to be children. Therefore, they may need to have their own playfulness delighted in and supported before they will understand its power in their children's development. In some cases, the parent may need to experience the therapist as a secure base or a safe haven in order to become one themselves. We use lots of humor and we value shared laughter as it becomes a shared experience of the release of dopamine and oxytocin between therapist and parent that can be replicated between parent and child. The NEAR therapist teaches, models, and coaches but always has as his or her core goal that of delighting in and holding the story of the parent as well as the child. Trauma mamas, who may be experiencing posttraumatic stress themselves, as they have endured the rages of their children while feeling helpless to impact them, need holding, coregulation, and coherent narrative building themselves before they will be able to give it to their hurt child. We soothe the parent before we ask the parent to become a soothing partner for the child.

Part of the coherent narrative building we do with parents involves inviting them to look at their own attachment history. Using a subset of questions from a clinical adaptation of the Adult Attachment Interview (AAI; George, Kaplan, & Main, 1996; Seigel & Hartzell, 2013), we offer titrated doses of reflection on their relationships with their own parents. For example, one of the original AAI questions asks the adult being interviewed to give five adjectives to describe the relationship between the interviewee's relationship with her mom during early childhood. After the participant lists five descriptors, the interviewer spends time on each adjective, asking for an example or a story to illustrate this descriptor of the participant's relationship with Mom. As in all parts of the model, a clinical focus on the parent's early attachment history would be prescribed if the parent appeared to be incoherent in their internal narrative. Returning to the premise of prescriptive play therapy, we may find that one family presents with a parent who appears to have a dismissive or ambivalent attachment style in adulthood that is hindering their ability to connect fully with their adoptive child, while another family may present with a parent who has already done a lot of their own therapeutic work, has both coherence and grounding in their current parenting practices, and is best supported by having us facilitate enhanced receiving by the adopted child of *in vivo* care and nurture. In the case where we decide to pursue deeper reflection with a parent on their own attachment history, we do it in a way that harnesses both left and right brain ways of knowing. We have parents write down and verbalize the five descriptors of their relationship with their mother, and then we offer a circular sandtray and invite the parent to choose a symbol to represent each descriptor. We work with these, moving back and forth between symbol (right hemisphere) and words (left hemisphere) to help bring integration (Kestly, 2015) to their experience.

Case Vignettes

Vignette 1: The Bunny Farm and the Baby Farm

Shawn is a 12-year-old male adopted from South Korea at age 3. At intake, mom describes their home as in constant chaos. She homeschools him and talks about how fixated Shawn can become on the next thing that he wants, thinking it will make him happy. If Mom has to say no about anything, he flies into a rage that may include hurting her or destroying property. Mom is quick to acknowledge that she often responds to his escalation with an escalation of her own. He is continually changing his look, has a momentary experience of being alright in his body, and then quickly devolves into the need to change his look again because he feels ugly and stupid. At the height of his rages, he will often say that Mom doesn't love him, that he should never have been born, that he was too ugly for his birth mother to keep him, and make other heartbreaking comments. During each of the two NHDAs, it becomes clear that Shawn performs in proscribed ways when he is in front of other people, while melting down at home, hinting at massive anxiety below the surface. During the second NHDA, Shawn had been perseverating on a bunny that the family was considering buying for him. They had agreed before coming for the session that they would go to the bunny farm afterward. The next week, as the therapist was taking Shawn back for his first individual assessment session, he blurted out that his bunny had died. The therapist had not known about the bunny joining the family the week before, and asked for the story. Shawn said, "Yeah, we got a bunny last week . . . and it only lived for, like, a day." The therapist reflected on this and offered that this might have been really hard for him. The therapist got a piece of paper and said, "Sounds like there is a story to what happened." The therapist began to write, "Once upon a time there was a bunny named . . . " Shawn filled in "Thumper." The therapist became his scribe, and he began to narrate. Below is his story:

> "Thumper was born on a rabbit farm with lots of other rabbits. He was used to the other rabbits and his rabbit cage. One day a young man came and chose him to be his pet. Thumper did not know that the young man wanted to take care of him, walk him on a leash, pet him, hold him, cuddle him. Thumper thought he was a predator and that he was being taken away from what he knew to be eaten. He got so nervous that he started making himself sick and throwing up blood. Rest in peace, Thumper. We wish you are good in heaven. We wish you had known that Shawn loved you."

When Shawn finished narrating, both he and the therapist were silent. Finally, we began to talk.

> THERAPIST: Thumper didn't understand that he would be safe in his new home when he left the rabbit farm.
>
> SHAWN: Yeah.
>
> THERAPIST: I wonder how long it would have taken him to learn that he would be safe?

SHAWN: Maybe years and years. I keep on bonding with him and he gets to trust me.

THERAPIST: You know, it sounds like some of what Thumper experienced is sort of like some of what you experienced. Would you like to start a story about yourself? [The therapist was prepared for the possibility that this invitation might result in an abrupt play disruption. This would be interpreted as a "no," and the therapist would track with his new choice of topic or play.]

Shawn became thoughtful and then started narrating out loud: "Shawn used to live in a baby farm with lots of other babies. One day a man and a woman came to choose him out of all the other babies to be their son." That's as far as we got before the session ended. We agreed that we would pick back up with the story when it was time.

The therapist let Mom know that some trauma-specific content had been stirred up, due to life events, earlier than a NEAR therapist would have normally begun to build connections between current behaviors and past trauma and attachment wounds, but the sudden death of Thumper needed to be brought into the room. Mom and therapist met for the first part of the next session. Mom explained that Shawn had been working at a crafts fair with his adoptive grandmother over the weekend. He had great trouble regulating, maintaining a façade while a customer was present, and then he melted down, telling Mom how she was unfair for not buying him whatever it was that he wanted, and berating first her and then himself. The therapist listened and then read Shawn's story to her. His experience of loss and the consequent grief, as well as the similarities between Thumper's story and his own, were palpable. Shawn's mom began to cry as she listened to the themes of abrupt change, difficulty trusting, and overwhelming fear that induced fatal psychosomatic symptoms for the bunny. In this case vignette, the new trauma caused by the death of a pet resulted in the need for a unique prescription of narrative-building work. This narrative work filled the mother's compassion well while helping her hear the fear underlying Shawn's rages in a new way.

The parents were then ready for psychoeducation, and therapy progressed along a track in which parent coaching sessions introduced the coregulation strategies encoded in SOOTHE and happened sporadically as we maintained a weekly pace of NEAR sessions. As these sessions began, Shawn had been picking at his arms and legs in ways that had left lots of scabs. The therapist led Mom and Dad in applying lotion and/or band-aids to the hurts. At Nurture House we keep a wide array of band-aids, and Shawn was particularly drawn to the Police Caution Tape band-aids. As we began a process of intentionally taking care of hurts, his arms began to heal. We also did some parts work in storytelling form, having the "oldest self" talk to "baby Shawn." Shawn drew both parts of self, neither of which was very defined to start with, and we began having these two parts dialogue with each other. Shawn was able to identify core negative beliefs about how he must have been bad or ugly since his birth mom didn't want him—and his oldest self would talk with baby Shawn and remind him that his mom was sick and unable to care for him.

The parents were also coached in soothing the younger parts of Shawn while telling Delighting-in stories from Shawn's early life out loud together while always taking time to narrate celebrations of his developing competencies. Shawn loved to hear Mom and Dad tell these stories about him and began to snuggle up to his parents with a different kind of stillness. Mom read books like *The Invisible String* out loud in session, and we visualized the string between them as strong and glowing, while this imagery was further installed with eye movement desensitization and reprocessing (EMDR). Reading *The Invisible String* and creating concrete representations in sand or art with real string are a standard part of our attachment-enhancement work. The child can then use the language of the string to express when they are feeling more or less connected. Love Connectors are also created for both parent and child and used as transitional objects when needed (Goodyear-Brown & Andersen, 2018).

Vignette 2: Connecting Somatic Reactions to Life Narrative

Johnny, a 5-year-old boy adopted domestically, was born fully addicted to methadone and had what his adoptive mother remembers as horrific withdrawal symptoms. The pain from his withdrawals was so intense that he was given morphine. Mom reports sweating, mottled skin, seizures, tremors, diarrhea, and an inability to suck. The withdrawal process took 7 weeks. His adoptive mother stayed the whole time but could not ease the physical pain he experienced. Johnny has no conscious memory of this time, but his body remembers (Ogden, Minton, & Pain, 2006; Rothschild, 2000). As we began the NEAR sessions, Johnny was highly resistant to having his hurts cared for. When a physical hurt on his body, a bruise or a scab, was remarked on by Mom, Dad, or myself and we would begin to apply a band-aid, he would grab the band-aid and put it on the Hug-A-Boo nearby. The therapist went with the resistance, delighting in his understanding that hurts need to be cared for whether or not we can see them. After he placed the first couple of band-aids on the Hug-a-Boo, Shawn allowed himself to be bandaged. In the first two sessions, he took them off almost immediately after we had put them on. In the third session, he allowed the band-aid to remain, and in the sixth session he said, "OW!" when the band-aid was applied and his body shook. It would have looked like resistance, rejection, or even the beginning of a tantrum to someone who didn't know his story. The therapist gave words to the somatic reaction, saying in a matter-of-fact tone, "You know, Dad, seeing Johnny's body jerk as I put the band-aid on makes me think about the story you told me about how he had to be in the hospital when he was really little. Sometimes his body would hurt, and even when the doctors would try to make it better, his body still hurt. His body is learning now that he can get help when he hurts, and he doesn't have to hurt alone." Johnny grabbed the nearest toy truck he could find and began zooming it up and down the cushions. The therapist understood that the titrated dose of this verbal story was enough for now, and the therapist and dyad moved into 5 minutes of special play time in which Johnny could be in charge while dad reflected, described, and practiced attuning to their son. NEAR therapists value nuance and titration of nurture, education, story, and skills practice in the hard work of healing.

Empirical Support for the Intervention

Since NEAR operates as an umbrella framework for the prescriptive integration of existing evidence-based models, it is most appropriate to cite the research for these models. Filial therapy has over 60 studies investigating its effectiveness (Bratton, Jones, Ray, & Rhine, 2005); CPRT has over 40 studies (Bratton & Landreth, 2010); and PCIT (Schuhmann et al., 1998; Nixon, Sweeney, Erickson, & Touyz, 2003; Linehan, Brabson, Highlander, Wallace, & McNeil, 2017) has been well researched. All of these, as well as the Circle of Security project and Theraplay, are on the Substance Abuse and Mental Health Services Administration list of evidence-based practices. This author, along with Patti van Eys and Linda Ashford, piloted this intervention, comparing a small group of families who were trained in the more comprehensive components of NEAR to a group of families who received PCIT proper. While the samples were too small to extrapolate much data, it was notable that those parents who received the NEAR intervention reported a larger decrease in their scores on the Parental Stress Inventory and an increased sense of competency at completion of treatment. We were concerned that attempting to augment the parents' behavior management toolkit while simultaneously offering attachment-centered principles would be confusing and overwhelming for parents. Most parents found the expanded skill set helpful. Overarchingly, the guiding question of "Is the child in his choosing mind?" served to help the parents become informal diagnosticians and encouraged them to provide nuanced parenting responses.

Conclusion

NEAR is a prescriptive play therapy model for working with attachment disturbances along a continuum of severity. While NEAR is often embedded within the larger TraumaPlay model in cases involving complex trauma or developmental trauma disorder, it can also serve as a stand-alone treatment for families in which attachment disruptions have led to other subsets of internalizing or externalizing symptoms. NEAR clinicians value the complexity of family systems, and assessment is a key component in deciding which treatment foci and specific intervention models, skill sets, and reflective activities may be needed with any specific family. The general goals of providing psychoeducation and coaching, facilitating in session Delighting-In experiences for parents and children, and creating coherence in their family narratives are all important pieces of the work, but the specific activities used to achieve these means encourages the playful creativity of the therapist to remain fully engaged and attuned to the family's needs at all points in the continuum of treatment.

REFERENCES

Ainsworth, M. S., & Bowlby, J. (1991). An ethological approach to personality development. *American Psychologist, 46*(4), 333–341.

American Psychiatric Association. (2013). *Diagnostic and statistical manual of mental disorders* (5th ed.). Arlington, VA: Author.

Anda, R. F., Felitti, V. J., Bremner, J. D., Walker, J. D., Whitfield, C. H., Perry, B. D., et al. (2006). The enduring effects of abuse and related adverse experiences in childhood. *European Archives of Psychiatry and Clinical Neuroscience, 256*(3), 174–186.

Bizzi, F., Cavanna, D., Castellano, R., & Pace, C. S. (2015). Children's mental representations with respect to caregivers and post-traumatic symptomatology in somatic symptom disorders and disruptive behavior disorders. *Frontiers in Psychology, 6,* 1125.

Booth, P. B., & Jernberg, A. M. (2009). *Theraplay: Helping parents and children build better relationships through attachment-based play.* Hoboken, NJ: Wiley.

Bratton, S. C., Jones, L., Ray, D., & Rhine, T. (2005). The efficacy of play therapy with children: A meta-analytic review of treatment outcomes. *Professional Psychology: Research and Practice, 36*(4), 376–390.

Bratton, S. C., & Landreth, G. L. (2010). Child parent relationship therapy: A review of controlled-outcome research. In S. C. Bratton, S. C. Ray, & J. Baggerly (Eds.), *Child-centered play therapy research: The evidence base for effective practice* (pp. 267–294). Hoboken, NJ: Wiley.

Chapman, G., & Campbell, R. (2008). *The five love languages of children.* Chicago: Moody.

Courtney, J. A., & Nolan, R. D. (2017). *Touch in child counseling and play therapy: An ethical and clinical guide.* New York: Routledge.

Dube, S. R., Felitti, V. J., Dong, M., Chapman, D. P., Giles, W. H., & Anda, R. F. (2003). Childhood abuse, neglect, and household dysfunction and the risk of illicit drug use: The adverse childhood experiences study. *Pediatrics, 111*(3), 564–572.

Dubois-Comtois, K., Moss, E., Cyr, C., & Pascuzzo, K. (2013). Behavior problems in middle childhood: The predictive role of maternal distress, child attachment, and mother–child interactions. *Journal of Abnormal Child Psychology, 41*(8), 1311–1324.

Fearon, R. P., Bakermans-Kranenburg, M. J., van IJzendoorn, M. H., Lapsley, A. M., & Roisman, G. I. (2010). The significance of insecure attachment and disorganization in the development of children's externalizing behavior: A meta-analytic study. *Child Development, 81*(2), 435–456.

Felitti, V. J., Anda, R. F., Nordenberg, D., Williamson, D. F., Spitz, A. M., Edwards, V., et al. (1998). The relationship of adult health status to childhood abuse and household dysfunction to many of the leading causes of death in adults: The Adverse Childhood Experience (ACE) study. *American Journal of Preventative Medicine, 14*(4), 245–258.

George, C., Kaplan, N., & Main, M. (1996). *Adult Attachment Interview* (3rd ed.). Unpublished manuscript, Department of Psychology, University of California, Berkeley, CA.

Goodyear-Brown, P. (2010). *Play therapy with traumatized children: A prescriptive approach.* New York: Wiley.

Goodyear-Brown, P. (2019). *Trauma and play therapy: Helping children heal.* New York: Routledge.

Goodyear-Brown, P., & Andersen, E. (2018). Play therapy for separation anxiety in children. In A. A. Drewes & C. Schaefer (Eds.), *Play-based interventions for childhood anxieties, fears, and phobias* (pp. 158–176). New York: Guilford Press.

Groh, A. M., Roisman, G. I., van IJzendoorn, M. H., Bakermans-Kranenburg, M. J., & Fearon, R. P. (2012). The significance of insecure and disorganized attachment for children's internalizing symptoms: A meta-analytic study. *Child Development, 83*(2), 591–610.

ICD-11 for Mortality and Morbidity Statistics. (2019). 6B44 Reactive attachment disorder. Retrieved September 3, 2018, from *https://icd.who.int/browse11/l-m/en#/http://id.who.int/icd/entity/1867081699.*

Kestly, T. (2015). *The interpersonal neurobiology of play: Brain-building interventions for emotional well-being.* New York: Norton.

Lecompte, V., & Moss, E. (2014). Disorganized and controlling patterns of attachment, role reversal, and caregiving helplessness: Links to adolescents' externalizing problems. *American Journal of Orthopsychiatry, 84*(5), 581–589.

Lieneman, C. C., Brabson, L. A., Highlander, A., Wallace, N. M., & McNeil, C. B. (2017). Parent–child interaction therapy: Current perspectives. *Psychology Research and Behavior Management, 10*, 239–256.

Lindaman, S. L., Booth, P. B., & Chambers, C. L. (2000). Assessing parent–child interactions with the Marschak interaction method (MIM). In K. Gitlin-

Weiner, A. Sandgrund, & C. Schaefer (Eds.), *Play diagnosis and assessment* (pp. 371–400). Hoboken, NJ: Wiley.

Madigan, S., Atkinson, L., Laurin, K., & Benoit, D. (2013). Attachment and internalizing behavior in early childhood: A meta-analysis. *Developmental Psychology, 49*(4), 672–689.

Main, M., & Hesse, E. (1990). Parents' unresolved traumatic experiences are related to infant disorganized attachment status: Is frightened and/or frightening parental behavior the linking mechanism? In M. T. Greenberg, D. Cicchetti, & E. M. Cummings (Eds.), *Attachment in the preschool years: Theory, research, and intervention* (pp. 161–182). Chicago: University of Chicago Press.

Marschak, M. (1960). A method for evaluating child–parent interaction under controlled conditions. *Journal of Genetic Psychology, 97*(1), 3–22.

Nixon, R., Sweeney, L., Erickson, D., & Touyz, S. (2003). Parent–child interaction therapy: A comparison of standard and abbreviated treatment for oppositional defiant preschoolers. *Journal of Consulting and Clinical Psychology, 71*(2), 251–260.

Ogden, P., Minton, K., & Pain, C. (2006). *Trauma and the body: A sensorimotor approach to psychotherapy.* New York: Norton.

Powell, B., Cooper, G., Hoffman, K., & Marvin, R. S. (2009). The circle of security. In C. H. Zeanah, Jr. (Ed.), *Handbook of infant mental health* (3rd ed., pp. 450–467). New York: Guilford Press.

Purvis, K. B., Cross, D. R., & Sunshine, W. L. (2007). *The connected child.* New York: McGraw-Hill.

Rothschild, B. (2000). *The body remembers: The psychophysiology of trauma and trauma treatment.* New York: Norton.

Schuhmann, E. M., Foote, R., Eyberg, S. M., et al. (1998). Efficacy of parent–child interaction therapy: Interim report of a randomized trial with short term maintenance. *Journal of Clinical Child and Adolescent Psychology, 27,* 34–45.

Siegel, D. J. (1999). *The developing mind: How relationships and the brain interact to shape who we are.* New York: Guilford Press.

Siegel, D. J., & Hartzell, M. (2013). *Parenting from the inside out: How a deeper self-understanding can help you raise children who thrive.* New York: TarcherPerigee.

van der Kolk, B. A. (2015). *The body keeps the score: Brain, mind, and body in the healing of trauma.* New York: Penguin Books.

CHAPTER 15

Play Therapy for Children with School Behavior Problems

Athena A. Drewes

Description of the Problem

Estimates show that one out of five children experience impairing emotional problems, although only one-third of these children are able to get the help they need (Mental Health America, 2009). The most common student referral is for disruptive classroom behaviors (Abidin & Robinson, 2002), and children's aggressive behavior is the most common presenting problem (Cochran, Cochran, Nordling, McAdam, & Miller, 2010). Disruptive and challenging behavior is defined as "any repeated pattern of behavior, or perception of behavior, that interferes with or is at risk of interfering with optimal learning, or engagement in prosocial interactions with peers and adults" (Smith & Fox, 2003, p. 5). Disruptive behaviors include externalizing behaviors that interfere with the teacher's ability to teach and for children to learn (Meany-Walen, Bratton, & Kottman, 2014). When a child becomes disruptive, the critical relationship between the teacher and student, as well as with other students, often becomes damaged and strained (Hamre, Pianta, Downer, & Mashburn, 2007; Myers & Pianta, 2008). Without intervention by a school counselor–play therapist, these disruptive behaviors often lead to serious problems over the child's lifespan, which include psychiatric diagnoses, antisocial behavior, violence, drug abuse, and juvenile delinquency (Barkley, 2007; Mental Health America, 2009), as well as school suspensions and school dropout

(Mayer, 1995). Furthermore, childhood conduct-disordered behaviors lead to academic failure, problems with socialization and peer rejection, poor educational and vocational adaptation in adolescence and adulthood, and adverse effects on their families, service providers, and their communities (Dunlap et al., 2006). In turn, there is increased risk for depressed mood and involvement in deviant peer groups (Cochran et al., 2010). Finally, when children with significant behavior problems are not identified in a timely way or given appropriate education and treatment, their problems tend to be long lasting and require more intensive services and resources over time (Dunlap et al., 2006).

Rationale for the Prescriptive Play Therapy

A child's school behavior problems often have as its genesis risk factors such as: lack of prenatal care, low birth weight, maternal depression, early temperament difficulties in infancy, developmental disabilities, early behavior and adjustment problems, and inconsistent and harsh parenting, making this a complex problem to treat (Huffman, Mehlinger, & Kerivan, 2000; Qi & Kaiser, 2003). Further, tolerance for aggression is low in elementary school. Poor teacher–student interactions negatively impact and exacerbate the child's behavior problems. Rather than ask for attention, the child "acts out" to solicit the adult's attention. Thus begins a negative relationship with the teacher who is susceptible to responding punitively in ways that may include expulsion, suspension, alternative school placement, removal from the classroom, or further alienation and ignoring.

Schools are in a unique position to identify children with emotional and behavioral difficulties and to provide the necessary early intervention and prevention of more severe problems (Meany-Walen, Bratton, & Kottman, 2014). In order to intervene and treat behavior problems in school, a multicomponent intervention needs to be implemented over time and across multiple relevant environments in order to produce generalizable increases in prosocial behavior and reductions in challenging disruptive behaviors. Thus, no single treatment approach is able to cover the complex, multifaceted aspects of a child's behavioral problems. Consequently, a prescriptive and integrative treatment approach is needed that includes family members, teachers, classroom and school environments, teaching strategies, and peer interactions, along with individual and group treatment approaches.

A multipronged treatment approach for behavior problems are typically based on cognitive-behavioral techniques and contingent management strategies (Boxer & Frick, 2008) that address significant information-processing deficits and distortions. Children with behavior problems and conduct disorder tend to view ambiguous stimuli in communication with others as hostile and attend to few social cues when making decisions (Ray, Blanco, Sullivan, & Holliman, 2009). They typically have difficulty taking another person's perspective and "reading" emotional cues (Frey, Hirschstein, & Guzzo, 2000), resulting in an unintentional act by another child being viewed as a hostile provocation. Deficits in social problem-solving skills lead to inaccurate encoding and interpretation of relevant social cues, generating and evaluating potential responses and behavioral enactment of a selected response. When the child experiences anger, attributed to hostile intent by others, anger lowers inhibitions that might otherwise moderate the child's aggressive responses. Thus, the child is unable to manage their emotions and emotion-related behavior, resulting in a strong likelihood of socially unacceptable ways (Frey et al., 2000). The use of cognitive-behavioral therapy (CBT) techniques such as verbal mediation or "self-talk" can be taught to help control impulses, think about consequences of actions, and reinforce the child's behavior. Play-based techniques can be utilized to help modify cognitive distortions, increase problem-solving and behavioral skill development, identify feelings and personal emotional "triggers" to situations that typically arouse intense, angry feelings, along with building a therapeutic relationship with the play therapist, all of which can lead to empathy enhancement and reduction of behavioral difficulties (Frey, Hirschstein, & Guzzo, 2000).

Child-centered play therapy (CCPT) and Adlerian play therapy also can facilitate a relationship and enhance coping skills. By allowing the expression of aggressive feelings or behaviors within the play therapy room, in the presence of an empathic and caring therapist who reflects and accepts and can limit strong emotions and negative behaviors, the child is able to learn socially acceptable behavior and ways to express them (Ray et al., 2009).

Adlerian theory, also known as individual psychology, holds that (1) people are social beings who are searching for a sense of belonging and connectedness in the world, (2) behavior is purposeful and goal directed, and (3) people are creative and unique (Adler, 1927/1998). Adlerian theory is among the play therapy theories most widely used by mental health professionals in their work with children (Lambert et al., 2007).

Children's behaviors are goal driven (Adler, 1927/1998), and they behave in ways that can be described as socially useful (e.g., helping others with homework or sharing resources) or socially un-useful (e.g., gang activity, aggressive behaviors, isolation). Both options will produce a response from their interactions in social situations. Children will interpret the responses they receive and consequently choose to maintain or change their patterns of behavior. Their interpretation is based on their *lifestyle,* which is how they make meaning of self, others, and the world. Part of the Adlerian play therapy process with behavior-disordered children is understanding the goals of the child's behavior and helping the child shift from socially un-useful goals to more useful goals (Kottman, 2003).

Children's misbehavior can be funneled into four goals: undue attention, struggle for power, retaliation and revenge, and complete inadequacy (Dreikers & Soltz, 1964). Thus, the goal of children's behavior is to meet a perceived need. Through Adlerian play therapy the child is able to practice socially useful behaviors and experiment with new thoughts and feelings within the safe, secure, and supportive therapeutic relationship. Further, the child can directly and indirectly learn and rehearse their changing perceptions, attitudes, and behaviors through language and/or metaphor (Kottman, 2003, 2011).

Besides individual therapy, consideration should be given to including dyadic sessions with a more competent behaving peer in order to watch, practice, and reinforce social and emotional skills and further develop social and emotional competencies. Inclusion in a group classroom violence-prevention curriculum that works toward reducing development of social, emotional, and behavioral problems and promoting the development of core competencies should also be considered. A program such as Second Step (Frey et al., 2000) fosters development of social–emotional skills necessary for successful and satisfying interactions with others. *Second Step* is a universal intervention for preschool through grade 8. It consists of a violence-prevention curriculum that teaches four essential skills to all students: (1) empathy, (2) impulse control, (3) problem solving, and (4) anger management/conflict resolution. This program contains both school and parent involvement components and is being widely adopted by school districts nationally. Teacher and peer reinforcement of socially competent behavior is more likely to occur if all the children use the same vocabulary and problem strategies that Second Step does within the classroom group setting.

It will also be important to work with the teacher and school environment on the handling of challenging emotional and behavioral disruptive behaviors. Although not all students who present with challenging behavior have a diagnosable disorder, emotional and behavioral problems, especially disruptive and violent behavior, certainly consume a great deal of teacher and school resources (Sugai, Sprague, Horner, & Walker, 2000). Traditionally, schools have addressed challenging behavior by increasing the number and intensity of punitive disciplinary procedures (Sugai et al., 2000; Utley, Kozleski, Smith, & Draper, 2002).

Punishment and aversive environments set the stage for the child's aggression, violence, and escape (Mayer, 1995). It will be important to work with the teacher on preventing use of coercive behavior management procedures, being inconsistent in setting rules, having poor communication, not implementing useful problem-solving skills, and administering harsh, inconsistent consequences (Mayer, 1995). Also, allowances for individual differences with respect to the student's academic and social skills and to the selection of reinforcers, punishers, or treatment strategies need to be utilized. Children who lack critical skills and might not have learned to persist on a task, comply with requests, pay attention, negotiate differences, handle criticism and teasing, or make appropriate decisions will require an educational program that can address these individual differences in learning as well as social skills, rather than being met with punishments.

Schoolwide interventions will be necessary to help the school provide a safe environment and effective programs to limit and prevent aggression and violence. School interventions for behavior-disordered and at-risk students from minority backgrounds are rarely contextualized in relation to the nuances of their cultural backgrounds. In addition, teacher interactions with minority at-risk students tend to be based on low-performance expectations, are critical rather than constructive, are short in duration, and also are often punishment oriented (Kumpfer & Alvarado, 2003). To achieve maximum efficacy, school interventions need to incorporate universal, schoolwide features that address the needs of all students as well as specific features that address the individual needs of those students who do not respond to the universal, schoolwide intervention through a team of committed staff members rather than just by individual teachers.

A final layer is working with parents, especially since parenting practices are highly correlated with antisocial behavior in early childhood (Mayer, 1995). A coercive or punitive interactive cycle can occur in the home as the child makes demands on the parent who lacks certain parenting skills. Thus, ineffective parent discipline and child antisocial behavior mutually maintain each other (Mayer, 1995). The most common predictor of children's externalizing behavior is associated with abusive, inconsistent, or chaotic home environments (Price, Chiapa, & Walsh, 2013). Therefore, inclusion of the parent is necessary to help address the home environment and parenting skills.

A weaving together of all these components, with some coming earlier than others, in a prescriptive and integrative way will help to reduce school behavior problems.

Step-by-Step Details of the Intervention

Throughout the treatment approach and interventions, an assortment of therapeutic powers of play are addressed and utilized: therapeutic relationship building, catharsis, direct and indirect teaching, perspective taking, creative problem solving, role playing and rehearsal, empathy (which negatively correlates with aggression), social competence, self-regulation, and self-esteem.

The school-based individual counseling sessions are broken into components that will allow for building the therapeutic alliance and relationship, utilizing CBT and Adlerian play-based activities for skill building and social competence, and allowing nondirective child-led time for use of metaphor along with control and power within the session. In the first few sessions, the play therapist works to build a collaborative therapeutic relationship. The play therapist, like a detective, searches for clues that will help to better understand the child's lifestyle and goals. This phase is active and directive in gathering developmental, environmental, familial, and situational information about the child. Strengths are noted, behavior in school and home and other social settings is explored, along with what the adults' perceptions and responses are. What the play therapist knows about the child from both history and observations is shared with the child and utilized to help create interventions so that the child will gain insight into their patterns of behavior, feelings, and thoughts. Play-based techniques that may be utilized during the more directive phase of the sessions include use of puppets, games, role plays, sandtray, problem-solving situations, and use of "homework" tasks to try outside of the session, all of which would help in challenging the child's thoughts and behaviors and assist in giving feedback to the child. In subsequent sessions, the first 5 minutes are used to review "homework," share information received from teachers, observations, parent calls, and follow up on anything from the previous session. This time helps to build and strengthen the therapeutic relationship through the transparency of the play therapist leading to the child getting to know and trust the play therapist.

All interventions are tailored prescriptively to the needs of each child. Using knowledge he or she has gleaned, the play therapist may direct the creation of a sandtray for a child who is more kinesthetic. Alternatively, the therapist may use bibliotherapy or metaphoric storytelling for a child who is more of an auditory learner, or use movement within therapy for a child who cannot tolerate sitting for long periods of time.

During the nondirective phase of the session, the child can select the activity or utilize metaphorical play, thereby helping him or her to feel empowered and in control. The play therapist utilizes nondirective skills such as tracking; restating content; reflecting feeling; playing actively with the child; role playing; and trying to understand the child's use of metaphors. The child may also choose to ask questions or use expressive arts, games, or sandtray during the session.

Throughout all the sessions, the play therapist utilizes limit-setting to help the child understand the rules within the office as well as the parameters of the child testing the therapist's limits or expression of aggressive and angry feelings. The play therapist clarifies the rules, reflects the feeling or possible goal of the behavior needing limit setting, and then helps to offer an acceptable alternative behavior that will help build the child's self-control and personal responsibility. The final few minutes of the session are spent on learning and practicing deep breathing, mindfulness, and anger-reducing activities that also help with the calm transition back to the classroom.

As sessions continue over the school year, they become more directive and didactic whereby the play therapist teaches the child new ways of looking at self, others, and the world in order to change his or her cognitive distortions and skewed world view; provides opportunities for the child to practice applying more constructive ways of thinking, feeling, and behaving; and helps the child acquire more constructive ways of building relationships and solving problems.

In between sessions, the play therapist maintains regular (once weekly to twice monthly) contact with the child's parent, with the hope of getting the parent to come in for some individual sessions. The goal of working with the parent is to help in assessing home behaviors, as well as parenting skills, which may require modification from a punitive approach to a more accepting one, sharing of counseling goals and techniques to use at home, as well as charting progress or change. In addition, the play therapist checks in regularly with the classroom teacher to assess behaviors as well as progress, but also to help in modifying punitive interactions and hostile environments. These interactions with teachers and parents help play therapists to gain a more positive picture of the child and his or her behavior and motivation. "Homework" may be given to the parent or even the teacher to help reinforce skill development and competence, and then success is followed up at the next meeting.

Separate dyadic sessions with another classroom peer who is higher functioning behaviorally may be scheduled intermittently to help in the use of modeling, role playing, *in vivo* exposure to emotional triggers, problem-solving situations, and to practice skill development and imitate the higher-functioning child's behaviors. Thus, a child who believes that he cannot connect with others and is unable to share power can learn to connect and share power with a new peer.

Prescriptively, the child's teacher would be helped to learn and utilize a classroom group curriculum for reduction of aggressive and negative behaviors. Second Step (Frey, Hirschstein, & Guzzo, 2000) provides classroom lessons twice a week, for 4–5 months, for school-age children. Second Step's goals are to have the teacher or counselor implement core competencies and behavior skills, work toward the generalization of individual skills, and to create consistency throughout the school, along with follow-up support, as well as to have a family component to encourage complementary home practices. The lessons utilize a cognitive-behavioral approach and are structured around large black-and-white photo cards depicting children in various social–emotional situations. The reverse side of the card provides the teacher with key concepts, objectives, and a suggested lesson script. The teacher reads the lesson story accompanying the photo and guides the whole group discussion. Lessons focus on empathy building, feelings identification, taking another's perspective, role playing, problem-solving scenarios of ambiguous situations, accurate encoding and interpretation of relevant social cues, practice of behavioral enactment of a selected response, use of "self-talk" to help control impulses, thinking about consequences of actions, and reinforcement of their own behavior.

There are also video-based lessons, skill-step posters to display in the classroom and throughout the school, and a family overview video to engage parental support. Grounded in social learning theory, this therapy emphasizes the importance of observation, self-reflection, performance and reinforcement, and the maintenance of learned skills (Frey, Hirschstein, & Guzzo, 2000).

Parent Involvement

Strong families and effective parents are critical to the prevention of youth problems. A positive family environment (e.g., positive parent–child relationships, parental supervision and consistent discipline, and communication of family values) is the major reason youth do not engage in delinquent or unhealthy behaviors. These protective family factors are even stronger predictors for minority youth and girls. The probability of a youth acquiring developmental problems increases rapidly as risk factors such as family conflict, lack of parent–child bonding, disorganization, ineffective parenting, stressors, parental depression, and others increase in comparison with protective or resilience factors. Hence, family protective mechanisms and individual resiliency processes need to be addressed, in addition to reducing family risk factors (Kumpfer & Alvarado, 2003). Consequently, it is critical to involve the parent in the child's therapy in order for changes to occur in the home environment. The play therapist works toward engagement with the parent through regular phone calls and invitations to come in to meet with the play therapist on a regular basis (as often as would be feasible for the parent), and offers feedback on the child's progress as well as teaching strategies for positive interactions and verbalizations.

Case Vignette: Dominick

Dominick is an 8-year-old third grader whose frequent defiant behaviors and angry outbursts were reported by his teacher. Frequently, Dominick would quickly get angry over difficulties with a classroom task, before a test, and whenever working with peers. His behaviors included turning over desks, throwing chairs, screaming, yelling, cursing, and pushing peers. Most recently, when he tried to leave the classroom and his teacher put up her arm to block his exit, Dominick bit her. Consequently, he has regularly been removed from the classroom and most recently was suspended from school. His teacher has reported frustration and dislike for Dominick and is glad for the "break" from dealing with him because of his school suspension.

Dominick's mother reported via a phone intake that he is extremely aggressive at home with younger siblings and has been defiant with her. Being a single mother, separated from a domestic violence partner, she fears at times for her physical safety from Dominick's outbursts. The home environment is chaotic and disorganized due to his mother's depression and inconsistent and often punitive limit-setting. Dominick's birth was also difficult, and he was premature. He often screamed when he was held and he could not be soothed easily, making bonding with him difficult. The play therapist also spoke at length with the referring teacher, who was extremely negative about Dominick and unable to come up with any positive attributes. She questioned whether he was purposefully defiant just to get out of the classroom and noted he was extremely unmotivated to learn. Her teaching style, she noted, was the same for all the children, and they were doing well in comparison to Dominick. She also stated that she was often unsure as to what set Dominick off and had not found anything that worked to calm him down. Peer interactions were always strained, and no one wanted to sit near him or play with him. Dominick's school had a zero-tolerance approach to any aggressive behaviors and no clear plans as to how to offer more positive reinforcement to lessen his aggressive behaviors.

After obtaining the necessary signed consents for assessment and counseling from the mother, the play therapist spent different times throughout the school week sitting in Dominick's classroom in order to make a functional behavioral analysis as well as learn more about the classroom environment and teaching approach. Dominick was also referred for a full psychological evaluation by the school psychologist to assess for learning disabilities.

Dominick was seen in weekly individual sessions, for 45 minutes each, over the course of the full school year, or a total of 30 sessions. In the first session with Dominick after his return from his school suspension, the play therapist shared what information she knew about why he was being seen and his history and explained the way the sessions would happen and when. The outline of the session with its various components was described, and he was told that the play therapist would decide activities but that he would also have a period of time to decide what play was to be chosen. Dominick quickly explored the room and the toys, and immediately started to test limits, trying to dump out containers of miniatures and getting sand on the floor. Limit-setting was enacted, which Dominick accepted.

The Gingerbread Person Feelings Map (Drewes, 2001) template was brought out for Dominick to add some feelings and to select the colors he wanted in order to shade in the body where he felt them. This "ice breaker" was used to see the extent of Dominick's feelings vocabulary and level of awareness of any physical reactions he felt when angry or upset. Dominick readily completed the task, chatting about situations that made him angry, including his recent suspension. Dominick stated that when he was younger, in preschool, he always got in trouble for biting peers. And when his teacher put up her arm to block him from leaving the classroom, he was expecting her to hit him "like my mother always does." Dominick shared that he had no other strategies he could have used in that moment, including telling his teacher why he needed to leave the classroom.

During the child-led portion of the session (about 20 minutes), Dominick chose to explore the sandtray, touching the sand, burying his hand and arm in it, and occasionally picking several miniatures to play with and also bury in the sand.

The last few minutes of the session were spent working together to clean up the room and having Dominick learn the Turtle Technique to use to help calm himself when someone was bothering him, teasing, or calling him names. The play therapist explained that turtles have a very useful tool they can use when they are upset or scared. They go inside their shell where it is safe, and no one can hurt it and it can't hurt anybody else. Then when they feel it is safe, they stick their heads out. Dominick was encouraged to imagine that he too had a shell and to think about what upsets him in class. Dominick stated that he disliked math and that when it was time to take a test, he started to think about how stupid he was, how unfair it was to take the test, and how dumb his teacher was for not helping him understand the math. The play therapist encouraged Dominick to wrap his arms around himself, to tuck his head into his chest, and to close his eyes. He was asked to imagine that he was pulling himself into his protective shell where no one could hurt him physically or with words. He was also asked to imagine a stop light with the red light shining. Then he was to slowly breathe in and out, safe in the shell, where he couldn't say or do anything that would get him into trouble, and he would have time to think about what he could do next. He was told to breathe in and out until calm, and the yellow light mentally appeared. Once he felt safe to come out and his anger had lessened or dissipated, then the green light would mentally appear, telling him he could come out of his "shell" (Eddy, Reid, & Fetrow, 2000).

Over the next 10 sessions, the therapeutic relationship evolved. The more open, truthful, and sharing the play therapist was in her response,

the more Dominick began to invite her into his play. He also would tenta-
tively test limits to see how the play therapist would respond and if it was
different from the punitive responses he would often get from his mother.
The balance of empathy, unconditional positive regard, and limits by the
play therapist seemed to give Dominick an opportunity to express enough
of his emotions to calm down, think, and choose more clearly. He was able
to develop self-control. Throughout the remainder of the school year, various CBT and Adlerian play-based techniques that dealt with feelings identification and expression, anger management, problem solving, and role-
playing responses in social situations were utilized. In addition, Dominick
tried out, in school and home when upset, the various calming techniques
learned and practiced at the end of the session whenever he began to feel
upset. He started to become insightful into the precipitants of his anger and
what was beneath it. He started to realize that when he felt embarrassed
and ashamed for not knowing something, his anger would flare up quickly.
During those times, he would then become physical rather than use his
words to say how he was feeling or try alternative ways to vent his anger.
Dominick learned ways to self-talk. He would tell himself that he was not
stupid, that he could pass the test or do the assignment, and that there were
other things he was good at. These repetitive "mantras" helped to calm him
down and get him through the task. While utilizing the Turtle Technique
to take time to calm down, Dominick would also repeat to himself one of
the above self-talk "mantras" which he felt quickened his release of anger.
Dominick's nondirective play also became more enlivened with fierce battles and catastrophes in the sandtray as well as enacted with the puppets.

By midyear, Dominick's negative classroom behaviors began to lessen,
and peers were more sociable toward him. For five sessions, spread out to
once per month, Dominick invited a classroom peer to his session where he
was able to play and practice his social skills, as well as begin to see how
his cognitive distortions and misreading of social cues would trigger his
negative behaviors.

The play therapist worked with the classroom teacher throughout the
school year to create a more positive classroom environment. She shared
observations from the behavioral analysis, what the communicative purpose of his misbehavior was, and the possible chain of events and triggers
that led to escalation of his behavior, along with the times when he actually was enjoying what he was learning. Strategies to increase the rate of
teacher-delivered praise and positive recognition for constructive classroom
behavior were shared with the teacher. She was given strategies for "catching Dominick being good," and she was encouraged to put a sticker on her
watch. Each time she happened to glance at it, she was to praise Dominick
for whatever he was doing that was positive, even if it was for just a minute
or two. For example, she was encouraged to say, "I like how you are sitting

at your desk, Dominick," or "You are working hard on your classroom work. Good job!" Rather than finding the negative behaviors to comment on, the teacher was helped to focus on the positives, as well as being specific on what behaviors she wanted. For example, she would tell Dominick, "I like it when you are working quietly and letting your classmates do their work," rather than "Stop talking or making noise. No one can work!"

The teacher and principal were helped to think about the use of "time-out" in a more positive way. A quiet area was set up in the room, where Dominick and other students could sit in a cozy corner on a bean bag and put on head phones with soft music playing, for a short break. Three cards were created for use during the day with "break time" on them, which could be "cashed in" whenever Dominick felt too upset to remain in class. Dominick would give the card to the teacher or put it on her desk and go directly to the library, which was two doors down and the designated break location, without disrupting the classroom or others in the building. He would go to the librarian and then take a book of his choice from her stack of his favorite books that she had for him, and he would spend 5 minutes looking at it. After 5 minutes of reading, and hopefully doing some mindfulness or deep breathing exercises, Dominick would return to the classroom in a calm and quiet manner. At first skeptical about this approach, his teacher and principal began to see the positive results.

The teacher was also helped to utilize the psychological testing results to create a more individualized learning approach for Dominick. Testing showed that Dominick was of average intelligence, had difficulties with auditorily presented material, and had a preference for visually based learning. As a result, the teacher started to break down directions into shorter components, giving them one at a time, rather than overload him with multiple directions at once. She used posters and pictures in the classroom that helped to support her verbal teaching. She also set up a system with Dominick that when she asked a question that she knew he could answer, she would approach his desk slowly, giving him time to think of an answer, and then she would call on him. When she knew he would not know the answer, or it was too hard, she would not go near his desk, helping to lessen his anxiety over being called on and being embarrassed that he did not know the answer. This was a secret "code" between them, which the other children were unaware of. Over time, Dominick began to feel more confident, spontaneously raising his hand to answer questions, and peers stopped teasing him about not knowing his work.

The teacher also was willing to learn the Second Step curriculum and utilize it within the classroom with all the children, including Dominick. She quickly felt more empowered in working with disordered behaviors and utilized the curriculum within her regular teaching methods, with positive results seen with all the children.

The school principal was open to the play therapist's suggestions to bring in Second Step into the classroom. He also was willing to work on how to make school and classroom rules and policies clear and positively focused, with allowances made for individual student differences, including consequences, social skills training, selection of academic materials, and instructional methodology. He also addressed increasing support for staff. Significant changes were seen throughout the building, as the play therapist used in-service conference days to explain ways to work more effectively and positively with children with disruptive behaviors. Teachers began to offer positive support to colleagues, and a "secret pal" program sprang up, with teachers anonymously leaving supportive notes in teachers' mailboxes.

Concomitantly, the play therapist worked with Dominick's mother. She would explain what was being done in the sessions, taught her some of the calming deep breathing strategies, and worked on more positive communication. She too was given wording and ways to concretely direct Dominick in how to behave, rather than being punitive. As time progressed, she began to see a positive shift in Dominick's behavior with herself and his siblings, thereby lessening the emotional stress and increasing positive time together. His mother was then more willing to come in to the school to meet with the play therapist, as well as accept a referral for her own private therapy. She also began to enroll Dominick in after-school activities where he could begin to feel competent and form more positive social relationships.

Empirical Support for the Intervention

For well over four decades, researchers from a variety of disciplines have conducted studies and meta-analyses concerning the impact and treatment of challenging children's behavior (Dunlap et al., 2006; Eyberg, Nelson, & Boggs, 2008; Wilson, Lipsey, & Derzon, 2003). Thus, there is more than adequate research support for the use of CBT, child-centered and Adlerian treatment, and Second Step, along with family, teacher, and school interventions for working with children's disruptive behavior problems in schools. A variety of cognitive processes have been studied, such as generating alternative solutions to interpersonal problems (e.g., different ways of handling social situations); identifying the means to obtain particular ends (e.g., making friends) or consequences of one's actions (e.g., what could happen after a particular behavior); attributing to others the motivation of their actions; perceiving how others feel; and recognizing the effects of one's own actions and those of others (Kazdin, 1997).

Research has shown that emotions account for much of the relationship between cognitive and aggressive behavior. Children experience anger when they attribute hostile intent to others, and anger lowers inhibitions that might otherwise moderate their aggressive responses. By managing his or her emotions and emotion-related behavior, the child is less likely to behave aggressively and more likely to behave in socially competent ways. Therefore, use of CBT anger management techniques, naturally paired with problem-solving and behavioral skill development, has been successful in reducing stress and managing anger and thereby decreasing disruptive and aggressive behavior in children (Frey et al., 2000; Kazdin, 1997; Wilson et al., 2003)

There is also an abundance of research in using CCPT to modify and lessen behavior disorders in school-age children (Baggerly, Ray, & Bratton, 2010; Wilson & Ray, 2018). Noteworthy is a meta-analysis and systemic review by Ray, Armstrong, Balkin, and Jayne (2015) that examined 23 studies evaluating the effectiveness of child-centered play therapy (CCPT) conducted in elementary schools. Results indicated that the CCPT studies provided support for its use in the schools.

Adlerian play therapy, an evidence-based treatment approach listed by the Substance Abuse and Mental Health Services Administration, integrates nondirective and directive play therapy techniques (Kottman, 2003, 2011) and is especially appropriate for children who have an increased need for power and control, have experienced traumatic life events, have a poor self-concept, are discouraged, and evidence poor cooperation skills, classroom misbehavior, and weak social skills (Meany-Walen et al., 2014). Researchers have begun building a foundation of research supporting the effectiveness of Adlerian play therapy with children who present with problematic behaviors. One notable randomized controlled study by Meany-Walen et al. (2014) demonstrated a statistically significant reduction in behavior problems with 58 school-age children who exhibited disruptive classroom behaviors. Adlerian play therapy demonstrated moderate to large treatment effects.

Evaluation studies (Frey et al., 2000) of the Second Step curriculum program indicate that perspective-taking and social problem-solving skills improved significantly following participation in the program. In a randomized controlled trial using intervention and controls groups, these authors found that Second Step decreased rates of aggressive behavior and increased prosocial behavior for intervention students compared to control students.

Research has shown that coercive parent–child interactions (reciprocal and escalating negative exchanges) and harsh parenting styles can contribute to an increased rate of aggressive behavior and externalizing behavior problems in young children (Dishion & Patterson, 2006). In addition, negative or coercive exchanges between siblings can also contribute to the development and maintenance of externalizing behavior problems (Ensor, Marks, Jacob, & Hughes, 2010). Further, dimensions of the physical and home environment have also been found to influence child conduct problems, both concurrently and longitudinally, due to the degree of disorganization and chaos in the home (e.g., excessive household noise, lack of family routines, an unclean and disorganized home) (Deater-Deckard et al., 2009). The effectiveness of parenting and family interventions to prevent many types of behavior problems (e.g., conduct disorders, violent and aggressive behaviors, delinquency, substance abuse, depression, suicide, teen pregnancy, HIV disease, school failure, and eating disorders) has considerable empirical support in the research literature (Liddle, Santisteban, Levant, & Bray, 2002; Lochman, 2000; Webster-Stratton & Taylor, 2001). Supplying the parents with behavioral techniques for teaching their child behavioral expectations and social skills, using positive reinforcement, teaching compliance, and addressing challenging behavior have resulted in impressive outcomes (Dunlap et al., 2006; Sanders & McFarland, 2000; Webster-Stratton & Taylor, 2001).

Conclusion

The most common student referral is for disruptive classroom behaviors, and children's aggressive behavior is the most common presenting problem. Compounding the child's school behavior problems are risk factors such as lack of prenatal care, low birth weight, maternal depression, early temperament difficulties in infancy, developmental disabilities, early behavior and adjustment problems, and inconsistent and harsh parenting, along with negative teacher–child interactions and punitive school responses.

Consequently, no single treatment approach is able to cover the complex, multifaceted aspects of a child's behavioral problems. Therefore, a prescriptive and integrative treatment approach is needed that includes family members, teachers, classroom and school environment, teaching strategies, and peer interactions, along with individual and group treatment approaches.

REFERENCES

Abidin, R., & Robinson, L. L. (2002). Stresses, biases, or professionalism: What drives teachers' referral judgments of students with challenging behaviors? *Journal of Emotional and Behavioral Disorders, 10*, 201–212.

Adler, A. (1998). *Understanding human nature.* Oxford, UK: Oneworld. (Original work published 1927)

Baggerly, J. N., Ray, D. C., & Bratton, S. C. (2010). *Child-centered play therapy research: The evidence base for effective practice.* Hoboken, NJ: Wiley.

Barkley, R. (2007). School interventions for attention deficit hyperactivity disorder: Where to from here? *School Psychology Review, 36*, 279–286.

Boxer, P., & Frick, P. (2008). Treating conduct problems, aggression, and antisocial behavior in children and adolescents: An integrated view. In R. Steele, T. Elkin, & M. Roberts (Eds.), *Handbook of evidence-based therapies for children and adolescents: Bridging science and practice* (pp. 241–259). New York: Springer.

Cochran, J. L., Cochran, N. H., Nordling, W. J., McAdam, A., & Miller, D. T. (2010). Two case studies of child-centered play therapy for children referred with highly disruptive behavior. *International Journal of Play Therapy, 19*(3), 130–143.

Deater-Deckard, K., Mullineaux, P. Y., Beckman, C., Petrill, S. A., Schatschneider, C., & Thompson, L. A. (2009). Conduct problems, IQ, and household chaos: A longitudinal multi-informant study. *Journal of Child Psychology and Psychiatry, 50*, 1301–1308.

Dishion, T. J., & Patterson, G. R. (2006). The development and ecology of antisocial behavior in children and adolescents. In D. Cicchetti & D. Cohen (Eds.), *Developmental psychopathology: Vol. 3. Risk, disorder, and adaptation* (pp. 503–541). Hoboken, NJ: Wiley.

Dreikurs, R., & Soltz, V. (1964). *Children: The challenge.* New York: Hawthorn/Dutton.

Drewes, A. A. (2001). The Gingerbread Person Feelings Map. In C. E. Schaefer & H. Kaduson (Eds.), *101 more favorite play therapy techniques* (pp. 92–97). Northvale, NJ: Jason Aronson.

Dunlap, G., Strain, P. S., Fox, L., Carta, J., Conroy, M., Smith, B. J., et al. (2006). Prevention and intervention with young children's challenging behavior: Perspectives regarding current knowledge. *Behavioral Disorders, 32*(1), 29–45.

Eddy, J. M., Reid, J. B., & Fetrow, R. A. (2000). An elementary school-based prevention program targeting modifiable antecedents of youth delinquency and violence: Linking the interests of families and teachers (LIFT). *Journal of Emotional and Behavioral Disorders, 8*(3), 165–176.

Ensor, R., Marks, A., Jacobs, L., & Hughes, C. (2010). Trajectories of antisocial behavior towards siblings predict antisocial behavior towards peers. *Journal of Child Psychology and Psychiatry, 51*, 1208–1216.

Eyberg, S. M., Nelson, M. M., & Boggs, S. R. (2008). Evidenced-based psychosocial treatments for children and adolescents with disruptive behavior. *Journal of Clinical Child and Adolescent Psychology, 37*(1), 215–237.

Frey, K. S., Hirschstein, M. K., & Guzzo, B. A. (2000). Second Step: Preventing aggression by promoting social competence. *Journal of Emotional and Behavioral Disorders, 8*(2), 102–112.

Hamre, B. K., Pianta, R. C., Downer, J. T., & Mashburn, A. J. (2007). Teachers' perceptions of conflict with young students: Looking beyond problem behaviors. *Social Development, 17*, 115–136.

Huffman, L. C., Mehlinger, S. L., & Kerivan, A. S. (2000). *Risk factors for academic and behavioral problems at the beginning of school.* Chapel Hill: University of North Carolina, FPG Child Development Center.

Kazdin, A. E. (1997). Practitioner review: Psychosocial treatments for conduct disorder in children. *Journal of Child Psychology and Psychiatry, 38*(2), 161–178.

Kottman, T. (2003). *Partners in play* (2nd ed.). Alexandria, VA: American Counseling Association.

Kottman, T. (2011). *Play therapy: Basics and beyond* (2nd ed.). Alexandria, VA: American Counseling Association.

Kumpfer, K. L., & Alvarado, R. (2003). Family-strengthening approaches for the prevention of youth problem behaviors. *American Psychologist, 58,* 457–465.

Lambert, S. F., LeBlanc, M., Mullen, J. A., Ray, D., Baggerly, J., White, J., et al. (2007, Winter). Learning more about those who play in session: The National Play Therapy in Counseling Practices Project (Phase 1). *Journal of Counseling and Development, 85,* 42–46.

Liddle, H. A., Santisteban, D. A., Levant, R. F., & Bray, J. H. (2002). *Family psychology: Science-based interventions.* Washington, DC: American Psychological Association.

Lochman, J. E. (2000). Parent and family skills training in targeted prevention programs for at-risk youth. *Journal of Primary Prevention, 21,* 253–266.

Mayer, G. R. (1995). Preventing antisocial behavior in the schools. *Journal of Applied Behavior Analysis, 28,* 467–478.

Meany-Walen, K. K., Bratton, S. C., & Kottman, T. (2014). Effects of Adlerian play therapy on reducing students' disruptive behaviors. *Journal of Counseling and Development, 92,* 47–56.

Mental Health America. (2009). Factsheet: Recognizing mental health problems in children. Retrieved from *www.mentalhealthamerica.net/farcry/go/information/get-info/children-s-mental-health/recognizing-mental-health-problems-in-children.*

Myers, S. S., & Pianta, R. C. (2008). Development commentary: Individual and contextual influences on student–teacher relationships and children's early problem behaviors. *Journal of Clinical Child and Adolescent Psychology, 17,* 600–608.

Price, J. M., Chiapa, A., & Walsh, N. E. (2013). *Journal of Genetic Psychology, 174*(4), 464–471.

Qi, C., & Kaiser, A. (2003). Behavior problems of preschool children from low-income families: Review of the literature. *Topics in Early Childhood Special Education, 23*(4), 188–216.

Ray, D. C., Armstrong, S. A., Balkin, R. S., & Jayne, K. M. (2015). Child-centered play therapy in the schools: Review and meta-analysis. *Psychology in the Schools, 52*(2), 107–123.

Ray, D. C., Blanco, P. J., Sullivan, J. M., & Holliman, R. (2009). An exploratory study of child-centered play therapy with aggressive children. *International Journal of Play Therapy, 18*(3), 162–175.

Sanders, M. R., & McFarland, M. L. (2000). The treatment of depressed mothers with disruptive children: A controlled evaluation of a cognitive behavioral family intervention. *Behavior Therapy, 31,* 89–112.

Smith, B. J., & Fox, L. (2003). Systems of service delivery: A synthesis of evidence relevant to young children at risk of or who have challenging behavior. Retrieved from *www.challengingbehavior.org.*

Sugai, G., Sprague, J. R., Horner, R. H., & Walker, H. M. (2000). Preventing school violence: The use of office discipline referrals to assess and monitor school-wide discipline interventions. *Journal of Emotional and Behavioral Disorders, 8,* 94–101.

Utley, C. A., Kozleski, E., Smith, A., & Draper, I. L. (2002). Positive behavior support: A proactive strategy for minimizing behavior problems in urban multicultural youth. *Journal of Positive Behavior Interventions, 4,* 196–207.

Webster-Stratton, C., & Taylor, T. (2001). Nipping early risk factors in the bud: Preventing substance abuse, delinquency, and violence in adolescence through interventions targeted at young children (0–8 years). *Prevention Science, 2,* 165–192.

Wilson, B. J., & Ray, D. C. (2018). Child-centered play therapy: Aggression, empathy, and self-regulation, *Journal of Counseling and Development, 96*(4), 399–409.

Wilson, S. J., Lipsey, M. W., & Derzon, J. H. (2003). The effects of school-based intervention programs on aggressive behavior: A meta-analysis. *Journal of Consulting and Clinical Psychology, 71*(1), 136–149.

Index

Note. *f* or *t* following a page number indicates a figure or a table.

HeartMath Solution for
Better Sleep

Resetting Your Body's Rhythms

Integrating emWave® and
Inner Balance™ Technologies

Deborah Rozman, Ph.D.
Rollin McCraty, Ph.D.

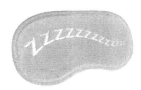

+💜 HeartMath.

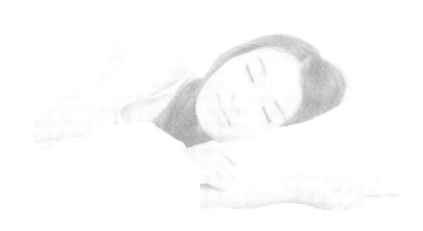

2075-0517

HeartMath Solution for Better Sleep

Welcome to the HeartMath Solution for Better Sleep. This Five Step Program is designed to help you change your response to stress and reset your body's rhythms so you can fall asleep more easily, sleep more soundly and wake up more refreshed.

Mental or emotional stress is often an overlooked cause of sleep problems. Yet stress is a key factor in sleeplessness and sleep disruption. HeartMath, a world leader in improving health and performance while reducing stress, developed the techniques provided in this *Better Sleep Guide*. Practicing these scientifically validated techniques will help you reduce stress, reset your response to stress, enjoy better sleep, and improve your life.

You will use three HeartMath techniques provided in this *Better Sleep Guide* to help you establish new mental, emotional and physiological rhythms that can dramatically improve sleep. While these techniques work by themselves, it's highly recommended that you integrate them with HeartMath's heart rhythm (HRV) coherence feedback technology (Inner Balance, emWave2 or emWave Pro)* so you can track when you really are in a coherent rhythm as you use the techniques to reset your body's rhythms.

I personally use the techniques you will be learning when I put my head on the pillow to drift into peaceful sleep or to fall back asleep if I wake up during the night. I also use the technology to release stress that may have built up during the day and to reset my body's rhythms at any time.

+♥ **HeartMath.**

If you follow the Five Step Program in *Better Sleep Guide,* you will improve the overall quality of your life.

Deborah Rozman Ph.D.
Boulder Creek, California

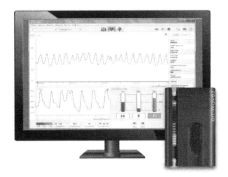
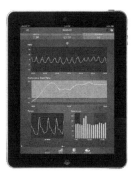
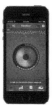

*You can purchase any of these technologies at www.heartmath.com

HeartMath Solution for Better Sleep

"It has now been about three and a half weeks that I have been enjoying about 6 hours of non-medicated sleep per night. What a difference this HeartMath program has made!! Sometimes I do wake up in the middle of the night, in which case I just repeat the before-bed process. At first I used the emWave for just five minutes before bed, now I'm finding that 15-20 minutes goes by with little effort, and then sleep just comes."

Natalie E., Singer, Songwriter, Performer

"I have PTSD and have had nightmares almost every night all my life. The first time I used emWave right before sleep, I had my first night's sleep with NO nightmares, and it still works every night! Also, having once been very articulate, I was very frustrated by memory problems affecting word recall. I struggled to find even simple every day words as I stammered, felt stupid and was often unable to express what I wanted. A few days after using emWave daily, I actually found myself discussing some fairly deep, abstract subjects fluently and effortlessly with NO word recall problem! It's also helped me with anxiety – it helps me calm before difficult tasks, calm after upsets, and get clearer to make important decisions. emWave has improved my life in many ways!"

Becky F., Psychiatric Social Worker

+♥ HeartMath.

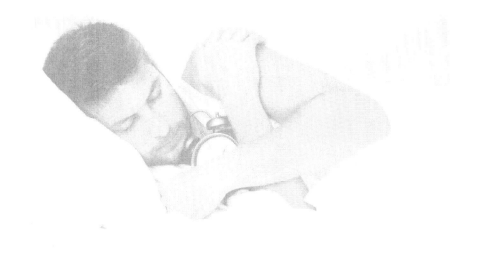

HeartMath Solution for Better Sleep

Contents

+♥ HeartMath.

Introduction

Getting a good night's sleep is important for many reasons—one of which is it replenishes the energy that you draw upon to handle your daily challenges and responsibilities. Each person is an "energy system" that has to both expend and renew energy to remain healthy and function well. You can think of this as how much energy you have stored up in an inner battery. This inner battery supplies the energy you have available to expend not only physically, but also mentally and emotionally.

When you have a fully charged inner battery, you have a greater capacity to stay in charge of yourself and a greater ability to remain calm, think clearly, and be in control of your emotions so you don't overreact. In other words, you can more easily "roll with the punches" and flow through challenges that come your way, rather than getting stressed out, which only drains your energy reserves.

One of the most important ways to renew energy or recharge your inner battery is to get enough uninterrupted sleep. Sleep is one of the most basic ways the body renews its energy levels. Another essential way not to waste your energy is to more intelligently self-regulate your emotions and stress reactions. This will greatly increase your ability to maintain mental focus and emotional composure, especially in challenging situations. You will drain less energy, build resilience to recharge your inner battery and perform better.

+♥ HeartMath.

Scientists have recently discovered that a lot more is going on in our brains while we sleep than previously thought. The brain on sleep mode acts like a computer sorting, updating and cleaning its files.

Coherence

Coherence is a term used to describe when your internal physiology is in-sync and balanced, which is essential for renewing and sustaining your energy. In a coherent state, heart, mind, emotions and nervous system, as well as hormonal and immune systems, are operating in a well-coordinated and optimal way. It's similar to driving a well maintained car; you get a smooth ride, have more available power and save fuel at the same time.

Coherence is an internal physiological state that you can learn to generate to give you a very real advantage in your health and performance. Research has shown that physiological coherence is linked to better sleep, significantly less fatigue and exhaustion, and improved mental capacities.

In this Five Step Program, you will learn to generate coherence with HeartMath techniques and emWave or Inner Balance coherence feedback technology, which measures your coherence level and displays when you are in that state.

When you are coherent, you save energy, are better able to take charge of yourself, and you make better decisions. All of us have many choices throughout a day and the decisions we make determine the quality of our lives.

Simply said, the more coherence you maintain, the more energy you build up in your system and store in your inner battery. You have more reserves to draw on—more fuel in your tank—and more clarity when you need it. Being in a coherent state is like having a rapid charger connected to your inner battery.

It's important to keep in mind that your energy can vary greatly from day to day. On low energy days, it's especially important to remember to practice the skills you will learn in this *Better Sleep Guide* to conserve energy and reset your system for a better night's sleep.

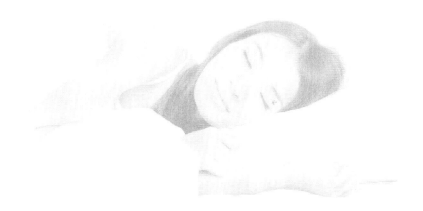

HeartMath Solution for Better Sleep

Part 1

Why It Can Be Harder to Fall Asleep or Stay Asleep in Today's World

If you are having trouble getting a good night's sleep, realize you are not alone. Surveys show that millions of people in countries across the world are experiencing more frequent sleep pattern disruptions and fatigue.

The U.S. Department of Health and Human Services reports that about 60 million Americans now suffer from insomnia. Insomnia is defined as "difficulty initiating or maintaining sleep, or both." The Centers for Disease Control and Prevention says that insufficient sleep has become a public-health epidemic. They state the consequences are sobering. It's harder to concentrate on tasks; we don't listen as well; we're quicker to overreact; and we may fall asleep at our desks.

The National Sleep Foundation (NSF) agrees that disordered sleep for several nights a week or more (difficulty falling asleep, light sleep or non-restorative sleep) affects nearly two-thirds of American adults. The NSF also found that this disordered sleep epidemic stems most commonly from stress. In fact, it is well known that one of the first symptoms of too much stress is sleep disruption.

Sleep disruption has been correlated to increased health risks, including anxiety, depression, hypertension, obesity, Type 2 diabetes, heart disease, stroke and even Alzheimer's disease.

+♥ **HeartMath**

All of these health issues are on the rise. A lack of sleep can have a major impact on weight gain. When people are awake at night they often eat snack, but more is occurring than that. A Mayo Clinic controlled sleep study found participants who got six hours or less of sleep per night were 23–73 percent more likely to be overweight. The sleep-deprived participants produced more ghrelin—the "hunger hormone," which increases appetite and had lower levels of the leptin—the "satiety hormone," which lowers appetite.

A Time Magazine article (March 31, 2017) describes sleep as "nature's panacea, more powerful than any drug in its ability to restore and rejuvenate the human brain and body. When we don't get enough sleep, our brain suffers. The article mentions the work of Dr. Sigrid Veasey, a sleep researcher and professor of medicine at Perelman School of Medicine at the University of Pennsylvania.

Dr. Veasey explains that when our brain doesn't spend enough time in sleep mode, our brain cells act "like overworked employees on consecutive double shifts and eventually, they collapse." Working with mice, she found that neurons that fire constantly to keep the brain alert spew out toxic free radicals as a by-product of making energy. During sleep, they produce antioxidants that mop up these potential poisons. When mice or people don't sleep enough, she says, "the cells are working hard but cannot make enough antioxidants, so they progressively build up free radicals and some of the neurons die off." Not getting enough sleep is aging us before our time, as nerve cells get less efficient at clearing away the toxins.

HeartMath Solution for Better Sleep

A 2014 study from Duke-NUS Graduate Medical School found that the less we sleep as we grow older the faster our brains age. In Alzheimer's patients, the brain ventricles widen as the brain shrinks, and the grooves and folds of the brain become more pronounced, creating gaps. Researchers have found that lack of sleep in older adults increased the pace of brain-ventricle enlargement and decreased cognitive performance, the very markers of brain aging associated with the onset of Alzheimer's.

More than half of older Americans have trouble sleeping and many believe that's just a natural part of aging. It's not. "Sleep problems in the elderly are not a normal part of aging," according to Dr. Julie Gammack, assistant professor of geriatrics at Saint Louis University.

Sleeplessness in today's world is affecting all age groups. A 2014 report by the American Psychological Association found that younger adults (millennials) are the most stressed generation. In the APA survey, a third responded that they can't sleep because they are thinking of all the things they need to do or did not get done or they have too much to do and not have enough time to do it all. Their parents often feel the same way. It has become a social norm to burn the midnight oil on chores, the internet or social media.

Many children and teens are also getting less sleep these days. In fact, difficulty falling asleep is the most common complaint among adolescents. According to a National Sleep Foundation survey, 45% of teens do not sleep the recommended hours on school nights

+💜 HeartMath.

that are required for the body and brain to regenerate. As a result, 25% of them report falling asleep in class at least once a week.

"It wasn't until I became a full time Mom that I truly understood the meaning of hard work and sleepless nights. Insomnia almost killed me. In fact, after my daughter was born I developed a chronic case of insomnia that became so severe my husband took me to every doctor and specialist we could find. Nothing worked for me. Not even pharmaceutical sleeping aids. Month after month I was getting by with less than three hours a night of sleep.

Anyone who has suffered from insomnia knows the darkness that descends when you're that sleep deprived. Then a doctor finally told me about emWave technology and it changed my life. emWave is a scientifically validated system for managing stress that can have a profound impact on stress symptoms like insomnia. Through a simple process that takes less than 5 minutes, you can learn how to control your heart rhythms. In minutes a day, I can now control my stress. I'm sleeping better. I have more patience and energy for my daughter. And I'm a thousand times more optimistic. I have the greatest compassion for those suffering from the debilitating effects of insomnia. That's why I recommend the emWave with all of my heart and soul."

—Traci W., Supermom Company co-founder

Waking Up

The good news is more people are "waking up" to the multifaceted consequences of sleep deprivation. Arianna Huffington is calling for a Sleep Revolution in her 2015 book of that title, where she describes the sleep deprivation epidemic and provides an exhaustive review of scientific studies on its deleterious effects on brain functioning, health, relationships, parenting, work or sports performance and more. She also offers many strategies and tips to help with sleep.

When Golden State Warriors basketball player, Andre Iguodala wanted to improve his performance, he discovered that regenerative sleep was the key. When he increased his sleep to eight hours a night, his points per minute went up 29 percent, his free-throw percentage increased by 8.9 percent, his three-point-shot percentage more than doubled, his turnovers decreased 37 percent per game, and his fouls dropped by 45 percent. When he was named the 2015 Finals MVP he gave a lot of the credit to better sleep.

Many people are also waking up to the limitations of sleeping pills to deal with their insomnia and looking for alternatives. In addition to their addictive nature and many side effects, studies have found that ongoing use of sleeping pills has a limited effect on total sleep time. As a result, the American Academy of Sleep Medicine no longer recommends sleeping pills as the first choice for chronic insomnia.

Wearable sensor-based products are now available with sleep tracking monitors that measure how much sleep we are getting and the quality of our sleep. It's surprising and inspiring how many companies and colleges are encouraging employees and students to take 20–30 minute nap breaks. They are providing nap rooms, napping pods or cots with timers. An app called Google Naps uses Google Maps to show you the best places near you to take a nap (parks, libraries, quiet park benches, etc.) and invites people to share their favorite napping places.

Even though Google didn't make this app, they told The Huffington Post. "As longtime supporters of napping, we're thrilled to see Google technology connecting the world's sleepiest citizens with places to catch some zzz's." According to a study by the Sorbonne University, short naps were found to lower stress and boost the immune system, and their data suggested a 30-minute nap can reverse the hormonal impact of a night of poor sleep.

If you search the internet, you will find many articles offering common sense, practical tips for better sleep. We will list some of the most effective here. If you're reading this *Better Sleep Guide,* you may have already tried some of these.

Practical Tips for Better Sleep

- Avoid caffeine, sugar, alcohol or strenuous exercise at least 3 hours before retiring.
- Avoid stimulating activity, such as emails, social media or stimulating TV shows at least 1 hour before retiring.
- Don't take your phone or tablet to bed with you and don't check them if you wake up during the night.
- Follow a consistent, calming bedtime routine.
- Make sure window shades are closed and the room is dark.
- Try to get up the same time each day.
- Try light exercise (not aerobic) such as stretching or a casual walk before sleep.

- Plan ways to enjoyably relax before bed. Find comforting things to do, such as reading a magazine or book, taking a hot bath, or listening to soft music.
- Ask your health care provider to check you for medical conditions that may be causing sleep problems and to recommend natural sleep aids or supplements.

*See Appendix for more tips

Many people who follow these common sense tips still find restful sleep elusive. We could go on and on citing causes and consequences of sleeplessness or interrupted sleep. But It's time to focus on the most common cause of sleeplessness and sleep disruption that is often skimmed over too quickly: daily stress and today's stress environment and how this HeartMath Program can help.

"In late 2012 my father began having terrible bouts with insomnia. He would sleep 1–2 hours a night, sometimes not at all, and it became evident that he was in a cycle that I had once been in — a cycle of stress leading to insomnia leading to depression leading to more stress, and of course more insomnia.

About 6 months before that, I had been experiencing insomnia almost every night, and I had just learned to live with it. I was very high stress, and would have frequent anxiety attacks. I began purchasing things recommended for breaking through stress. I noticed a blogger's #1 recommendation was the emWave2, so I purchased one and began my coherence training. Needless to say, today as I write this story, I'm a different person than I was that day.

+💜 HeartMath.

When my father came to me with his insomnia problem he had already developed high blood pressure from the stress and was taking medication for it. The doctors had given him a leading prescription sleep sedative and a host of other unsavory drugs to help him get to sleep. At one point he was taking more than one sedative a night and still not sleeping.

I had mentioned the emWave technology to him multiple times and how it helped me, but he was skeptical and labeled it a 'holistic' approach. The issue persisted for months with my dad going back to the hospital multiple times a week for sleep studies, blood tests, MRI's—the whole medical nine yards. Nothing was working.

My family and I became tremendously worried. My father is 67 years old and his health was only getting worse. He became disillusioned with the treatment options he was given, but I implored him one night and showed him the HeartMath diagram that outlines stress and explains how coherence training works.

He purchased an emWave device that night and began his coherence training. Two weeks later, he had reduced the amount of the sedative he was taking to one a night. Two months later he was cutting that in half. I visited him earlier this week and I'm happy to say he's completely independent of this sedative.

The only variable that had changed was the emWave technology. I'd like to give my warmest thanks to the Institute of HeartMath for this. Your work gave my father back his life and made me a better person. I try to tell people about HRV coherence training with the emWave whenever I can, *because it has had such a profound impact on my life and the lives of my family members. I feel as though this technology could literally reshape the world if more people knew about it. Sincerely and coherently."*

—Peter M., Network Technician for a wireless provider

The Stress Epidemic

While there are many causes of sleeplessness and many tips and remedies to improve sleep, HeartMath research suggests that stress is often the overlooked factor. Unless **stress is adequately managed** other remedies may not be that effective.

Stressors contributing to sleeplessness range across a wide array of issues, including major life changes such as divorce, job loss, or trauma. However, it's the accumulation of stress from work over-load, financial challenges, relationship problems, health concerns, or global issues that create uncertainty about the future that are contributing to an epidemic of anxiety, worry and depression.

Unresolved emotional stress often causes sleeplessness; and lack of sleep contributes to ongoing emotional stress. This can create a vicious cycle: You can't quiet your restless mind or you wake up during the night, realizing you are wide-awake when you should be sleeping and become anxious. Anxiety causes adrenaline to flood the system, and adrenaline prompts the mind or body into action— the opposite of what's needed to sleep effectively.

Understanding the Stress Response

People talk about positive stress, which is associated with a fun or motivating challenge, and negative stress, which is most often a

distressing feeling or emotion. It can be a feeling that
you don't have enough
time, leading to frustration
or angst; or a feeling of
impatience because things
are not going the way you
want; or a feeling of not
being in control. Any of
these disturbing feelings can
lead to stronger emotions
like anger or anxiety and
drain energy. *It's important
to realize that what you feel
throughout the day affects
how you sleep at night.* This
is because emotions (even if
we are not always aware of
them) affect the activity in
our nervous system and are
one of the primary factors
that activate the release of
hormones.

A Note about prescription sleep medication by Dr. Paul Rosch, Chairman of
the Board of the American Institute of
Stress,:

Physicians today are prescribing more
sleeping pills than ever before. Sales of
insomnia prescription drugs were nearly
$3B/ year in the USA in 2011 and have
been rising ever since.

But prescription sleeping pills are addictive and can have significant gastroin-
testinal, neurological and psychological
side- effects. Prescription sleeping pills
are also associated with a 44% higher
risk of developing sinusitis, phyrgitis,
upper respiratory tract infections, influ-
enza, herpes, and other viral infections.
Furthermore, many people find that
after a while sleeping pills aren't working even if they increase the dose; they
still wake up in the middle of the night
tossing and turning with worry, anxiety,
judgments or blame and can't turn their
mind off. This doesn't mean people
should never take them but they should
address the stress causing the problem.

It's no surprise that chronic insomnia is associated with elevated
levels of the stress hormone cortisol. Even a few minutes of being
frustrated or irritated can significantly increase the release of cortisol, and once released, it stays active in the body for many hours.

If you allow stress related hormonal releases to build in your system during the day, it throws off your body's natural metabolic and nervous system rhythms, which disrupts your sleep rhythms. A study in *Sleep Medicine Review* found that insomniacs are at greater risk for chronic anxiety and depression and recommends that insomniacs take steps to decrease their overall level of emotional arousal during the day to improve their nighttime sleep. Otherwise the effects of stressful emotions accumulate during the day and they take it to bed with them. The body's systems just can't shut down, leading to difficulty in sleeping or staying asleep

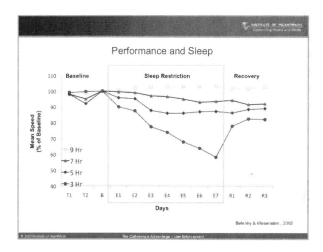

This graph shows the effects of not getting enough sleep over a one week period. A study at the Walter Reed Army Research Institute tested the reaction times of groups of participants who got nine, seven, five or three hours of sleep each night over a week. The performance of the group that got nine hours in bed gradually increased during the week. The graph shows what happened with the seven, five and three hour groups. The study clearly shows that the fewer hours of sleep, the lower the performance. Researchers found that their performance still hadn't recovered after three nights of having eight hours to sleep. They found that it took them two weeks to recover. Yet, when asked about their perception of their performance, they thought they were good to go and performing normally. They were not aware of their impairment.

+♥ HeartMath.

The impact of not getting enough sleep on performance was shown in a study conducted at the Walter Reed Army Research Institute (see graph above). The study clearly shows that the fewer hours of sleep, the lower the performance. When the study was first designed the researchers thought that following the study three nights of sleep would be enough time for the participants to recover their energy and return to normal functioning levels. They were wrong.

They found that it took them two weeks to recover! What was especially concerning was that when the researchers asked the participants about their perception of their performance, they thought they were good to go and performing normally. In other words, they were not aware of their impairments nor how significant they actually were.

In his article *Stress and Insomnia – Surprising Solutions* (Health and Stress Newsletter) Dr. Paul Rosch reports that numerous research studies show—across the board—that stress is the common trigger for both short-term and acute insomnia. Stress drains your emotional and physical energy reserves until you feel like you are operating on raw nerve energy. Stress related emotions can also cause headaches, indigestion, hormonal imbalances, susceptibility to colds, flu and infections, and more.

The bottom line is this, *when you don't manage stressful thoughts and feelings during the day, they can disrupt your sleep patterns at night and when sleep isn't restful, you wake up tired.* A few nights of restless sleep in a row can in turn make you more susceptible

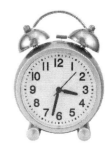

to frequent stress reactions during the day, which makes it even harder to turn off your mind and sleep at night, leading to a downward spiral that can have a major impact on your health, relationships, mental abilities and performance.

The good news is we don't have to become a victim of stress and sleeplessness, yet it's important to identify what factors are contributing to our stress so we can take charge of them and manage our reactions to them.

The HeartMath Solution for Better Sleep is an innovative and scientifically validated approach for managing and reducing stress while increasing energy and improving sleep, cognitive function, health, performance and overall well-being.

"HeartMath techniques have been demonstrated to provide powerful stress-reduction benefits in carefully designed scientific studies that are supported by a documented reduction in damaging stress hormones."
—Paul Rosch, President, The American Institute of Stress

"I had the opportunity to visit with our Sailors in Afghanistan last fall and the leadership told me that the HeartMath program is clearly helping the Sailors that use it and they had a number of compelling examples. A common theme was improved sleep, and the ability to sustain their composure in high stress interactions with the detainees.
—CAPT Laraway, Operation Stress Control Officer, US Navy

"I first learned about HeartMath and the emWave technology in the fall of 2006. I researched it, and discovered it was backed by proven science

and clinical research. I had been struggling to overcome anxiety and being a Type A personality doesn't help. I am a medical student and during my education, for almost the past two years,

I have used emWave to help me with exam related stress and to improve my sleep. The HeartMath techniques with the emWave monitor have given me the ability to improve my concentration and academic performance as well as my sleep.

I use the emWave unit for roughly 10–15 minutes while lying in bed right before I go to sleep for a more restful sleep. Stress is in everyone's lives more than ever these days, and if you are at your 'wit's end' with stress, then I strongly suggest you use the emWave regularly. You will find your mind in a clearer state, concentration, memory processing, and emotional stability will all improve, at least from my experience. I can honestly say that HeartMath has changed my life in such a positive way that I don't know where I'd be without it. Thank you to everyone at HeartMath."

—Robert S., a medical student

The Stress Environment

In today's rapidly changing interconnected world, all of us are exposed to more stressors and we often develop unhealthy habits to cope with them. See which ones may apply to you:

Information Overload—Most of us have to process and deal with increasing amounts of information. This can lead to overwhelm and overload — more information coming in than our mental and emotional systems can keep up with. Some of us even get addicted to the mental stimulation of constant information input, whether checking email all the time, texting, surfing the net, staying glued to social media or playing video games into the wee hours of the night. Between the hours of midnight and 3:00 a.m., over 20 million Americans are watching TV. Add to this the number of those still surfing the net or on social media and you get the idea. This over-stimulation or constant absorption with our electronic devices creates a type of mental stress and burns energy. Over time, this can take a toll, disrupting our body's mental, emotional and physical rhythms. We all need to learn to step back to ask, "Do I really want or need to be doing this now?"

Speed of Change—The #1 stressor we hear about in our HeartMath training programs is the feeling that time is speeding up and that there is too much to do and not enough time to do it all. This can create an emotional tension, mental fog, high levels of cortisol (the stress hormone) and nervous system burnout, all of which disrupt sleeping rhythms.

It's obvious the pace of change has sped up dramatically—and people's emotional reactions have sped up with it. The speed of change creates an atmosphere that feels like life is on fast-forward. Anxieties become amplified and so do impatience and irritation. A culture of speed pushes us to multitask, doing two, three, or more things at the same time.

It's important to learn how to take a few minutes to effectively rebalance before the next task or the next download of information—before your energy starts to drain and your body's natural rhythms become disrupted—creating the stressful feeling of overload.

Stimulation Fatigue—To keep up with the pace of life and all that has to get done, many people drink more coffee or energy drinks or take other types of stimulants, especially if they are not getting enough sleep. Constant energy expenditures fueled by caffeine or other stimulants can lead to a deeper chronic fatigue which can affect overall health. This is sometimes called stimulation fatigue or adrenal fatigue, and is associated with diminished hormonal responses and imbalances, which further disrupt the sleep cycle.

Environmental Stressors—Being overloaded means the mind and emotions can't keep up, so you feel more reactive, irritable or worried. If you're also tired, the smallest interruptions can set you off. Now multiply your reactivity by all the people around you who are overloaded as well. This collective emotional overload can create an exhausting stress environment at work, at home, and in society that can affect your ability to sleep. A frenetic stress atmosphere can create a background energy that affects the nervous system in ways that can make it difficult to fall asleep or sleep through the night.

Another energetic stressor that can disrupt sleep is over-exposure to the stress waves broadcast by the news media. If watching too much news is affecting your sleep, then it's important to limit your exposure to all the fear and negativity.

Sensitive people often are affected by full moon energies or by solar flares that disturb the earth's magnetic fields and ionosphere which vibrate at the same frequencies as our heart rhythms and brain waves. Even if you can't perceive these energetic disruptions, they can be affecting your hormonal and nervous systems, causing mental fogginess or forgetfulness, mood changes, unexplainable feelings of sadness, anxiety or angst, as well as sleeplessness.

There are other environmental stressors that many people are sensitive to, including electro-magnetic and microwave radiation. Some are sensitive to blue light from smartphones and tablets and are advised not to sleep with these electronics on or near their bed.

Practicing the Five Step Program in this *Better Sleep Guide* can help you find more inner balance and better manage these environmental stressors. Have compassion for yourself through the process.

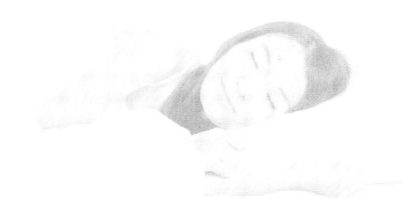

+♥ HeartMath.

Changing Your Body's Rhythms

Your body has various natural rhythms, including mental rhythms, emotional rhythms, metabolic, hormonal and sleep rhythms. The rhythm most associated with sleep is the circadian rhythm. The circadian rhythm is a repeating cycle that occurs once every 24 hours.

We often think that during sleep the body is just resting, but as we described earlier, it is actually very busy rebuilding and repairing itself. It is also accumulating energy and charging your inner battery. Your immune system is more active at night and you have higher levels of many hormones that are working to replenish your system so you are ready to take on the activities and challenges of the next day.

If your circadian rhythm pattern is disrupted (from prescription medications, excessive alcohol consumption, energy drinks, caffeine, changing shifts at work, jet lag, environmental stressors or dealing with daily stress), it throws off the nervous system rhythm and the body does not receive the normal amount of repairs and energy accumulation during sleep. When you don't sleep well for a number of nights, the energy depletion affects your mental, emotional and physical rhythms. These rhythm disturbances often result in poor concentration, lack of focus, getting overwhelmed, feeling anxious, irritable, dull or forgetful, and feeling less coordinated.

Within the 24 hour circadian rhythm there are many faster rhythms. An example is the rhythm of your mental capabilities and the rhythm of your moods and emotions. Research has shown that people tend to have more negative moods in the morning hours (this is probably where the saying, "I woke up on the wrong side of the bed" comes from) and more positive moods and feelings in the late morning (around 11 a.m.) and into the afternoon and evening. Most people are also familiar with the rhythm of an afternoon slump in their mental abilities.

Taking Charge of Your Energy

There are steps that you can take to recover and replenish your energy during the day, especially in your mental and emotional systems. It can take a little time to refill your energy reserves and reset your natural rhythms if they've been out of whack for a while.

First, it's important to identify and plug the sources of unnecessary energy drains, and this requires taking action to better manage your thoughts, attitudes and emotional reactions to stressful situations. The second important step is to reset your circadian (sleep) rhythms so you get adequate renewal and restoration while you are sleeping—and your heart rhythm is key to this process.

Your Heart Rhythm

Your heart rhythm reflects your emotional state. Stressful emotions (irritation, impatience, anger, frustration, anxiety, etc.) create jagged, irregular patterns in your heart rhythm. On the other hand, calming or uplifting positive emotions create order and smoothness in your heart rhythm. Your heart rhythm is called the master rhythm because it has a major impact on the brain and the body's other rhythms.

HeartMath Solution for Better Sleep

If your heart rhythm pattern is smooth and ordered (a coherent wave-form), as shown in the bottom graph on page 37, it facilities your brain functions. You feel more at ease and mentally clear. On the other hand, if your heart rhythm pattern is jerky and disordered (an incoherent waveform) as shown on the top graph on page 37, it impairs brain functions, especially in the area called the executive center. This is the part of the brain that controls your ability to self-regulate your emotions, impulses and behaviors, as well as make good decisions. When this part of the brain is not functioning optimally, you can be overreactive, can't think clearly, and may say or do something you later regret. And if you go to bed with that stressed, jagged heart rhythm pattern, it can disrupt your sleeping rhythm.

The HeartMath Solution for Better Sleep provides you with scientifically validated HeartMath techniques to use with heart rhythm coherence feedback to help you plug energy drains, manage your energy draining responses to stressors and reset your body's rhythms.

Even if you don't sleep like a baby on the first night, you will start to accrue benefits from the practice of this Five Step Program.

The emWave and Inner Balance technologies won't change your heart rhythm pattern for you—they help you do it for yourself. They give you real-time feedback on the incoherence or coherence of your heart rhythm, your body's master rhythm. As you use the HeartMath techniques, the technology will show you when you have shifted into a more coherent state and prompt you to increase your coherence level.

+♥ HeartMath.

The emWave® technology won the Last Gadget Standing People's Choice Award at the 2009 International Consumer Electronics Show as "the stress relief technology needed for these times". HeartMath also developed an emWave Pro desktop technology for health professionals and the Inner Balance app and sensor for smartphones and tablets. Using the techniques and technology to shift into a coherent rhythm a few times during the day and before you go to sleep will help you release and deal more effectively with stress, adds energy to your system, and resets your body's rhythms for more restful sleep at night.

Heart Rhythm Monitoring

Heart rate is measured by how many times the heart beats in one minute. Heart rate actually changes with every heartbeat, and the measurement of these beat to beat changes over time is called Heart Rate Variability (HRV). The pattern of these beat-to-beat changes is called a heart rhythm pattern. Your heart rhythm pattern reflects interactions between your heart and brain, the activity occurring in important brain centers, and in your autonomic nervous system.

Understanding HRV is significant, as it is a key indicator of physiological resilience, vitality, and mental and emotional flexibility—your capacity to respond effectively to stressors and challenges. Stressful emotions, such as anxiety, fear, anger, frustration and irritation, cause the HRV (heart rhythm) pattern to become disordered (top graph on page 37) indicating you are out of sync. It's a lot like driving your car with one foot on the gas pedal with the other riding the brake and burning more gas. The good news is that positive, renewing emotions, such as gratitude, appreciation, love, care and compassion, cause the heart rhythm pattern to become ordered in a smooth coherent waveform called "heart rhythm coherence"—indicating that you are in sync, adding energy to all of your systems, physical, mental and emotional.

Heart Rhythm Patterns

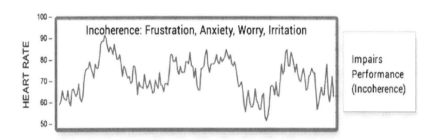

Stressful "negative, depleting" attitudes and emotions, like frustration and anxiety cause chaotic heart rhythm patterns which impair mental functions and lead to increased cortisol levels which can disrupt sleep rhythms.

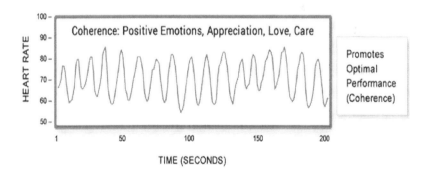

Positive and renewing attitudes and emotions, like appreciation or care create smooth coherent heart rhythm patterns which enhance mental functions and lead to more restful and revitalizing sleep.

+♥ HeartMath.

The emWave and Inner Balance technologies measure the degree of coherence, harmony, and stability occurring in your HRV or heart rhythm pattern. A more coherent pattern reflects efficient or optimal function, which relates to the ease and flow of energy and information in your nervous system and between your heart and brain. An erratic, incoherent pattern reflects stress and energy drain. The heart rhythm pattern tells the brain how the body feels and affects brain centers involved in your ability to deflect stress or maintain composure.

A wide range of benefits comes from the practice of being in a heart coherent state (even for short periods). These benefits have been validated in numerous independent studies and include the following:

Benefits of Heart Rhythm Coherence

- Improves sleep – falling asleep faster and staying asleep.
- Helps you be in charge of your reactions and maintain composure in challenging situations
- Neutralizes stressful reactions that erode health and mental and emotional composure
- Increases vitality and builds resilience for faster recovery from physical, mental and emotional stressors
- Enhances the ability to think clearly, find more efficient solutions to problems and improve performance
- Activates more intuition throughout the day

Validated Outcomes—Mental Functions and Capacities

- 40% improvement in long-term memory

- 24% improvement in short-term memory
- Improved decision-making

Validated Outcomes—Personal Health
- Reduced fatigue and exhaustion
- Reductions in stress hormones
- Reduced anxiety
- Reduced physical stress symptoms

Validated Outcomes—Workplace
- Reduced stress, drama, and time and energy waste
- Improved communication
- Increased productivity
- Reduced health care costs

Validated Outcomes – Sports Performance
Coherence training is used by Navy Seals and numerous medal winning Olympic athletes as well as professional athletes and sports teams to improve and sustain high performance, including:

- Increased endurance
- Improved concentration and focus under pressure
- Improved motor coordination and reaction time speeds
- Reduced muscle tremors (yips)
- Increased self-regulation of performance anxiety
- Regenerative sleep

In summary, HRV or heart rhythm coherence is a highly efficient state where less energy is wasted. It is an optimal state in which the

+♥ **HeartMath.**

heart, mind and emotions are aligned and in-sync. Practicing heart coherence techniques with heart rhythm coherence monitoring increases resilience for deflecting stress or bouncing back quicker after challenging situations. Resilience is an energy that gives you increased mental, emotional and physical flexibility and well-being—and promotes deep, restful sleep.

Benefits of Restful Sleep

- Wake up feeling rested, refreshed and ready for new day
- Increased mental awareness, concentration, focus
- Body energized, alert; less potential for accidents
- Improved memory
- Reduced risk of illness, disease

So, lets get started.

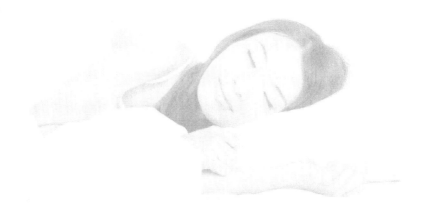

Part 3

The Five Step Program

In this Program you will use three scientifically validated HeartMath techniques along with your emWave or Inner Balance technology to improve the quality and coherence of your heart rhythms. This will help you reset your response to stress and your body's rhythms for better sleep. As your heart rhythms become more coherent (smooth and ordered), your brain and nervous system synchronize to the heart's coherent rhythm, which helps to release mental and emotional stress accumulation.

> **Note:**
> Keep in mind there may be other causes for your sleep problems besides stress. This Better Sleep Guide can be used in conjunction with other aids. For example, if you have sleep apnea, which disrupts your breathing rhythm, then you may need a breathing aid while you sleep. If you are undergoing a life change (e.g. marriage, divorce, job change, move, travel) your sleep rhythms can be disrupted. Pregnancy, perimenopause, or menopause can also disrupt hormonal rhythms. If you have a long-term chemical imbalance or have extensively used sleeping pills, you may need certain organic compounds to help rebalance your body's biochemistry. It's important to see your health care provider for diagnosis and treatment of any medical concerns you may have and for advice on implementing lifestyle changes such as diet, supplements, exercise, etc.

This Program will show you how to calm your mind and emotions at any time. It will help you deal with the stress of time pressures, and overload, so your body is better prepared for sleep at the end of the day. Read on.

+♥ **HeartMath.**

For many people, the Five Step Program is all they will need to progressively improve sleep.

You can use the coherence techniques provided in this program to manage and reduce stress and improve performance. However, it's highly recommended that you integrate your practice of the techniques with the emWave or Inner Balance technology to monitor and track your heart rhythm coherence.

Step 1—Learn to Operate your emWave or Inner Balance technology

For best results, start by learning how to operate your emWave or your Inner Balance technology. These heart rhythm coherence training technologies have been developed from over 20 years of scientific research conducted by Doc Childre and the HeartMath Institute. They have earned the Seal of Approval from the American Institute of Stress and rated as one of the top approaches for improving cognitive functions by the *Sharp Brains Guide to Brain Fitness*.

- Remove the contents from the box and read the instructions. We also recommend you take the short e-training program for the product you have (www.heartmath.com) or attend the free telephone orientation classes offered each week.
- Attach the pulse sensor to the fleshy part of your ear lobe and move it around until you get a good pulse signal on your device. Play with your emWave or Inner Balance Trainer and get comfortable using it.

Step 2—Learn the Quick Coherence® Technique

The first HeartMath technique you will be using is the Quick Coherence Technique. Practice this technique until you can get into coherence with the technology before you add the other techniques. You can use this technique to increase heart rhythm coherence at any time, with or without the technology.

Quick Coherence® Technique

Step 1:

Focus your attention in the area of the heart. Imagine your breath is flowing in and out of your heart or chest area, breathing a little slower and deeper than usual.

Suggestion: Inhale 5 seconds, exhale 5 seconds (or whatever rhythm is comfortable).

Putting your attention around the heart area helps you center and get coherent.

Step 2:

Make a sincere attempt to experience a regenerative feeling such as appreciation or care for someone or something in your life.

Suggestion: Try to re-experience the feeling you have for someone you love, a pet, a special place, an accomplishment, etc., or focus on a feeling of calm or ease.

+♥ **HeartMath.**

You can learn more about this simple technique in several ways:

1. Read about the Quick Coherence Technique in the Inner Balance app Quick Start Guide or in the HeartMath tab on your device. The Inner Balance app will also guide you through the technique. Go to Settings, Tutorial Audio in the app to make sure it is turned on.

2. If you have the emWave handheld, download the software that accompanies it onto your computer, then click on the Coherence Coach® (it's already installed in the emWave Pro) to learn or be guided through the technique.

Step 3—Practice the Quick Coherence Technique while using your emWave or Inner Balance Technology.

Once you have learned the technique, you are ready to use it along with your device. Your goal in using the Quick Coherence Technique with the technology is to get the red light on your emWave (red dot on your Inner Balance app) to turn from red (low coherence) which is normal, to blue (medium coherence) which is much improved, to green (high coherence) which is the optimal state. Sustain blue or green as long as you can. Make it a gentle process and continue to feel appreciation.

If you practice the technique with your eyes closed, which can be helpful when you are learning, you'll be able to tell when you have shifted into medium or high coherence by listening to the change in audio tones on your device if you have the sound turned on. Note how you feel after you practice the Quick Coherence Technique.

"Using the emWave handheld before going to bed has enabled me to quiet the noise from the day, and focus my attention in my heart and on things I appreciate. Doing so has created more consistent, peaceful sleep and overtime has anchored this sleep pattern as my norm".

—Holly T. Nurse

Step 4—Preventing and Releasing Stress Accumulation

It's important to remember that how you manage your energy and what you do during the day can affect how you sleep at night. In order to effectively deal with sleeplessness it is essential to learn how to release stress as it occurs during the day and not let it build up.

Using the Quick Coherence Technique with the emWave or Inner Balance Trainer several times during the day will help you more quickly release stress accumulation and regain balance, calm and composure. This increases energy and reduces fatigue. Getting in high coherence (in the green) aligns your heart and brain to bring you important perception shifts, so you can see a bigger picture or intuitive solutions to time pressures or stressful issues that you couldn't see before.

You can always take a one-minute coherence time out between activities, at your desk, on a break, or anywhere. Shift focus to your heart (look at picture of a loved one, remember a favorite pet, or recall a time in nature) and feel appreciation or gratitude. It's important that the appreciation be heartfelt (not just from the mind) to activate heart rhythm coherence and the hormones that help bring harmony and stability to your mental and

+♥ **HeartMath.**

emotional processes. Breathe a genuine feeling or attitude of appreciation through the area of your heart for a minute (without mentally multi-tasking as you do this). Taking coherence breaks builds resilience and helps you listen to your heart's intuitive guidance on what else you need to do to prevent or release stress build-up.

"HeartMath practice has helped with my insomnia but also quelling some free floating anxious feelings."

—Danielle F.

Prep and Reset

There are several key times you'll want to use the Quick Coherence Technique and "get in the green" with the emWave or Inner Balance technology. It's helpful to use coherence feedback so that you know when you really have made the shift to inner balance. It's easy when stressed to think you're back in balance when you're not. The technology keeps you honest and on track. Two of the key times are what we call at HeartMath "Prep" and "Reset". Prep means to get into inner balance and coherence before events that may be stressful and Reset means to get back into inner balance and coherence after a stressful episode.

Times to Prep (prepare) especially for potentially stressful events

- First thing in the morning before you start your workday
- Before a commute where you are likely to face traffic jams
- Before speaking with someone you know could be difficult

- Before a meeting that could be challenging
- Before responding to an email that you reacted to
- Before any situation that is likely to trigger your emotions
- Before public speaking
- Before a fitness workout
- Before a creative project
- Before sleep

Other (fill in the blank) _____

Times to Reset (recover) especially after stressful episodes

- After a difficult conversation when you are stressing over what was said or what you should have said
- After feeling overloaded by work or time pressure
- After feeling anxious about something that didn't go the way you wanted
- After anything that triggered you emotionally
- After expending a lot of energy and wanting to recover more quickly
- After work and before you go home
- When you didn't sleep well and wake up tired
- Other (fill in the blank) _____

"I had not slept well and awoke feeling very tired. My heart prompted me to go get my emWave device. I did, and while lying in bed I started my heart breathing, heart focus and sending love and appreciation to those I love. I felt my body let go into a deeper relaxed mode. After finishing the exercise I felt rejuvenated, even better than as if I had a full night's sleep."

—Catherine – Commercial bus driver

+♥ HeartMath.

The Carryover Effect

Using emWave or Inner Balance technology to Prep or Reset has a carryover effect. As you practice sitting in coherence even for a few minutes, your mental, emotional and physical energies come into balance. This adds energy to your system and opens a connection to new insight that carries over into your next perceptions and choices.

Just like a battery retains its charge, the accumulation of coherence in your mental and emotional system carries over into your activities and interactions, even when you're not walking around in physiological coherence (in the green). It gives you more objectivity to make better decisions. You'll find it easier to let go of irritations, easier to be patient, to listen more deeply, to move with ease and find a flow in your communications.

The more often you use the Quick Coherence Technique or "get in the green" with the technology for even a few minutes, the quicker you will be able to change your stress set point. And as you learn to clear stress as you go, you reduce the amount of cortisol (stress hormone) you are adding to your system, which can help you sleep better at night.

The 30-Minute Game

Try this self-empowerment game and see if it doesn't carryover into your day. As soon as you know you are awake in the morning, start using the Quick Coherence technique, breathing a feeling of calm, ease or appreciation. Continue breathing calm, ease or appreciation as often as you can remember as you get out of bed, use the bathroom, get dressed, etc. for 30 minutes. If you forget for a min-ute or two, then just start up again as soon as you remember. This can also help offset the tendency to wake up in a negative mood or be more susceptible to negative moods during the first few hours of the morning.

Observe how long the carryover effect lasts into your morning and "reboot" with the Quick Coherence Technique when you feel it fad-ing. If you had a sleepless night, playing the 30 minute game can jump start your day and help prevent stressful energy draining episodes.

Step 5—Get into Heart Coherence before Sleep

Using your emWave or Inner Balance technology to get into coher-ence right before sleep not only can help you slide into deep sleep, it's important in resetting your natural sleep rhythm.

Sometimes it's harder to quiet the mind before sleep. You may have "recurring thought loops" about a person or situation. Your mind rehashes a situation and your emotions react to what you are thinking with worry, anger or other stressful feeling. These stressful thoughts and feelings generate incoherence in your heart's rhythms and make it much harder to fall asleep or stay asleep. You can wake up in the middle of the night or in the morning and start right up where you left off with feelings of worry or projecting negative outcomes. Or you can "wake up on the wrong side of the bed" as the saying goes, feeling grumpy or anxious without knowing why.

The second HeartMath technique you will learn, called the Heart Lock-In® Technique will help you sustain coherence for longer periods and help quiet stubborn recurring mental and emotional loops. You can practice the Heart Lock-In Technique with your emWave or Inner Balance technology (instead of the Quick Coherence Technique) before sleep or any time to assist emotional healing. Turn on the audio and let the tones guide you into coherence and help you sustain coherence. Listening to the tones with eyes closed can help you stay with the positive feeling as you drift off to sleep. If you wake up in the middle of the night, gently unfocus and float as you use the Heart Lock-In Technique with or without the technology to help you fall back to sleep.

Heart Lock-In® Technique:
Step 1.
Focus your attention in the area of the heart. Imagine your breath is flowing in and out of your heart or chest area, breathing a little slower and deeper than usual.

Step 2.
Activate and sustain a regenerative feeling such as appreciation, care or compassion.

Step 3.
Radiate that renewing feeling to yourself and others.

In Step 3, just radiate positive, renewing feelings from the heart. Gently feel as if these positive emotions are going out to others, to the world or to yourself. If stressful thoughts or preoccupations try to take over, bring your focus and your breathing gently back to the area around the heart. Try to feel a caring softness in your heart area and reconnect with feelings of care, appreciation, compassion or love for someone or something in your life.

Before you go to Sleep

Sit or lie in bed and practice the Heart Lock-In Technique with your emWave or Inner Balance technology for 10 to 15 minutes at Challenge Level 1. (If you are using emWave Pro, practice doing a 10–15 min session at your computer before going to bed.) Turn on the audio tone to guide you into coherence (unless it will bother someone else) so you can close your eyes. Do this each night for one to two weeks. Many people have noticed a significant difference in sleep quality right away or within two weeks. Remember not to disrupt your body's rhythms with caffeine or other stimulants before bed.

If you find it very easy to stay in high coherence yet still have trouble falling sleep, you can move to Challenge Level 2, which will help you further increase coherence in your heart rhythm pattern.

"Despite having practiced HeartMath tools for several years, I still deal with occasional occurrences of 'overcare' either due to worry about problems, or over-stimulation from technical challenges at work. The symptoms are that I can't fall asleep because I'm churning the issues over and over, or I will wake up in the middle of the night and have a hard time falling back asleep, since I continue thinking about the issues. Just using Quick Coherence and similar techniques is not always enough. So I have my emWave device on my night stand, I set the lights to low and the sound is off so my wife doesn't wake up. By being able to practice the

+♥ **HeartMath.**

HeartMath techniques with the help of the emWave, it helps me really get to coherence and not just hope I'll get there. The emWave also distracts my focus from the conscious thoughts or worries.

Five minutes of watching the green light are usually enough to slip back into my restful sleep pattern. Since I have used emWave in this way, now just its appearance on my night stand when I wake up actually helps trigger this restful rhythm response."

—Harvey S. Software Engineer, San Jose CA.

When you Wake Up in the Night and Can't Fall Back Asleep

Keep your emWave or Inner Balance technology near your bed where you can easily reach it with minimum movement if you awaken during the night and can't get back to sleep no matter what you do. First, try the Quick Coherence or Heart Lock-In Technique without the technology. If you're still awake, then use the technology with the Heart Lock-In Technique until you fall back asleep. Even if you don't fall into a deep sleep, continue to softly radiate care, appreciation, compassion or love as this will give your mind something productive to do and regenerate your system.

"If I wake up in the middle of the night thinking or worrying about something so I have trouble getting back to sleep, I take out my emWave device and use it. By using the Quick Coherence Technique, my heart intelligence will tell me what the real cause of the upset is, and often provide valuable information about how to resolve it. Sometimes the use of additional HeartMath techniques like Heart Lock-In is indicated. But

I always feel so much better, more resolved and at ease and ready for sleep and then for the next day ahead."

—Melinda D. Corporate Controller

The Five Step Program works best if you practice daily and allow yourself time to reset your rhythms. Resetting habit patterns and rhythms is a process. It usually takes six to nine weeks to reset a neural habit. There will be modulations. Don't expect perfection or start judging yourself when your energies modulate. Be patient and compassionate with yourself. Like a Silicon Valley corporative executive's story below, if you allow your body time to reset its rhythms you'll start to notice a difference both in how you feel during the day and in the quality of your sleep at night. Even if there are nights of restless sleep, you should see your overall sleep quality improving, especially if you are also improving your sleep hygiene by following the common sense practical tips on page 18 and the helpful tips in Part 4.

"After several months of very few hours of sleep per night, it became critical for me to find a solution. I didn't want to take a sleeping pill, but my doctor reassured me that it wouldn't make me dependent. It seemed a lifesaver to begin with – ah, the magic of a good night's sleep. However, there were a few side effects and after a while, I didn't want to take it. Now that I'd caught up on some sleep, I didn't think that I would need the sleeping aid anymore. So, I figured I could just stop taking it – no problem. Well that is when the problems really began. I wasn't able to sleep at all. The withdrawal symptoms were worse than the original sleeplessness. I went back to the pill and tried to cut back more slowly, but that didn't work either.

+💜 **HeartMath**

Luckily, a friend showed me the emWave portable device. I'm a take-charge executive. I work long hours and always have a lot on my plate, so I was looking forward to the stress relief benefits as well as sleeping better. I used the emWave with the herb Valerian to help wean me from the sleeping pills. It took nearly five somewhat sleepless nights, but I could feel it progressively working. Now, I use the emWave before bed and am sleeping well.

Here's what I do:

First, I get comfortable in bed, under the covers, resting against the pillow with the light on and eyes open. I relax as if I were going to read an inspirational book. Second, I hold the emWave device in my hand with my thumb on the sensor (alternately, I could easily use the ear sensor). Third, I begin heart focus, heart breathing and heart feeling as I watch the light change from red to blue to green. I focus on the region around my heart and breathe evenly in and out as in meditation or yoga. I recall when I felt care for someone or something or felt appreciated during the day.

I feel what it's like when seeing the face of a loved one or experiencing a wonderful moment. I anchor that positive feeling and feel the warmth surround me. Occasionally, I watch the blue LED lights rise and fall to aid my breathing and watch the progress made (bars increasing). Once I get into the green, I listen to the tones, which reinforce the feeling that it is working and help to celebrate the success. I use the emWave device for 5–10 minutes this way and then retain the feeling of this coherent state for 5 minutes more without the emWave. (Note: This process works even if I am not able to retain a green or blue state for the full time of 5–10 minutes.) During that time, I begin to feel ready to go to sleep. I set the emWave device down, turn the light off, slide down into bed, and, go to sleep!

HeartMath Solution for Better Sleep

During the first few weeks of coming off the sleeping pill and using the emWave before bed, I'd wake up in the night and find it hard to go back to sleep. I'd wake up and in would flood some unresolved issues and worries, that in my vulnerability in the middle of the night I'd make into big deals, or ideas would come to mind that I didn't want to forget. If I got up to write them down, it would wake me up more. When this happened, I'd get frustrated that I couldn't get back to sleep and worry about waking up tired and dragging around the next day. I finally realized I could use the emWave technology with The Quick Coherence or Attitude Breathing techniques at those times to ease me back into my sleep mode.

Now, when I wake up in the middle of the night with any accumulated stress, I don't allow myself to go there. I apply the heart focus and quietly say, 'stop' to the turbulent thoughts. I slowly heart- breathe and feel appreciation or recall that place I go to when I'm 'in green' on the emWave device. I get my whole body relaxed into the pillow and mattress as if I were in deep sleep and just calmly ease into heart breathing in my comfortable sleep position. I heart lock-in on that feeling and sustain a really positive feeling such as being on a beach. This usually works to get my sleeping rhythm to take over and most of the time I slip back off to sleep right away.

If I wake up and think of something important I want to remember or something I forgot to do, I find it's better to just let it go. If I do decide to write it down, then I stay in a peaceful heart and go back to sleep mode—the feeling I get when I'm totally relaxed and ready to slip into sleep. I just write down a few key words and not get into the head stuff about it, as that's what will wake me up.

+♥ HeartMath.

I understand it's a process resetting your rhythms. When I first started using these techniques, it took a little longer than I liked to fall back to sleep after I'd wake up in the middle of the night, but progressively the time got shorter. The sleep pattern gradually improves. Now I have longer periods being asleep and shorter and fewer periods awake. I feel more refreshed and function better in the day. I also use the Attitude Breathing Technique with the emWave device during the day to clear unresolved issues so I don't wake up with them at night. This is what works for me. It is truly amazing and worth trying for yourself. The emWave has made a huge difference. Thank you HeartMath."

-Katie C, Corporate Executive, Redwood City CA

Summary of the Five Step Program

1. Learn to operate your emWave or Inner Balance technology.
2. Learn the simple Quick Coherence Technique.
3. Practice the Quick Coherence Technique with the technology to get in medium coherence (blue) then high coherence (green) and stay in high coherence for longer periods.
4. Prevent and release stress accumulation by using the Quick Coherence Technique with the emWave or Inner Balance technology for a few minutes to "Prep" before a potentially stressful situation and to "Reset" after a stressful experience. Enjoy the carryover effect as you move with more ease and flow and make better choices.
5. Get into heart rhythm coherence before sleep. Use the Heart Lock-In Technique with your emWave or Inner Balance technology and "get in the green" for 10–15 minutes just before going to bed and again if you wake up during the night and have difficulty falling back asleep. The combination of learning

to "Prep and Reset" during the day, the carryover effect, and getting into heart coherence before bed is a natural way to help you fall asleep more readily, sleep more deeply, and wake up feeling more refreshed.

Bonus: Inner-Ease™ Technique

Once you are comfortable using the Five Step Program and increasing your heart coherence, you can add a third HeartMath technique, called the Inner-Ease Technique which you can use with or without the technology.

The Inner-Ease Technique is designed to help you self-regulate the balance and cooperation between your heart, mind and emotions **as you move through activities.**

Using the Inner-Ease Technique is a bonus because it helps you create more ease and flow while on the go, especially when you feel rushed, time-deprived, tension or angst—in meetings, on the phone, anywhere. It helps you move in a state of ease, where you are composed and balanced on the inside, but ready for intelligent action. This can create a much easier transit through challenges, bringing you more creativity and intuitive guidance for effective reasoning, discernment and communication.

The Inner-Ease Technique

Acknowledge your feelings as soon as you sense that you are out of sync or feeling common stressors such as frustration, impatience, anxiety, overload, anger, mental gridlock, being judgmental, etc., then practice the Inner-Ease Technique:

Step 1: Heart-Focused Breathing

Focus your attention in the area of the heart. Imagine your breath is flowing in and out of your heart or chest area, breathing a little slower and deeper than usual.

Suggestion: Inhale 5 seconds, exhale 5 seconds (or whatever rhythm is comfortable).

Step 2: Draw in the Feeling of Inner-Ease

With each breath, draw in the feeling of inner ease to balance your mental and emotional energy.

Step 3: Anchor and Maintain the Feeling

Set a meaningful intent to anchor the feeling of inner ease as you engage in your projects, challenges or daily interactions.

Once you have learned the technique you can just remember to use these Quick Steps while on the go.

Inner-Ease Quick Steps

- Heart-Focused Breathing
- Draw in the feeling of inner ease
- Anchor and maintain the feeling

Soon you will be able to shift to the attitude of ease just by remembering to breathing it in.

There are more scientifically developed HeartMath techniques for clearing stress accumulation, improving decision-making and increasing intuitive discernment. If you would like further training, private coaching or additional assistance please call us and speak with one of our HeartMath specialists at 1-800-450-9111.

Results You Can Expect

HeartMath has provided hundreds of training programs for thousands of individuals, health care professionals, corporations, government and health care organizations, schools, and the U.S. military. In HeartMath's work with the U.S. Navy, we were able to reduce the number of sailors (deployed on a high stress mission) taking sleep medications from 80% to 5%.

Many HeartMath training programs in organizations include pre and post assessments called the POQA (Personal and Organizational Quality Assessment). The following data was compiled from over 15,000 men and women. As you practice HeartMath techniques with the emWave or Inner Balance technology, you can expect similar results.

In just six to nine weeks, HeartMath programs consistently achieved the following outcomes in people who said they had these symptoms often, very often, or always. In addition, post-assessments after six months and one year showed sustained improvements.

- 58% reduction in metabolic syndrome (3 or more of 5 major health risk factors*)
- 44% drop in feeling tired
- 52% drop in feeling exhausted
- 52% drop in anxiety

+♥ **HeartMath.**

- 60% drop in depression
- 61% drop in feeling annoyed
- 33% improvement in sleep

*high blood pressure; low HDL cholesterol; high glucose levels, high triglycerides, large waist circumference

The POQA is a normed and validated assessment instrument that is taken prior to HeartMath training and again 6–9 weeks after (in class or online). The survey takes 10–15 minutes to complete. Participants gain more insight into the scope of stress and the links between physical, emotional and behavioral symptoms they are experiencing.

Surveys are confidential and are sent directly to the HeartMath Institute for analysis. For organizations, an aggregate analysis and group report is provided. The 52-question POQA survey measures physical stress symptoms, psychological health, resilience, emotional competencies and organizational quality organized into four factors: Emotional Vitality, Emotional Stress, Organizational Stress and Physical Stress. Each of the four factors has been constructed into a robust, statistically valid and reliable scale with subscales to provide a fine-grained picture of the organization's workforce. Questions include a seven point response scale (e.g. not at all, once in a while, sometimes, fairly often, often, very often, always).

There are a number of peer-reviewed, published studies on the effectiveness of heart coherence training on reducing stress and improving sleep and health. Here is a summary of one study published in Psychology 2014. Vol.5, No.1, 78 "Stress Management Based on Trait-Anxiety Levels and Sleep Quality in Middle-Aged Employees Confronted with Psychosocial Chronic Stress."

"A stress management program using cardiac coherence was implemented after an organizational downsizing. The study was conducted in nine voluntary workers in order to evaluate the efficiency of the program. A baseline evaluation was conducted on psychological variables (anxiety, perceived-stress, well- being and sleep), endocrine assessments (urinary cortisol excretion, alpha-amylase and salivary concentrations) and physiological recordings (sleep and heart rate variability). The low number of participants was due to the intrusive approach in collecting physiological and endocrine variables.

"The program consisted of ten sessions of cardiac coherence training during a 3-month follow-up period. At the end of the training sequence, subjects were once again exposed to the same evaluation battery. A decrease in perceived stress and a subsequent increase in well-being were observed. Sleep quality improved as suggested by the results of the subjective and objective measurements.

"For the entirety of the results, improvements were higher in subjects with high vs. low trait-anxiety scoring. The pattern of results for subjects prone to a high level of trait-anxiety suggested that stress and sleep are related to each other in a bidirectional way:

+♥ HeartMath.

increased anxiety is associated to poor sleep and stress reduction improves both anxiety and sleep. On the basis of these results, we suggest that trait-anxiety can be used as an indicator of which employees should be given priority for stress management intervention."

Part 4

More Helpful Tips

#1 The number one tip for better sleep: Put stress in check.
One of the first symptoms of stress overload is disrupted sleep. Stressful feelings throw our inner rhythms out of sync and have a negative carryover effect on hormonal and nervous systems – making it difficult to sleep. You can use other sleep tips, but if managing stress isn't a priority, other strategies have less chance of helping you get the quality sleep you need.

#2 Eat right and get regular exercise
Light exercise in the evening can help release tension without over stimulating the body. Try simple yoga postures or gentle stretching exercises to help you unwind. As little as ten minutes can be beneficial and help promote sleep.

Save the caffeine for morning. Believe it or not, caffeine can cause sleep problems for some people up to ten hours after drinking it. Experiment with eliminating caffeine after dinner or after lunch.

Avoid large meals at night. Try having your dinner earlier in the evening and avoid heavy, rich foods and sugar within two to three hours of bed as they use a lot of energy to digest.

Try an herbal nightcap. Instead of alcohol before bed try some chamomile tea, which has relaxing and soothing properties.

+♥ **HeartMath.**

Alcohol can reduce sleep quality and possibly even contribute to waking you up later in the night.

#3 Regulate your sleep schedule

Keep a regular sleep schedule. This is an important strategy for good sleep hygiene. Try to go to bed and get up at the same time each day. Try to maintain your usual sleep time and wake-time even on weekends so you build consistency into your routine.

Recharge with a power nap. Limit naps to 20–30 minutes and try and get them in in the earlier part of the afternoon so you don't throw off your sleep routine.

#4 Create a relaxing night time routine

Carve out some wind down time. At an hour or two before bed stop stimulating activities such as being on the computer, tablet or watching TV. Instead, opt for quieter things such as reading, knitting, taking a bath or listening to soothing music.

Soothing sounds help prepare you for quiet. If you live in a noisy area with sirens, barking dogs, city traffic, etc., camouflage the noise with a fan or perhaps listening to nature sounds. You might also try a sound machine with white noise. Good-old-fashion earplugs can also be helpful.

Check your thermostat. The ideal sleeping temperature for your bedroom should be around 65° F. A room that is too warm or too cold can affect your quality of sleep. Also make sure you have good air flow and ventilation. A fan on low can keep the air gently moving, which prevents the room from getting stuffy.

#5 Take charge of your well-being

Remember that sleep deprivation reduces HRV (heart rate variability) and low HRV is a significant risk factor for chronic diseases, heart attacks and even all-cause mortality.

A Harvard study that followed 122,000 women for over ten years found that those who slept five or less hours a night were 82 percent more likely to have a heart attack compared to the control group who slept eight or more hours.

Even women who got six hours of sleep nightly had 30 percent higher heart attack rates.

Another study of almost 5000 people 59 and younger who slept less than six hours a night had more than double the risk of high blood pressure, compared to control group who slept more than six hours.

Cortisol levels are generally high upon waking, increase over the next hour or two, and fall to much lower values at bedtime. Stress can alter this normal health pattern in several ways. One study showed that when older adults went to bed feeling lonely, sad or overwhelmed, they had much higher levels of cortisol than normal shortly after waking up in the morning.

As with stress, depression can be both a cause and consequence of insomnia. One sleep survey found that over 40% of patients

+ ❤ **HeartMath.**

reported symptoms of insomnia before the development of a mood disorder.

Another found that patients with persistent insomnia were 3.5 times more likely to develop depression over the next 12 months com-pared to controls with no sleep complaints. Insomniacs were also five times more likely to experience strong paranoid thoughts than others without sleep complaints and were more prone to addiction problems. Chronic sleep deprivation is also associated with higher rates of ADHD. Increasing total sleep time can improve mood, emotional responses, concentration, and memory, scholastic and athletic performance.

Short naps of 15–30 minutes have been shown to be effective in improving alertness as well as productivity and more companies are recognizing this and providing rooms for employees to use to take "power naps".

Increasing your HRV coherence baseline through managing your energies and resetting your body's rhythms can improve overall HRV and your mental, emotional, and physical health.

For detailed summaries of HeartMath Institute's years of innovative research on HRV and coherence, read *The Science of the Heart*.

Notes

+♥ **HeartMath.**

Your Sleep Companion: emWave® or Inner Balance™

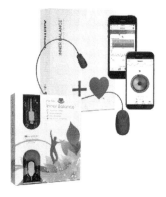

HeartMath's Heart Rate Variability (HRV) technology is a scientifically validated system that trains you into an optimal high performance state in which the heart, brain and nervous system are operating in sync and in balance. We call this state coherence. HeartMath's HRV products measure your coherence level, store your data and connect you to the HeartCloud™ for community support and rewards. As you increase your coherence level, your ability to focus and take charge of emotional reactions improves and you have greater access to your heart's intuitive guidance system for making effective choices.

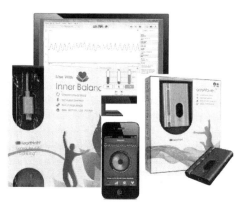

The emWave2 or Inner Balance

Portable and convenient ways to reduce stress, balance your emotions, increase your cognitive functions and enhance performance. Used just a few minutes a day, this simple-to-use technology helps to transform anger, anxiety or frustration into inner peace, ease and mental clarity. Health, communication and relationships improve.

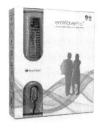

emWave Pro for PC & Mac

Using a pulse sensor plugged into a USB port, emWave Pro collects and translates HRV (heart rate variability) coherence data into user-friendly graphics. It provides a Coherence Coach®, fun visualizers and games that respond to your coherence level. emWave Pro and emWave Pro Plus are multiuser and ideal for classrooms and for health professionals to keep track of client data and progress.

www.heartmath.com or call 1-800-450-9111

HeartMath Solution for Better Sleep

Training and Certification Programs

Add Heart™ Daily Calls

Dial in or log in to join a 10 minute call with a HeartMath staff trainer to increase your mental and emotional fitness and practice the Heart Lock-In® Technique together.

Become an Add Heart™ Facilitator

Become an approved facilitator to learn and share with others some of the science that underpins the HeartMath system, an effective three-step technique for getting into coherence, and how to use the Inner Balance Trainer. In this online course, you learn how to share what you are learning in personal and professional situations.

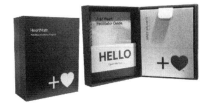

Become a HeartMath® Certified Coach/Mentor

Learn via an 8 week telephone course HeartMath's scientifically–validated tool set and how to teach these tools to clients. HeartMath Coach/Mentors are licensed to teach the HeartMath System in a one-on-one setting or small groups of 10 or less.

Become a HeartMath® Certified Trainer

Attend a full immersion 4.5 day certification program. HeartMath Certified Trainers are licensed to provide HeartMath workshops in a 6 hour program, and in shorter modules, or to embed HeartMath modules, techniques, tools and scientific concepts into other training programs.

Become a Licensed HeartMath® Health Professional

The HeartMath Interventions Certification Program includes 6 one hour interactive webinars and video presentations. Health professionals learn how to use HeartMath techniques and technology with patients in various therapeutic and clinical applications.

HeartMath Institute

HeartMath Institute (HMI) is nonprofit organization that researches and develops scientifically based tools to help people bridge the connection between their hearts and minds. It also provides HeartMath programs to social service agencies, and curricula for children and schools pre K-college. **www.heartmath.org.**

Call 1-800-450-9111 or visit www.heartmath.com

　　　　　　　　　　　　　　　　　　　♥ HeartMath.

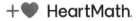

Heart Intelligence: Connecting with the Intuitive Guidance of the Heart
By Doc Childre, Howard Martin, Deborah Rozman Ph.D. and Rollin McCraty Ph.D.

Our newest book, Heart Intelligence, provides breakthrough research linking the physical heart to the spiritual (energetic) heart. This book provides simple techniques for accessing our heart's intuitive intelligence for moment-to-moment guidance and discernment

Transforming Anxiety: The HeartMath Solution for Overcoming Fear and Worry and Creating Serenity
by Doc Childre and Deborah Rozman, Ph.D.

Transforming Stress: The HeartMath Solution For Relieving Worry, Fatigue, and Tension
by Doc Childre and Deborah Rozman, Ph.D.

Transforming Depression: The HeartMath® Solution to Feeling Overwhelmed, Sad, and Stressed
by Doc Childre and Deborah Rozman, Ph.D.

Transforming Anger, The HeartMath Solution for Letting Go of Rage, Frustration and Irritation
by Doc Childre and Deborah Rozman, Ph.D.

The HeartMath Solution
by Doc Childre and Howard Martin

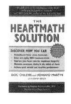

www.heartmath.com or call 1-800-450-9111

HeartMath is a registered trademark of Quantum Intech, Inc.
For all HeartMath trademarks go to www.heartmath.com/trademarks

Notes

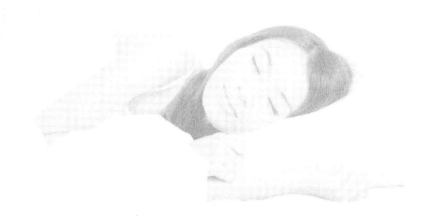

+ ♥ HeartMath.